A WORKING
HERBAL DISPENSARY

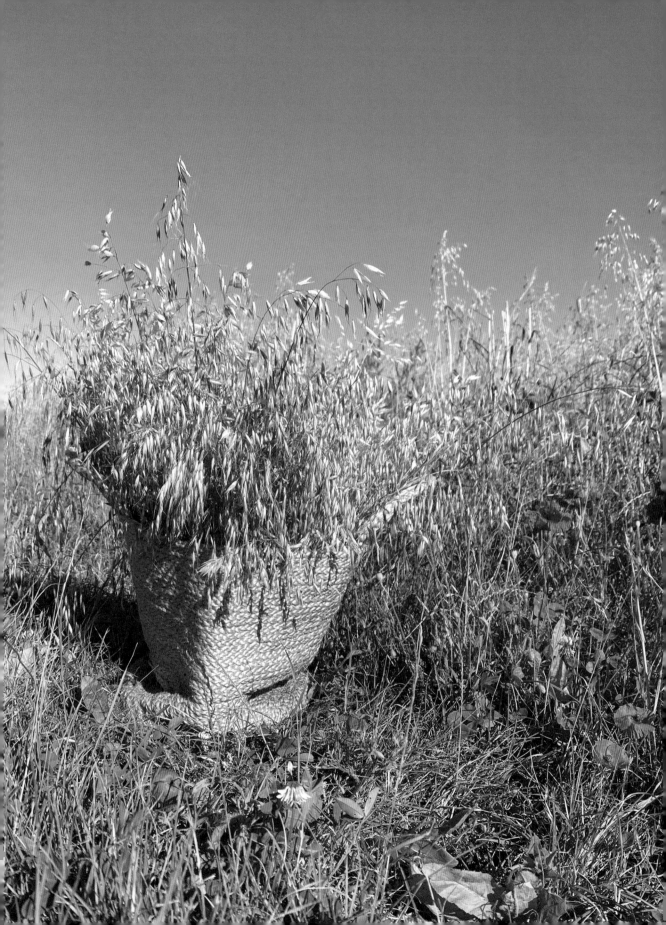

A WORKING HERBAL DISPENSARY
Respecting Herbs as Individuals

Lucy Jones

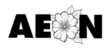

First published in 2023 by
Aeon Books Ltd

British Library Cataloguing in Publication Data

A C.I.P. for this book is available from the British Library

ISBN: 978–1–80152–042–3

Printed in Great Britain by Bell and Bain Ltd, Glasgow

www.aeonbooks.co.uk

Contents

Herbs by common name

Herbs by Latin name

Acknowledgements

This book could never have come about without the years of teaching and encouragement from my spiritual teacher, the late Chöjé Akong Tulku Rinpoché. Everything about him demonstrated immense wisdom, compassion, and interconnectedness, ideals that, as healers, we can only hope to aspire to. Without his support, I would never have been able to study Tibetan Medicine, and I would not have had the drive and determination to complete many more years of study in order to integrate Western herbal medicine with it. I am always grateful for his very positive influence and inspiring example. My ability to live up to it is very much a work in progress, but I do keep trying.

I would like to extend my humble thanks to my Tibetan teachers, Khenpo Troru Tsenam, Sonam Chimé, and Thubten Phuntsok, who overcame significant obstacles and travelled many miles in order to bring the very precious Tibetan medicine teachings and lineage to our little group of Western students. Their teaching was truly life-changing, and its benefits continue to radiate out far beyond our own personal horizons.

I am also greatly indebted to my Western herbal medicine teachers, especially the late Edith Barlow, Barbara Howe, and Ifanca James, without whom I would not have been able to tread this path. Edith, in particular, was a very great support to me throughout my time in herbal practice. I am enormously grateful to her for generously sharing her knowledge and experience.

With much love and appreciation to my husband, Mark, and my children, Andrew and Bex, who have encouraged, helped, and supported me throughout my herbal journey and my writing. There have been times when it felt too big a responsibility to write coherently about my herbal practice and the herbs that I work with, but they unfailingly believed in me and lifted my spirits if they were flagging.

I am also very fortunate to have had so much help and support from the wonderful team at Aeon Books. Without them I could not have brought my ideas and enthusiasm into a form that could be shared with so many others.

I want to specifically thank my very capable herbal assistant, Alice Martin. Not only is she indispensable in helping me to juggle running a busy practice with writing, but she has also enthusiastically discussed thoughts and ideas with me and has helped me to source items and set up layouts for many of the photographs.

Grateful thanks to Abbey Morris for taking the time and trouble to photograph some Hops for me, and, likewise, to Alice Betony from Sacred Seeds for giving up her valuable time to do the same with some of her gorgeous Passion Flower harvest.

I also want to extend my thanks to my colleagues in the wider herbal community, from whom I learn and am inspired by every day.

I am truly blessed.

A WORKING
HERBAL DISPENSARY

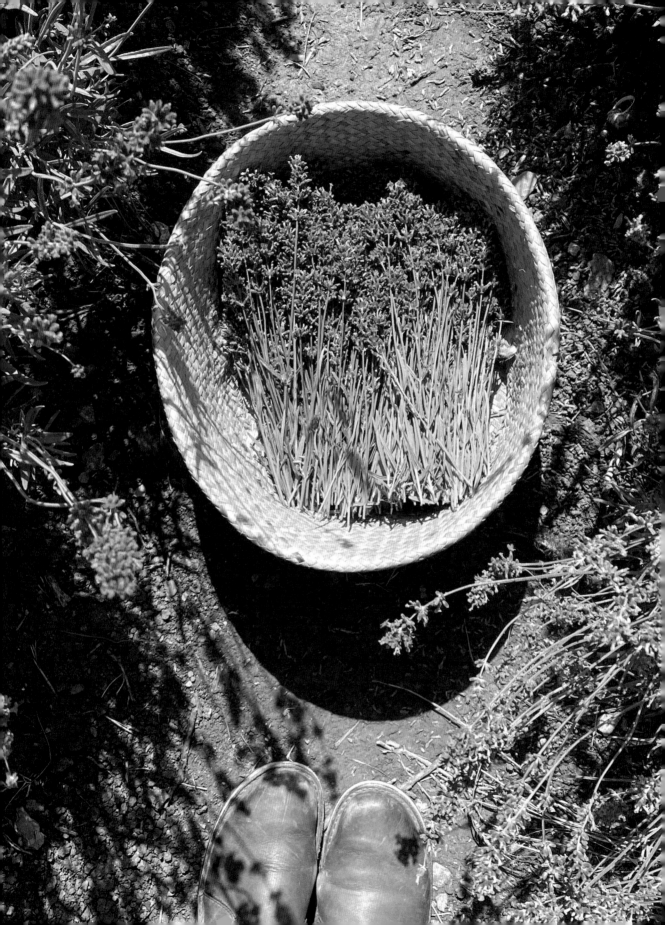

Introduction

This is a book in which herbs themselves play a starring role. Since they are unable to write a book themselves, the thoughts that I share here are inevitably influenced by my own experiences with them. Your experience with these herbs may well be different from mine, but I hope that my words will reveal some common threads and will act as inspiration for further learning and connection.

At the time of writing, I have been working as a full-time medical herbalist for over seventeen years. During that time, you could say that the herbs and I have been on a journey together. When I first started my herbal dispensary as a newly qualified student, I had the idea that I was 'using herbs to help my patients get well again'. As my practice grew, and I started to see just how transformative holistic herbal medicine could be, I realized that to describe my relationship with herbs in that way felt rather uncomfortable. It did not take account of the interconnectedness between practitioner, patients, and medicinal plants. It felt somehow exploitative to say that I was 'using them'. I began to feel that I was 'working with the herbs to help people feel better'. That seemed much more respectful. Nowadays, I would prefer to describe my relationship with the herbs as 'working for them' rather than 'working with them'. Strange as it may at first seem, I feel as though I am a catalyst, and they are working through me. The herbs are the 'experts', but sometimes they need a human intermediary. I respect their inherent natural wisdom, and I aim to help them reach the people who need them.

In many ways I admit that this book was conceived and written in response to what I have noticed as a growing tendency to view herbs in a way that

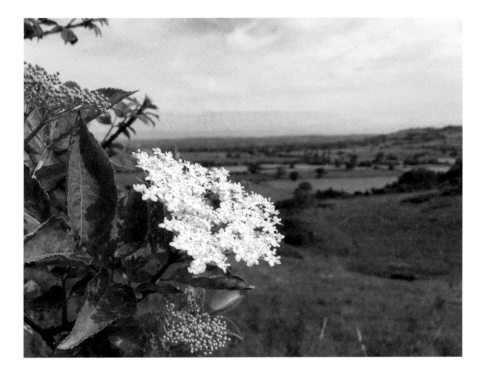

centres around 'what condition they can be used for' or 'what chemical constituents they contain'. I know that these pieces of information can seem quite
helpful, especially to those who are beginning their herbal journey; however,
I rail against seeing and describing herbs primarily in this way. I believe that
our relationship with herbs is reciprocal. Viewing herbs primarily in terms of
'how they can be used' does not recognize and honour them as individual
beings, with their own healing intelligence.

In this tour of my dispensary, I have included 108 of the key herbs that
I work with. These herbs are mostly Western herbs, but there also some
herbs and spices more commonly associated with Tibetan medicine. At
the request of my spiritual teacher, Akong Rinpoché, I studied Tibetan
medicine before Western herbal medicine, and I have been combining the
two traditions in my clinic ever since I first started to treat patients. I view
health, illness, the body, mind, and spirit through the lens of Tibetan medicine but tend to formulate prescriptions largely based on locally sourced
herbs. When writing about the herbs that I work with, it is therefore inevita-
ble that I will include a Western therapeutic understanding of their virtues
as well as a Tibetan one.

It is said that it takes more than one lifetime to learn about herbs properly, and, while I am doing my best, I accept that my own knowledge and experience can only ever be a tiny fraction of the enormous, interconnected herbal whole. I think that we would all agree that our worldwide human family has a myriad sophisticated herbal medicine traditions, each with its own fascinating pharmacopoeia. I do not consider my knowledge of herbs to be fully ripened, yet over the years I have already seen how herbs and herbal medicine can totally transform people's lives. I would like to think that I have gained some pretty interesting insights along the way; I would love to share some of these with you. Perhaps my words will help to confirm your own experiences, or they may encourage you to look at familiar herbal friends in a new light. Either way, I hope you feel inspired to carry on deepening your own relationships with the herbs with which you intend to work, taking into account your own ancestral traditions and the nature of the land where you find yourself living.

Whatever your connection to herbs, and whether or not you are a formally trained medical herbalist, I welcome you most warmly to this tour of my dispensary. Herbs are for everyone. I am keen to show you the herbs that I share my life and work with. I hope that by sharing their stories and some of the stories that they and I have created together, I will be able to convey their individuality and the ways that we, as herbalists, can work with them in a spirit of respect and appreciation.

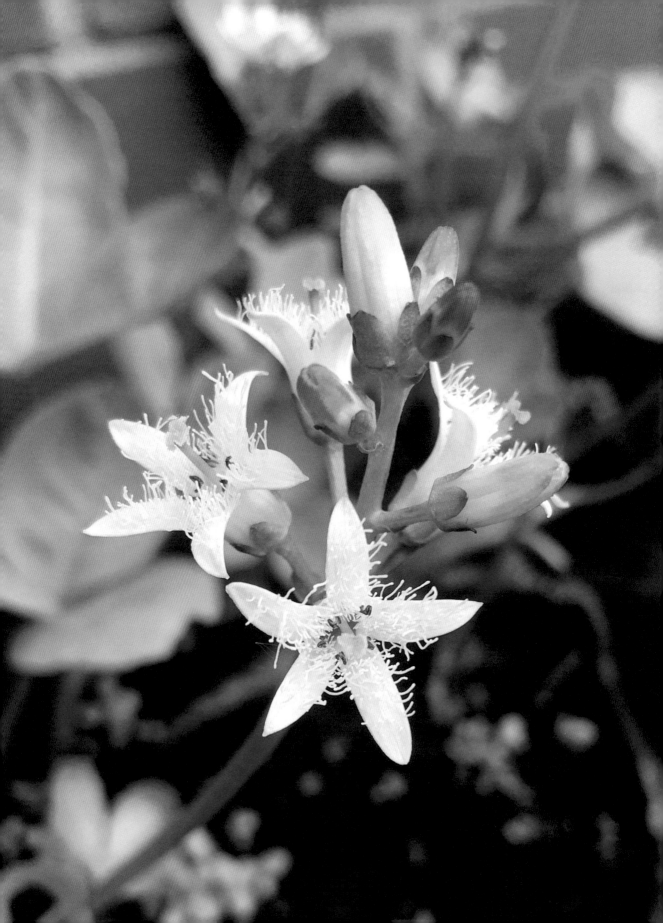

Part One

A RECIPROCAL RELATIONSHIP

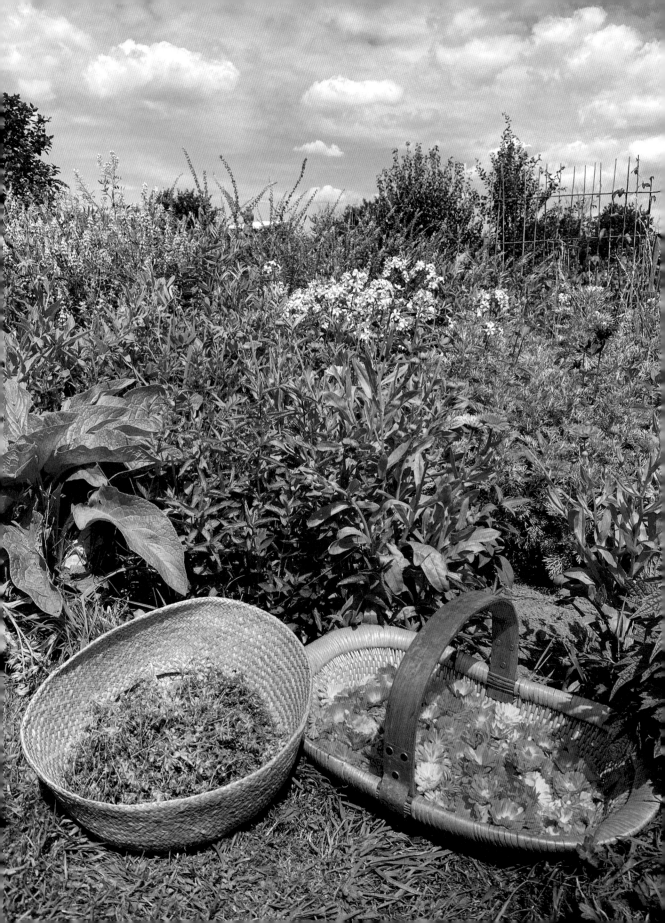

1

The importance of understanding herbs as individuals

Herbs are amazing. They can nurture, support, and heal whole systems of the body, often in many ways at the same time. When we turn to herbs for help, we are not just 'taking a medicine'. We are entering into a relationship with them. We have to 'work with them' by being committed to playing our part in the healing process. The herbs positively influence our healing, but under normal therapeutic circumstances they cannot 'control' our body or override unhelpful lifestyle and dietary choices. Herbal medicine is a healing partnership.

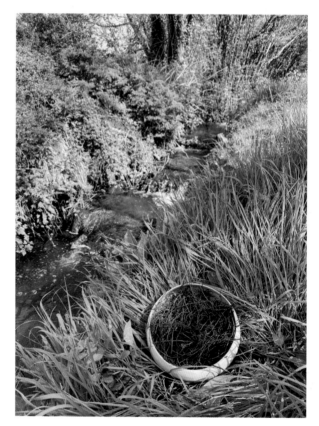

Herbs act on different levels: they nourish us as food, they physiologically influence particular body systems (all of which are interconnected, of course), they balance our body energetically in terms of the elemental principles of Earth, Air, Fire, and Water, and they offer support for our emotional health. For centuries herbs have also been considered to have magical and ritual properties.

Herbal practitioners usually work with whole herbs rather than isolated constituents. Chemical constituents have been

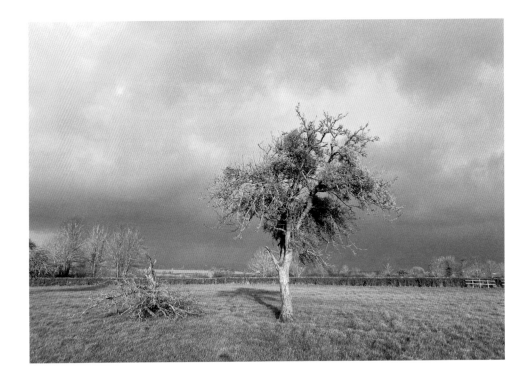

isolated from many herbs, and learning about these can help us to understand the main actions of those herbs; however, when prescribed on their own, these isolated constituents do not work in the same way as the whole herb. They may sometimes be faster-acting or may behave more like an allopathic drug, meaning that there is a greater chance that the treatment could create further imbalance in the body. Whole herbs are, in my opinion, much more sustainable, both in terms of their biological actions and the environmental impact of sourcing them.

In many cases we do not actually know the exact mechanism by which a herb works. We may know about certain 'headline' constituents, such as alkaloids or tannins, but each whole herb has a myriad other compounds alongside these that support and moderate its action in the body. It would be incredibly complicated and hugely time-consuming to try to isolate all of the chemical compounds in each herb, let alone to test how each of them affects the body. It gets even more complicated when we add in the fact that herbs work in relationship with us, since each human being has an individual constitution, lifestyle, diet, habitual thought pattern, and past medical history. To investigate all herbs based on their individual chemical components and actions would be a very long and costly job, in terms both of financial invest-ment and of carbon footprint. Generally, our sector does not prioritize such an approach. Instead, we have years – often many centuries – of empirical evidence to show the efficacy of a herb in certain medical conditions.

As herbalists, we strive to learn the individual characteristics of each herb and how it can support us in various different circumstances. In practice, we aim to match herbs to the needs of individual patients, rather than seeing herbs in terms of which 'condition' they fix. To do this matchmaking well, we need to understand herbs as unique beings.

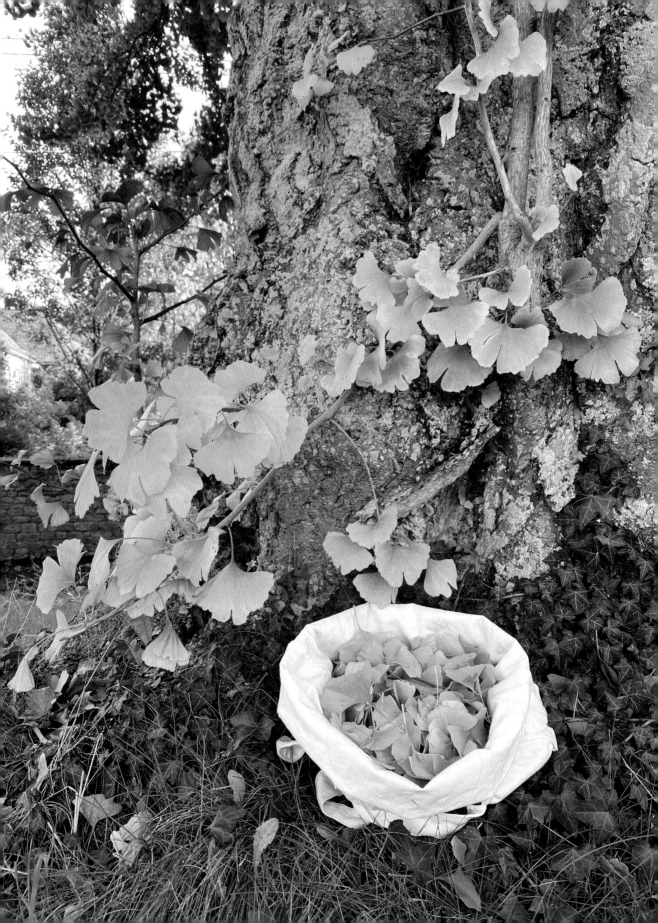

2

The actions of herbs in physiological healing

When I was a student studying herbal *materia medica*, the herbs we were being taught were divided into herbs for different systems of the body and also those that shared 'similar' actions. For example, we studied herbs for the digestive system, the respiratory system, the circulatory system, the skin, the nervous system, the reproductive system, the urinary system, the musculo-skeletal system, and the endocrine system. There was a great deal of information to absorb and learn, so it was essential that it was broken down in some way; yet, even at that early stage, I remember really struggling to classify these herbs into having actions on just one body system or to choose one primary mode of action for each.

As a study aid, I created revision cards, each with a little drawing of a herb and some key facts about its actions, its nature, and how it could be prescribed. I decided to colour-code the cards by body system: for example, yellow for the digestive system, or purple for the nervous system. I wanted to add a symbol in the corner to indicate each herb's primary mode of action: diuretic or cholagogue, for example. I soon found that it was totally impossible to place herbs into neat categories, as each herb had virtues that spanned many body systems and usually also had multiple ways of acting on our bodies. Most of the cards ended up with having borders of many colours and several different symbols crammed into their top right corners.

Since my days of preparing revision cards, I have come to understand that learning about herbs in terms of their actions and the body systems they support is just one step on the path of studying herbs. It is an important step,

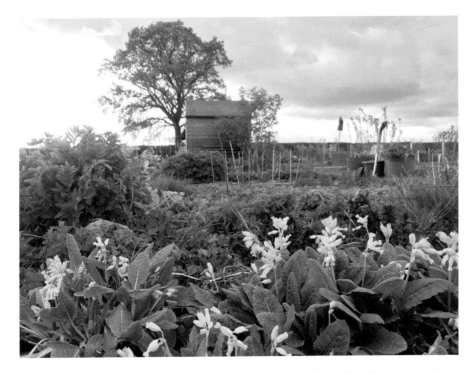

but as we continue our herbal learning journey, it is one that we will move on from. We may try to solidify the role of each herb in our minds and their place in our dispensaries, but as we connect with them more deeply, we find we cannot comfortably do this. Just when we think that we understand how they work, we discover that there is a whole dimension of additional therapeutic knowledge that has slipped through our fingers. This is when we understand that asking 'What does that herb do?' or 'How do you use that herb?' is not the simple question that it may at first seem.

Holistic herbal medicine treats each person as an individual. My tutor, Ifanca, used to tell me that 'herbs treat people, not conditions'. This was not a passing comment: she seemed to say it virtually every time I saw her, and, in case I might forget it, she often wrote it in red pen on the clinical case studies that I had submitted to her. She said it so often that I think it is engraved on my psyche. I am very grateful though. She taught me well.

If we are to treat someone effectively with herbal medicine, we need to understand the underlying root cause of that person's health condition. A treatment protocol suitable for one person with a particular 'health condition' may not be at all appropriate for another with the same condition. If we choose our therapeutic approach skilfully and prescribe for the person rather than 'the condition', the herbal treatment will usually only be a temporary support and will result in a fully sustainable cure.

Having said that, when learning about herbs, it is, of course, very helpful to understand their actions within the human body and the names that we have given those actions. For those not familiar with this terminology, I describe briefly the main physiological herbal actions as I see them.

Adaptogenic herbs

Adaptogenic herbs are considered to help the body to deal more effectively with stress, whether that is physiological, environmental, or emotional. Stress unbalances our body systems, affecting our blood sugar balance, our circulatory system, our reproductive hormones, our digestion, and our mood, to name just a few. When we experience prolonged stress, we can lose our ability to feel 'safe' and 'at home' in our body. Adaptogenic herbs nourish and support us, improving our resilience and helping us to recover more quickly from stressful events. Over time, an improvement in our physiological stability will help us to see the bigger picture and enable us to start to navigate our way out of the circumstances that are causing us stress and draining our health. Ashwagandha is an example of an adaptogenic herb.

Alterative herbs

One of the old ways of describing alteratives is that they 'clean the blood'. In reality it is difficult to describe what they do, other than that they support us in a general way, improving elimination and digestion. Herbalists often choose alteratives when patients are affected by long-term degenerative conditions such as chronic skin conditions or inflammatory joint issues. Burdock and Cleavers are examples of alterative herbs.

Anticatarrhal herbs

Anticatarrhal herbs help our body to remove excessive mucus. Mucus tends to build up when the digestive system is weaker than it should be, often when our diet is too rich in difficult-to-digest 'mucus-forming' foods. Mucus is also formed in response to inflammation or infection. Some anticatarrhal herbs help us to eliminate mucus by making it less viscous. Others dry up the secretions directly. Goldenrod, Elderflower, and Eyebright are examples of anticatarrhal herbs.

Anti-inflammatory herbs

Anti-inflammatory herbs are helpful to alleviate the discomfort of inflammation, but holistic practitioners see inflammation as a natural process, which should be supported rather than suppressed. Where there is inflammation, we should aim to treat the underlying reason for it, rather than just the inflammation. Very many herbs are anti-inflammatory, but Meadowsweet, Slippery Elm, and Ginger are some examples.

Antimicrobial herbs

Antimicrobial herbs may be directly antibacterial, antiviral, or antifungal, or they may support our immune response so that we are better able to overcome an infection from one of these infectious challenges. Examples of antimicrobial herbs are Garlic, Goldenseal, and Thyme.

Antispasmodic herbs

Antispasmodic herbs relax tension in the body and ease spasms and cramps. They tend to promote a feeling of relaxation without being heavily sedative. Some examples of antispasmodic herbs are Cramp Bark, Caraway, and Vervain.

Aperient herbs

Aperient herbs act as a mild laxative. Examples of herbs that are aperient are Dandelion, Cleavers, and Chickweed.

Astringent herbs

Astringent herbs tighten and tone tissues, reducing inflammation and drying up secretions. They can also stop bleeding when applied topically. Many herbs are astringents alongside their other actions. Astringency is caused by the presence of tannins, a class of constituents named after the process of tanning leather. Examples of astringent herbs are Horse Chestnut, Shepherd's Purse, and Raspberry Leaf. While astringents are very helpful in cases of diarrhoea, over-prescribing them can lead to constipation or reduced absorption from the digestive tract.

Bitter herbs

Bitters are very important for our health. When we taste them, they directly stimulate our digestive systems. For example, by encouraging better bile secretion, bitters can improve detoxification through the liver and help to produce a more regular stool. Supporting the liver can, in turn, have benefits in numerous health presentations, including hormone imbalances, skin conditions, low immunity, and depression. Bitters also help to improve our blood sugar balance through their effects on the secretion of pancreatic hormones. We have bitter receptors in many of our systems, not just in the digestive system. Bitters have multiple virtues, which include stimulating appetite, promoting better absorption, helping to heal the gut, and supporting thyroid health. They can be mild – for example, Chamomile, Yarrow, and Dandelion – or they can be more intense, such as Vervain, Oregon Grape, and Wormwood.

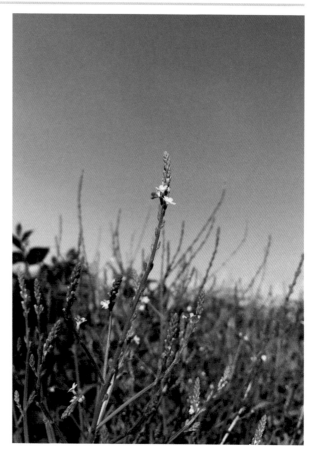

Cardiotonic herbs

Cardiotonic herbs support and benefit the heart and circulatory system, but they do not actively affect the function of the heart, like those herbs that are described as cardioactive. Cardiotonic herbs appear to work in a gentler, indirect way, being thought to strengthen and improve the integrity of the blood vessels and support the natural action of the heart. Herbs such as Hawthorn, Lemon Balm, and Motherwort come into this category.

Cardioactive herbs

Cardioactive herbs contain a group of compounds called cardiac glycosides, and these have a much more active role than cardiotonic herbs in influencing the function of the heart, strengthening its contractions and decreasing its rate. Some allopathic heart drugs are based on the compounds originally discovered in plants – for example, digoxin from Foxglove. Even though whole herbal preparations are generally more balanced than isolated constituents, herbs that contain cardiac glycosides should be prescribed with care. The cardiac glycosides are eliminated relatively slowly from the body, and there is a risk that their levels could accumulate and cause serious effects. Cardioactive herbs include Lily-of-the-Valley and Figwort.

Carminative herbs

Carminative herbs contain aromatic ingredients that relax the smooth muscle in the gut. They ease griping and colic, as well as the discomfort caused by trapped wind. Examples of herbs that have a carminative action are Caraway, Fennel, Peppermint, and Sage.

Cholagogue herbs

Cholagogues encourage more bile to be produced by the liver or released by the gallbladder. You will probably have already figured out by now that cholagogues are also bitters. Cholagogues can be helpful when patients have a deficiency of bile being delivered to their digestive tract, as can happen if they have had their gallbladder removed or if their gallbladder is dysfunctional in some way. It can also happen if the amount of bile produced by the liver is insufficient, at least for the diet that is being consumed. Cholagogues can play a part in the treatment of jaundice or mild hepatitis. Caution is required if patients have painful gallstones, obstructive jaundice, or severe liver disease. Examples of cholagogues are Greater Celandine, Oregon Grape, Artichoke, Culver's Root, and Fringe Tree.

Circulatory stimulants

Circulatory stimulants enliven the circulation, and, through that, they can have far-reaching effects on many different systems of the body. They support improved blood flow throughout the body, and their actions range from a gentle relaxation of the peripheral vessels to the more forceful stimulating action of some of the more heating herbs. Circulatory stimulants can be helpful in cases of hypertension, cold hands and feet, poor venous return, and intermittent claudication, for example, but they do need to be prescribed with care when there is cardiovascular disease. As ever, understanding the underlying cause and treating that is much safer and more effective than just considering the name of the condition and the 'category' of herbal action. Examples of circulatory stimulant herbs are Yarrow, Elderflower, Rosemary, Ginkgo, Chilli, Horseradish, and Ginger. Many of these are also diaphoretics, which help to induce sweating and lower fevers.

Demulcent herbs

Herbs that are demulcent contain mucilage that soothes and protects tissues. We see this most clearly when demulcent herbs come into direct contact with the mucous membranes of the digestive tract, but herbalists have long known that consuming demulcents can benefit inflamed tissues in other locations, such as the urinary system or the respiratory system. The precise mechanism for this indirect action is not certain. We know that mucilage is broken down in the gut, but it is thought that the gut must be communicating with the rest of the body via the nervous system or hormonal secretions. The action of

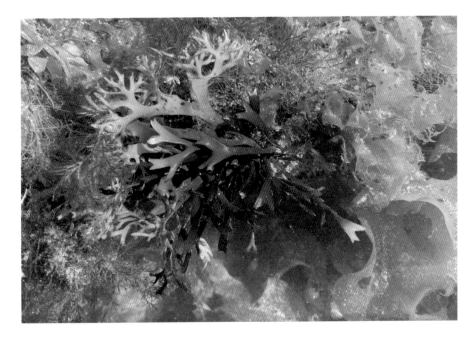

demulcent herbs away from the digestive tract is a beautiful demonstration of the body's inherent wisdom. It also shows how herbs and our bodies have an interconnectedness that goes beyond our current capability to analyse things in a reductionist way. When demulcent herbs are applied topically, they are often described as emollients. Examples of demulcent herbs are Slippery Elm, Marshmallow, and Irish Moss.

Diaphoretic herbs

These are herbs that help to induce sweating and can help in fever management (see circulatory stimulants for some examples). Consider diaphoretics when a patient reports that they never sweat, or when it is desirable to make a feverish patient feel more comfortable. In holistic medicine, fevers should, ideally, be supported rather than suppressed.

Diuretic herbs

Diuretic herbs increase the production of urine. This can be through increasing the blood flow through the kidneys, or it might be through encouraging the kidneys to reabsorb less water, leading to increased urine output. Diuretics can be helpful in cases of oedema, hypertension, urinary system infections, urinary retention, or, in some cases, kidney stones or gravel. Examples of diuretic herbs are Dandelion leaf, Couch Grass, and Pellitory-of-the-Wall. Urinary system demulcents are a subcategory here, with Cornsilk being an example.

Emmenagogue herbs

The traditional definition of emmenagogue is a herb that stimulates menstruation. The term is often broadened to any herb that has an action on the female reproductive system, but this is, in my view, a much less helpful grouping (see uterine tonics as a separate category). Examples of herbs that can stimulate menstruation are Mugwort and Yarrow.

Expectorant herbs

Expectorant herbs support the removal of mucus from the lungs. They are usually divided into either stimulating or relaxing. Stimulating expectorants encourage the respiratory system's natural mucus-expelling processes and make the mucus less viscous. Relaxing expectorants assist mucus expulsion by reducing tension in the respiratory passages and reducing inflammation. Some stimulating expectorants contain saponins, which are soap-like compounds. When ingested, these mildly irritate the stomach, which shares a common nerve root with the respiratory system. This means that the respiratory system is also mildly stimulated, in a process called reflex expectoration. This is why saponin-rich herbs can cause a feeling of nausea if too high a dose is taken. Examples of saponin-containing expectorants are Soapwort, Cowslip, and Daisy. Other stimulating expectorants may be rich in aromatic oils; examples of these are Elecampane and Poplar buds. Relaxing expectorants may be soothing demulcents, such as Irish Moss and Marshmallow, or they may be antispasmodic in nature, such as Thyme and Wild Cherry bark. Some herbal expectorants actually combine the qualities of stimulating and relaxing, delivering the support that is needed by the body in a wide range of respiratory situations. Examples of these amphoteric expectorants are Elderflower, Garlic, and Mullein.

Hepatic herbs

As their name suggests, herbs that are hepatics support the liver. There is a great deal of cross-over with bitters and cholagogues, but in herbal medicine there are many ways of supporting the liver, and stimulating greater bile production is only one of them. For example, in traditional herbal medicine it is considered common for some patients to hold tension in their livers, especially when they are trying to present a calm and happy image to the outside world. Hiding tension in the digestive tract, in particular the liver, is considered to reduce its efficiency, perhaps due to a slightly reduced blood flow. Relaxing hepatics, such as Agrimony, can be very helpful in these cases.

Hypnotic herbs

Hypnotic herbs relax us and help us to sleep more easily and deeply. They range from quite mild relaxing herbs, such as Lemon Balm and Lime flower, to potentially stronger sedatives, such as Wild Lettuce, California Poppy, Valerian, and Mistletoe.

Hypotensive herbs

Hypotensive herbs act to reduce blood pressure when it is too high. They may work by encouraging diuresis, such as in the case of Dandelion leaf, or they may be herbs such as Hawthorn, Cramp Bark, and Lime flower, which directly influence the cardiovascular system and help it to reach a healthier equilibrium.

Nervine herbs

Nervine herbs have a beneficial effect on the nervous system. They may be directly calming, as is the case with Skullcap, Chamomile, and Mugwort, for example, or they may be a healing tonic to the nerve tissue, as is the case with Wild Oat. Many of the calming Western nervine herbs are bitter in nature, and, while they can be very helpful to ease the symptoms of nervous disorders, it is important that the underlying cause is addressed alongside alleviating symptoms. According to Tibetan medicine, if the bitter influence in a prescription is too great, it can worsen nervous symptoms such as anxiety and sleeplessness. This means that while short-term or balanced prescribing of bitter nervines can be a helpful support, long-term or unbalanced prescriptions can create dependence rather than effect a sustainable cure. (I talk more about the importance of balancing prescriptions energetically in chapter 3.)

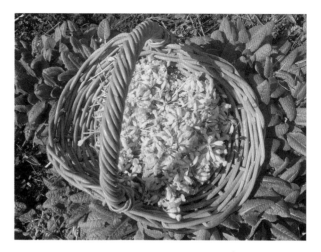

Uterine tonics

Uterine tonics strengthen and nourish the uterus and tone the entire female reproductive system. Raspberry leaf is a well-known herb in this category.

Uterine astringent herbs

Uterine astringent herbs help to reduce blood loss from the uterus. They are helpful in cases of menorrhagia or post-partum haemorrhage. Examples are Shepherd's Purse and Lady's Mantle.

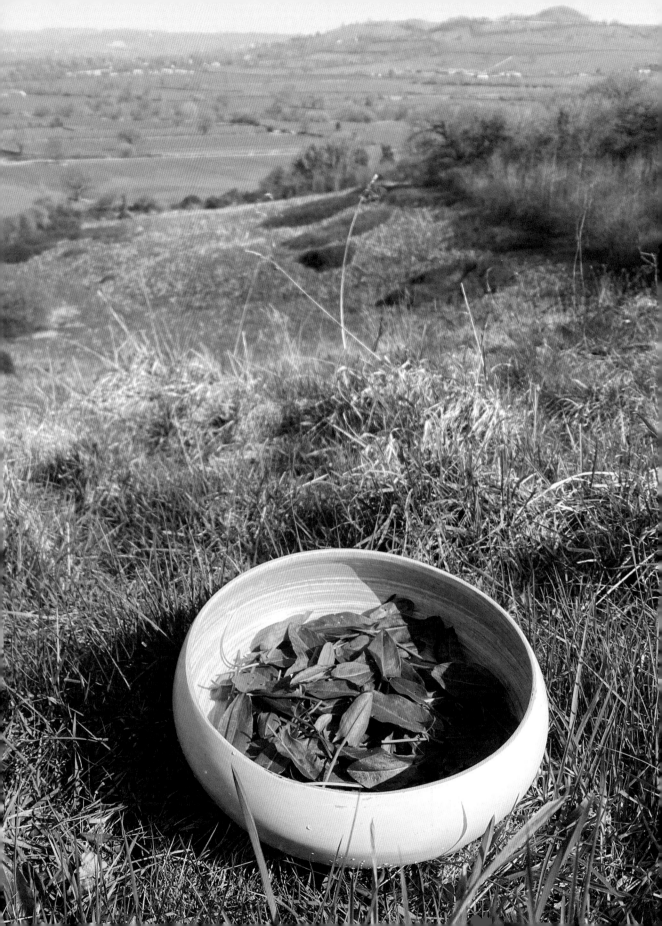

3

Energetic actions: Tibetan medicine and the interplay with the elements

A brief introduction to Tibetan medical principles will help you to see the herbs through my eyes and give you access to an extra layer of information within my herbal descriptions.

In my practice I treat my patients with the use of Tibetan diagnostic principles and a Tibetan medical framework. My prescriptions, made mostly with Western herbs, are formulated taking into account the principles of Tibetan medicine. I also regularly make and prescribe a few Tibetan formulae made from herbs and spices to which I have access.

When I studied Tibetan medicine with Khenpo Troru Tsenam, he emphasized how much he hoped that Western practitioners would learn to integrate the principles of Tibetan medicine into their work. He said: 'Western practitioners will need to understand the tastes and potencies of herbs. They should use the power of logic to deduce what would be good in different situations. This is how we can formulate new compounds with Western herbs.'

Tibetan medicine sees health, illness, and medicinal substances in terms of the elements. There are three humoural principles, based on the elements of Earth, Air, Fire, and Water, and these vary according to the patient's inherited constitution, their age, the season, the weather, their behaviour, thought patterns, and dietary choices. Each humour is associated with a particular element or pair of elements.

Those familiar with the Western Galenic system of humours – sanguine, choleric, phlegmatic, and melancholic – should put this framework temporarily to one side while reading my introduction to the Tibetan approach.

Although in some areas there is a good correspondence between the Western and the Tibetan systems, in others there are some rather confusing differences. I admit to having spent years trying to comfortably merge the two approaches; I have now concluded that I prefer to understand my cases energetically through the lens of Tibetan medicine.

In Tibetan medicine, the three humoural principles – or *nyepa sum* – are related to the elements in the following ways: Air is linked to the wind humour, which is called *rLung*; Fire is linked to the bile humour, which is called *Tripa*; and Earth and Water together are linked to the phlegm humour, which is called *Pekén*. We are all influenced by the three humours, which ebb and flow in relationship to each other at all times, whether we are 'healthy' or diseased. The closer we are to a balanced state, the healthier we are, but for each of us that point of balance will be different. Nothing is solid and fixed. The humours can be altered by factors outside our control – the season, for example – but if we understand which foods, behaviours, and herbal support will help us move back into balance, we will be better able to take care of our own health.

When a patient seeks my help, I am looking far beyond the name of the condition that ails them. In hearing about their health challenges and past diagnoses, I am tuning into the nature of their constitution and the elemental balance in their body. Are they someone who is experiencing an excess of Air, or is their condition one of Fiery heat? Is the patient sitting in front of me suffering from too much Earth and Water, or, as is most common, is their condition caused by a combination of two or three humoural imbalances?

Tibetan medicine demonstrates interconnectedness at the most fundamental level. I was taught that the deepest healing takes place when we realize that interconnectedness. Both illness and remedy are seen as a continuum, explained by the beautiful and sophisticated dance of the elements, both within the body and in the external environment. Although seeing ill health and creating herbal formulations based on the elements and energetics may seem like something from a bygone age, I think that it is a very valuable approach, especially when used alongside a more modern physiological and system-based approach. To understand our health in terms of the humours is empowering and helps us to change our inner health narrative. We can move from being powerless and bewildered to feeling in control and understanding

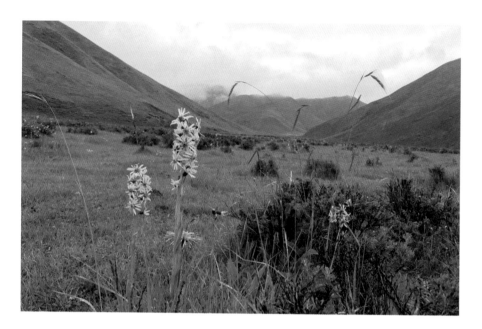

how we can best support our own health. I have lost count of the number of patients who have told me that it all makes so much sense when they view their health in this way.

The humours

Let us talk a little about the qualities of the three humours, so that we can understand the qualities of the herbs that we need to choose to balance them.

rLung

rLung is the Air humour. It is characterized by instability and excessive movement. There are many manifestations of a *rLung* imbalance, and most often it manifests in combination with one or both of the other humours. When we suffer from an excess of the Air humour, we may feel ungrounded and anxious. Our mind is likely to have a tendency to run away with us. Overthinking and over-analysis is the norm. We may suffer from a physical need to move, finding it hard to sit still. We may need to talk very quickly, because the ideas bubbling up in our mind are so rapid we can hardly express them fast enough. Our mood may be changeable, our blood sugar unstable, and our hormones feel unpredictable and alien. We may tremble and yawn. In severe cases we will experience retching or dry heaves. Any symptoms that we have are likely to change and shift rapidly. It can be bewildering and exhausting to suffer from a *rLung* disorder.

Overall, our ability to feel settled and comfortable in our body is much reduced. I have heard patients describing themselves as 'feeling hollow' or 'invisible', or lacking in substance. Some tell me they no longer recognize the body they are inhabiting, because it feels out of control. They report that their health imbalances feel confusing and unbearable. Often the illnesses that these people experience are not 'acknowledged' by the allopathic health professionals, because nothing shows up in physiological tests. They are told to relax or to take antidepressants, which causes them to feel even more alone and hopeless. Others, often those especially drawn to spiritual practice, may start to feel that their physical body is an impediment. They do not see the point of taking care of it. Some say that they feel as though they could float away. All of these experiences make perfect sense within the Tibetan medical framework. There are practical steps that can be taken to balance the excess of the Air element with more Earth, Water, and Fire through diet, lifestyle, and herbal prescriptions, according to the individual needs of each case.

People with more Air in their constitution tend to be sensitive and thoughtful. They are often intuitive and empathetic. They may have a strong calling to help others and are able to empathize with their patients and friends. Sometimes this sensitivity feels like a burden, because they can feel drained by the disturbed energy of those around them. People who have a *rLung* constitution can experience enormous overpowering enthusiasms for new projects and initiatives. They are very good at getting things started, but, unfortunately, they have a tendency to get burnt out and run out of energy before they can see a project through to fruition.

Energetically, *rLung* has the characteristics of being rough, light, cold. The characteristics of the medicines and behaviours that remedy excess *rLung* are smooth, heavy, warm, oily, and stable. *rLung* tends to increase any imbalance in the body, and it can be considered to be either cold or hot, depending on the circumstances. It is also understood to be dry in its influence on the body. This is very different from the Western Galenic understanding of the Air humour (sanguine), which is considered as being warm and moist.

The elemental nature of the treatments that should be chosen for a patient with excess *rLung* is that they should be sweet, sour, and salty. The characteristics or potencies of those treatments should be rich, oily, and nutritious. On a spiritual level, the cultivation of acceptance is the best way of counter-acting *rLung*, since it is made worse by wanting things to be different from how they are.

Tripa

Tripa is the Fire humour. It is characterised by growth and ripening. In pathological manifestations it can be seen as driving over-activity. There may be inflammation, fever, diarrhoea, irritability or rage, joint pains, and redness. We see *Tripa* in excess when there are angry skin conditions, inflam-mation of the digestive tract, joint swellings and gout, acute fevers, tonsillitis, rhinitis, arthritis, cellulitis, bronchitis, and many other conditions ending in '–itis', which means inflammation. *Tripa* is associated with jaundice and 'hot-natured' diarrhoea.

People with a fiery constitutional tendency are often driven and ambitious. They can be confident, 'go-for-it', impulsive people. They are natural lead-ers and movers and shakers. The downside of this is that people with a *Tripa* nature can be impatient and get irritated by others who either do not keep up with their own ideas or disagree with how things should be done.

Tripa has the characteristics of being oily, fast-acting, hot, light, odorous, laxative, and wet, so the remedies that counteract it have the opposite quali-ties of being lean, slow-acting, cool, heavy, liquid, and dry. The nature of the treatments that should be chosen for a patient with an excess of *Tripa* are sweet, bitter, and astringent, with smooth, slow-acting, cooling potencies. On the deepest level, *Tripa* is calmed by transforming anger into compassion.

Pekén

Pekén is the Earth and Water humour. It has the characteristics of being oily, cool, heavy, slow-acting, stable, smooth, and sticky. The treatment strategies to counteract excess *Pekén* are to encourage more Fire and Air in the system. In terms of herbal prescribing, we should aim to treat *Pekén* excess with hot, sour, and astringent herbs. The herbs chosen should have the characteristics of being warming, drying, fast-acting, light, mobile, and rough.

Someone with an excess of *Pekén* can find it hard to initiate new treatment protocols, because making changes is much harder for them. They may suffer from poor circulation and a slow metabolism. The chances are that they will have a slow digestion and be prone to mucus and phlegm. They may find that they suffer from water retention and feel soggy. Excess weight may be hard to shift, and their disinclination to get moving is an obstacle to making positive therapeutic changes. A rise in *Pekén* can be one of the ways of understanding the awful deep dark depression that can overtake some people, sapping their motivation as well as their happiness.

On the plus side, people who naturally have more Earth and Water in their constitution are stable, grounded, and loyal. They are calm in a crisis and will see projects through to completion once they have started them. In fact, they can sometimes be quite stubborn about changing tack. Excess *Pekén* that is causing ill health is counteracted by meditation on precious human life and impermanence.

Prescribing energetically

When prescribing energetically, the herbal prescription is by no means the only therapeutic influence. Diet and lifestyle are fundamental areas to consider if we are to encourage healing. In fact, in Tibetan medicine it is considered unethical to prescribe herbs without treating diet and lifestyle first. We can be much more flexible about the elemental nature of the herbs we prescribe if we are able to encourage our patients to support their healing by changing their diet and lifestyle in a way that is appropriate to their condition.

The other thing we need to consider is that within Tibetan medicine it is very rare to prescribe single herbs. Herbs are prescribed within beautifully sophisticated formulae that are designed to provide balance to the humours as well as targeted support for physiological actions within the body, as needed.

Herbs according to Tibetan medicine

When it comes to choosing Western herbs according to Tibetan medicinal principles, this is an enormous subject and one that we can explore for ourselves over many years. Apart from some very pronounced examples, such as the bitterness of Vervain or the sweetness of Liquorice, the way we view the taste qualities of individual Western herbs is often a matter of experience and opinion. We generally come to our own conclusions based on working with those herbs ourselves.

Tibetan medicine teaches us that the elemental correspondences of the six tastes are as follows:

- **Sweet:** Earth and Water
- **Sour:** Fire and Earth
- **Salty:** Fire and Water
- **Bitter:** Water and Air
- **Astringent:** Earth and Air
- **Hot:** Fire and Air

When choosing herbs to calm excess *rLung*, we need a warming, nourishing, stabilising influence. Herbs that have Air within their taste makeup should ideally be balanced by those that are heavier and more stable. In practice, this means being careful with bitter, astringent, and hot herbs.

When choosing herbs to calm excess *Tripa*, we need to choose cooling and anti-inflammatory herbs, such as bitters, astringent herbs, and nourishing sweet herbs. We should be careful with hot, sour, and salty herbs because these contain the element of Fire and could aggravate the *Tripa* state.

When choosing herbs to calm excess *Pekén*, we need to introduce warmth and movement. Hot, sour, and astringent herbs are usually most indicated. We need to be careful with cooling herbs or herbs that are oily and heavy.

This is only a very brief and simple explanation. I hope that it gives you a starting point to explore the actions of familiar herbs in a new way. In practice it is very rare to see a single humoural imbalance: we are most often faced with complicated combinational imbalances that can shift in terms of the proportions of each element on a daily basis. We need to decide on the proportions of the herbs we prescribe based on many factors, including our instincts.

By seeing medicines, the environment, our diet, behaviour, our own selves, and our patients in terms of the elements, we are practising a deep understanding of interconnectedness. It becomes much easier to create a more positive and understandable health narrative and to be empowered to look after our own health in terms of our daily choices and thoughts.

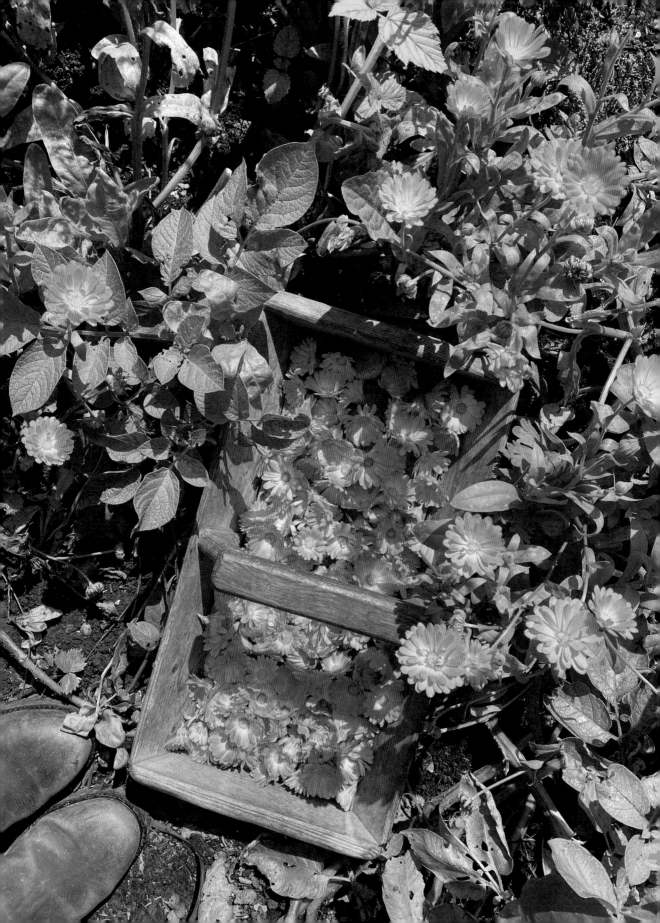

4

Healing the emotions and encouraging connection to the whole

Bodily systems can never be completely independent of each other, and, likewise, the physiological processes within our body have a direct impact on our emotional state. I was taught that in order to process our emotions, we need to digest them – and, indeed, most patients report much better emotional health when their digestive system returns to health after a period of imbalance.

If we are to treat truly holistically, we must be open to the way that physiological processes can influence our emotional wellbeing. For example, if our body feels tense, we cannot help but be less flexible in our thought processes; if our lymphatic system is congested, we tend to feel muddle-headed and cluttered. I have noticed that those with weaker blood-vessel boundaries, seen in capillary fragility or varicose veins, find it more difficult to manifest boundaries in their life. If they consistently find it difficult to say 'no', they will gradually feel taken advantage of, depleted, and probably quite angry. Herbs that support healthier boundaries within the body seem to support us in manifesting healthy boundaries within our day-to-day life. Herbs that help us to breathe more easily can help us to say what we really want to say and also to process grief. These examples are interconnectedness in action.

Many of the herbs that we work with in our dispensaries have traditional emotional correspondences that may not be explained by science. We think of Borage for courage and Motherwort to heal our relationship with mothering or being mothered. Most of us know that Rose is associated with opening the heart and helping us to move through grief. Hawthorn encourages us to put into place firm, healthy boundaries, and Cramp Bark makes us more flexible in our attitudes. Tibetan medicine explains this by pointing out that our experience of the wider world and our attitude to it is hugely influenced by the state of our physical body and the state of our mind. Changes that are brought to bear within the physical body will therefore have an influence on our attitudes and emotions.

I often include within a prescription herbs that will help to shift mental and emotional attitudes. Of course, the patient will be making dietary and lifestyle changes and will most likely be taking herbs to support physical healing at the root cause, but to support the emotions and help to support a shift in habitual thought patterns is very helpful for the overall healing process. Over the years I have repeatedly observed how effective this strategy is, and I am very grateful that the herbs offer themselves to patients in this way alongside their physiological properties.

As well as prescribing herbs based on their emotional correspondences, I also take account of the so-called 'mind poisons' that are likely to be a factor in a patient's ill health, based on their humoural imbalances. *Tripa* is associated with the mind poison of anger, and we know that a liver that is in need of support is often associated with a tendency to irritability or anger. In this case choosing herbs that support the liver, within the context of the overall prescription, will help the patient to overcome their tendency to anger. It can also be helpful for this type of patient to cultivate the development of compassion. The best meditative practice to counteract *Tripa* is to work on transforming anger into compassion. *Pekén* is associated with the mind poison of apathy and this can be helped by reflecting on impermanence and how precious our life is. Patients with an excess of *Pekén* often have a weak digestion and have a hard time digesting emotions and experiences. This can lead to crippling indecision, which can, in turn, lead to stagnation. It seems easier to keep things as they are than to risk making the 'wrong' decision. When these patients are given herbs that support the digestion, they very often find that they have an increased zest for life and become more focused. *rLung* is associated with attachment, usually manifested by wanting aspects of our life to be different from how they are and constantly thinking about that rather than being able to accept the situation. This elemental imbalance is often linked to problems in the large intestine, an organ that functions best when we learn to 'let go' rather than 'hold on' to things. By helping the large intestine to function better and encouraging an ability to accept and let go, a patient's overall health is often greatly improved.

In holistic herbal medicine we cannot separate mind, body, and spirit. There is a clear link between organ systems, energetic principles, and emotional states, but we should also recognize that our habitual thought patterns influence our organ systems and can unbalance our health. It is no good eating the healthiest diet in the world if we feed our minds with a daily diet of angry, negative, or fearful thoughts. When herbalists choose herbs to support a patient's physiological processes, they can overlay an intention for emotional healing within the same prescription. I always explain this by saying that if another herbalist looks at a prescription on a purely body-systems basis, this should make perfect sense, but the herbs that I have chosen may also have another layer of action that should be helpful.

I am going to add a little warning here. When treating patients in this very complete way considering different levels of herbal action at the same time, it may be difficult to treat family members or close friends. Discussing habitual thought patterns and emotional tendencies can be a tricky conversation, and it is always important to prescribe herbs in a way that is going to be helpful given where a patient is at the time and your relationship with them. The good thing is that emotional healing happens when the physiological healing happens, even if has not been directly discussed. For example, if someone is very irritable and angry due to liver congestion, supporting their liver will make them feel much calmer and less easily angered. Also, if someone with a chronic respiratory issue struggles to say what they think or to be heard, treating them with respiratory-system-supporting herbs can help them to find their voice alongside improving their physiological condition. One last example is the case of someone with varicose veins and haemorrhoids, who also finds it very difficult to set healthy boundaries in their life. If they are treated with herbs that support the integrity of their veins (creating a stronger boundary within their system), they usually start to enforce healthy boundaries without being prompted. These emotional or 'non-physiological' effects have made themselves very clear to me over the years. When I was first in practice, I honestly did not expect them, but now I have seen again and again how herbs really support our health on different levels at the same time. I think of it as each herb or combination of herbs reflecting the perfect balance of the 'whole'. When we take herbal medicine that has been carefully formulated for our unique circumstances and we support the process by adapting our lifestyle and creating a more positive health narrative, our bodies are stimulated into regaining a healthful balance. That is true herbal magic!

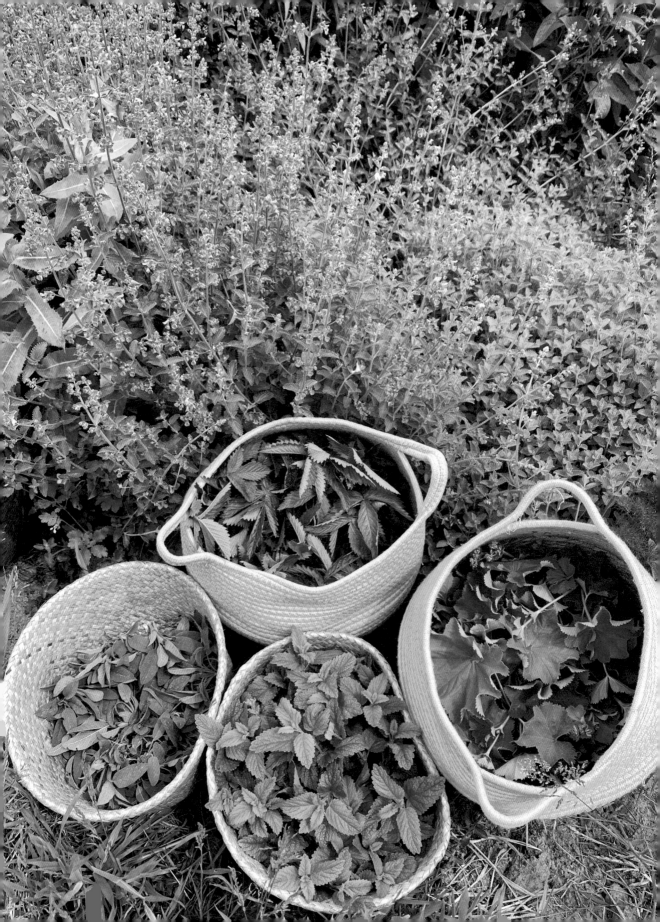

Part Two

THE HERBS

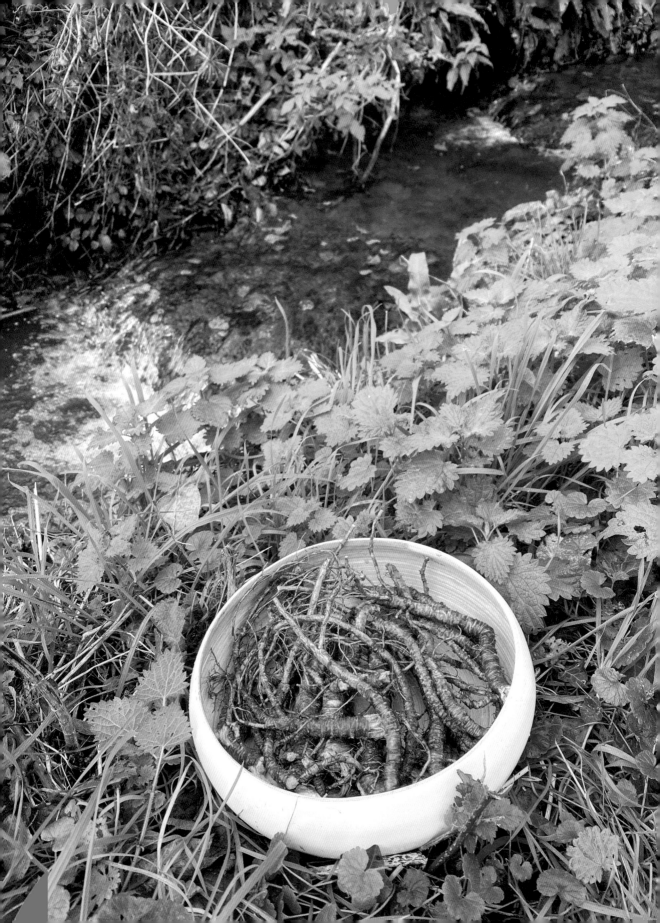

5

Introducing the herbs

This book is about understanding and respecting herbs as individuals. In my description of each herb, I discuss physiological actions, energetic characteristics, and emotional aspects where these apply. I also unashamedly include historical information, since, in many cases, historical sources point towards valid therapeutic strategies that have now fallen out of favour. I have added some informal anonymized case studies from my clinic in order to illustrate my way of prescribing and the way that I view herbal actions within the context of my work. Herbal medicine is about so much more than just 'treating conditions'.

I would love to support you in your quest to build up a working herbal dispensary of your own, so I have included some herbal recipes. These recipes are for products aimed at acute conditions or general health support. I have chosen them very carefully so that they are a helpful addition to the home apothecary and will help to deepen your own relationship with herbs. They may provide relief for chronic conditions too, but in order to properly treat the underlying cause of chronic conditions I believe patients require a much more in-depth and individual approach.

It almost goes without saying that for a safe and effective herbal treatment of patients we need to understand the different ways that good health manifests in people of differing constitutions, as well as the wide range of ways that the body and mind can behave when things are out of balance. In a time when a great many people are taking allopathic medication, we also need to accept that herbal medicine can, in some cases, interact with these medications adversely. If we are prescribing or suggesting herbs to others, it is very important that we have the knowledge to avoid that. Medical herbalists are trained rigorously in these aspects, and each of us is bound by a solemn vow to protect life and avoid harm. We are taught to spot dangerous symptoms, and we know when to advise a patient to take a dramatically different course of action from the one that they are expecting from us. If you are in any doubt about how to work with herbs in your own or your family's situation, please, take advice from a professional. This plea is not motivated by a disrespect of those with genuine experience or a heartfelt connection with herbs, or, for that matter, a wish to 'generate more business' for medical herbalists. It is offered with the intention of keeping people safe, reducing the suffering of those who are unwell, and helping herbs to do their work most effectively. We all need to recognize our limitations, medical herbalists included, and patient safety must come first.

Agrimony 🌿 *Agrimonia eupatoria*

'Agrimony encourages us to reset the balance between tension and relaxation in our bodies.'

I deliberately do not have 'favourite' herbs, because I respect and love all of the herbs that I work with, but if I had to choose a dozen, Agrimony would definitely be included. Before it flowers, Agrimony is a mass of gentle, lemony fragrant, calming leaves. It exudes relaxation. When it flowers, it seems tall and tense and spiky. It bears numerous seed heads, which cling to your clothes and hair. It is almost as though it has an attention-seeking, tense side. If this is the case, I fully embrace both of its aspects, although I prefer to harvest the leaves early in the season when the yield is more abundant and the stalks are easier to cut.

Agrimony was named after King Mithridates VI Eupator because of his interest in herbs. He was especially fond of Agrimony as an eye treatment. The generic name 'Agrimonia' comes from the Greek word '*argemone*', which means cataract. Its folk names – 'Church Steeples', 'Cocklebur', 'Garclife' (meaning 'Spear Cleavers' in Anglo-Saxon) – refer to its growth habit.

Its slightly lemony fragrant scent reveals Agrimony's relaxing and calming qualities. The aromatics responsible for this are cleverly packaged with gentle bitterness and astringency, making it also very helpful for toning tissues that have become too relaxed or inflamed. This combination of a calming, relaxing influence with a toning and tightening action is a very valuable attribute.

When I dry Agrimony for prescribing throughout the year, it is reassuring to know that the lemony scent is captured fully. This is very obvious when you open the storage box. I have never noticed the same when smelling Agrimony from large-scale production, but, to

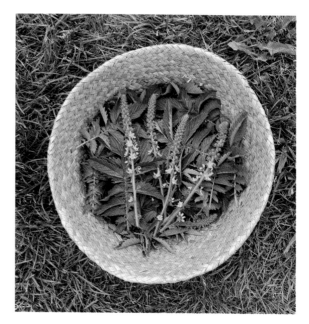

be fair, I do not buy it in these days, and it seems rude when visiting herbal friends to ask if I can sniff their Agrimony!

Agrimony leaps out, asking to be included in prescriptions for patients who 'put on a brave face', who 'hide their worries behind a happy countenance', and who drive their tension deep inside their body, so that the surface seems relaxed and calm. They also invariably hold their breath when they are in pain. Another sign that Agrimony is needed is when people are addicted to activities that get their adrenaline flowing or that they can indulge in to excess. These people may like driving too fast, doing extreme sports, drinking too much, or partying hard. They have the ability to hold everything in and keep control, but every so often they need a release valve. Agrimony is ideal for them, because it balances tension and relaxation.

When people are hiding their tension, it tends to accumulate in the digestive tract, gradually eroding efficient digestion and causing poor absorption and the start of irritations, inflammation, and leaky gut, for example. You cannot digest food – or emotions, for that matter – if your gut and liver are too tense.

Medicinal parts

▷ Aerial parts

Physiological actions

Summary

▷ Hepatic
▷ Antispasmodic
▷ Astringent
▷ Bitter
▷ Diuretic
▷ Anti-inflammatory
▷ Vulnerary
▷ Antimicrobial

Physiological virtues

Agrimony is most often described primarily as an hepatic herb, recommended for chronic liver disease, cholocystosis, and to increase the secretion of bile in general. It does have some bitterness that helps to stimulate the production of bile through the taste reflex and through its action on bitter receptors in the gut. That is by no means the whole story though. This herb helps liver function in quite a different way from traditional liver/gallbladder herbs, such as, for example, Milk Thistle, Oregon Grape, or Greater Celandine. Agrimony, especially when home-grown and small-batch-produced, is very aromatic. It smells gorgeous and lemony and is very relaxing to be around. The aromatic compounds help to relax the digestive system as well as gently relaxing the blood vessels supplying the gut and associated organs, including the liver. Livers need a good supply of blood to do

their work most efficiently, and those who are chronically tense may be causing this flow to be lessened. We can therefore see that Agrimony especially supports the liver through its ability to relax tension. This has wide implications in relieving digestive disturbances, blood-sugar imbalances, poor fat digestion, jaundice, and cyclical hormonal symptoms such as premenstrual tension, dysmenorrhea, and menorrhagia.

Agrimony is also significantly astringent, a property that means that it has, since old times, been traditionally considered an anti-inflammatory and wound-healing herb. Astringency is a quality associated with tightening and toning and is in some ways the opposite of relaxation. Alongside this toning action, Agrimony acts as an antispasmodic and anti-inflammatory within the digestive tract in general. This can be very helpful in cases of diarrhoea, malabsorption, gastritis, and irritable bowel syndrome (IBS). In this latter condition we often see alternating constipation and diarrhoea, a symptom pattern associated with periods of excessive tension and excessive relaxation. Agrimony is a master of balancing tension with relaxation, so it is not surprising that is so helpful for those with IBS.

Consider prescribing Agrimony to a breast-feeding mother in order to gently treat diarrhoea in her baby or giving it as a cooled tea to small children with upset tummies. Agrimony's attributes as an astringent, relaxing diuretic are also excellent to support the urinary system. It helps to resolve cystitis, irritable bladder, urinary stones, and incontinence.

Just because Agrimony is so valuable as an internal treatment, we should not dismiss its powers as a topical application. It can be made into a fomentation to relieve muscle spasms and an eye wash for inflammatory problems of the eyes, such as conjunctivitis and blepharitis. As well as being healing and anti-inflammatory, it is directly antimicrobial. It is a useful choice for a mouthwash for inflamed gums and a gargle for a sore throat. As a douche it will relieve vaginal infections. It is an excellent overall styptic and wound healer, not only due to its astringency and antimicrobial properties, but perhaps also because it has a high silica content.

Agrimony is one of those herbs that is a medicine chest in itself. It really is a remarkable herb in so many situations. It surprises me that it is not prescribed more widely by herbalists, but then I remember how different home-grown Agrimony is compared to large-scale bought-in plant material. If you grow just one medicinal herb in your garden, I would say make it Agrimony.

Like many herbs, it can thin the blood, so avoid therapeutic doses when taking antiscoagulants and for a week prior to scheduled surgery.

Energetics

Agrimony is astringent, bitter, and warming. It is specific for people who like to put on a brave face, hiding their stress and worry deep inside. This is the classic British 'stiff-upper-lip' syndrome. We do not want to bother someone else with our troubles and prefer to keep up a pretence of all being well. This dual reality sets up a lot of tension inside the body, so much so that a release valve can be needed. Often this is achieved by the person falling prey to addictive behaviours, such as excessive drug-taking or alcohol consumption, or thrill-seeking behaviour patterns such as driving too fast or other dangerous activities that patients say 'gives them a buzz'. This can sometimes also be manifested as an addiction to very intense exercise.

Perhaps Agrimony understands that sometimes tension is needed in order to 'get a job done' or to cope with adversity? If this is the case, we should see this tension as a means to an end, not a default state of being in the body. If we need excessive tension to cope with our way of living, we really need to look at making some significant changes if we want to stay healthy.

In Tibetan medicine

Agrimony tastes astringent and bitter and has a slightly warming potency. It is quite a balanced herb in terms of its tastes, especially when grown and prepared in small batches so that its aromatic properties are properly preserved.

In my dispensary

Agrimony is a very important crop for me, because I know how superior home-grown or small-scale-produced Agrimony is compared with that from large-scale production. In small-scale production, it is possible to better preserve the aromatic constituents that provide an antispasmodic and warming influence to the action of the herb. This is remarkably helpful for people with nervous digestive disorders or chronic held-in tension. In the Western world this symptom picture is sadly a very common state of affairs, so I admit that I often reach for Agrimony in my prescription blends.

I like Agrimony as a topical wound treatment too. It is one of four herbs in my general all-purpose healing ointment, something that is a staple of my home apothecary or travel first-aid kit.

The following case illustrates a patient who very clearly needed Agrimony and how helpful it was to her.

'Julia' was 63 years old. For the last nine months she had been experiencing dry, itchy skin, and it was getting worse. She said that she had tried many different topical creams, and none of them made a difference. She also told me that, at night, the itching was always worse on the side on which she was lying. There was no visible rash, and her GP had said that it was not shingles. Julia was going through quite a stressful time in her life in general and had an elderly relative for whom she was a main carer. She had a lot of tension and was clearly someone who had to hide it and maintain a calm exterior. She also mentioned that she had recently bought a sports car, which she loved driving very much. As quite often happens, I had already written 'Agrimony' in the margin of her notes within 10 minutes of starting the consultation.

She suffered with anxiety, her mouth and eyes were dry as well as her skin; this was probably partly due to the fact that she drank six cups of tea and only one cup of water each day. Drinking less tea and more water was therefore my first recommendation. She also suffered with alternating constipation and diarrhoea, classic symptoms of IBS, so I knew that Agrimony was indicated on a physiological level as well as an energetic one. I prescribed an individual tincture blend with Agrimony as the main herb, with Mugwort, Vervain, Blessed Thistle, Wild Oat, and Calendula as supporters. Within four weeks the itchiness had disappeared, her skin, mouth and eyes were less dry, her energy level had improved, her bowels were more stable, and her anxiety had lessened, although it was still present. She said that her nerves did not feel as 'jangly'. She continued to benefit from the tincture over the next few months and felt much more balanced and better able to cope with her ongoing stress as a result.

Historical applications

Dioscorides considered Agrimony to be a snake-bite medicine, recommending it to be made into a salve with Plantain and Bistort. Before applying the salve, the bite area was ringed with Agrimony in order to confine the poison. Agrimony was also one of the 57 herbs in the Anglo-Saxon 'Holy Salve', which was considered effective against goblins, evil, and poisons. I have always included Agrimony in my general healing salve, but I must admit that I have never thought to mention its additional action against goblins!

John Parkinson wrote that Galen '*saith, it is of thinne parts, and hath a cleansing and cutting facility, without any manifest heate: it is also moderately drying and binding.*' He went on to say: '*It openeth the obstructions of the Liver, and clenseth it, it helpeth the jaundice, and strengthneth the inward parts, and is very beneficial to the bowels, and health their inward woundings and bruises or hurts, and qualifieth all inward distempers, that grow therein. . . . A decoction of the herbe, made with wine and drunke, is good against the sting, and bitings of Serpents.*'

He also said that Agrimony is '*good for the strangury, and helpeth them to make water. . . It clenseth the breast, and helpeth the cough: it is accounted also a good help to ridde a quartaine as well as a tertian ague, by taking draught of the decoction warm before the fit which by altering them, will in time ridde them.*'

Dioscorides wrote that '*the leaves and seeds stayeth the bloody flixe, being taken in wine.*'. . . . '*Outwardly applyed it helpeth old sores, cancers, and ulcers that are of hard curation, being stamped with old Swines grease and applyed, for it clenseth and afterwards healeth them. In the same manner also applied, it doth draw forth the thornes or splinters, nayles, or any other such thing, that is gotten into the flesh. . . . It helpeth to strengthen members that be out of joynt. It helpeth also foule impostumed eares, being bruised and applied, or the juyce dropped into them.*'

John Gerard charmingly writes that '*a decoction of the leaves is good for them that have naughty livers.*'

In the fifteenth century Agrimony was the main ingredient in '*arquebusade water*'. This formula was a staple of the battlefield medicine chest for wounds caused by an 'arquebus': a fifteenth-century long-barrelled gun. This highlights Agrimony's significant styptic action.

Nicholas Culpeper recommends it for gout, as well as all of the other applications already mentioned. He said that it could be applied as '*an oil or ointment or taken inwardly, in an electuary or syrup, or concreted juice*'.

In his *Universal Herbal* of 1832, Thomas Green writes that Agrimony root '*appears to possess the properties of Peruvian Bark in a very considerable degree, without manifesting any of its inconvenient qualities, and if taken in pretty large doses, either in decoction or powder, seldom fails to cure the ague*'.

Magical

Agrimony is considered to banish unwanted spirits. It can be burned as incense to keep away astral intruders or added to protection sachets and spells to banish negative energies and spirits. It has the reputation of being able to break hexes (and reverse them). In the Tyrol, Agrimony was used to detect the presence of witches by being combined in an amulet with Broom, Rue, Maidenhair Fern, and Ground Ivy. It enabled the bearer to see witches or prevent them from entering the house. This way of working with Agrimony apparently continued well into the nineteenth century.

It is said that placing some Agrimony under the head will allow a person to sleep soundly. An old English medical manuscript mentions this magical property of Agrimony as follows:

> '*If it be leyd under mann's heed,*
> *He shal sleepyn as he were deed:*
> *He shal never drede ne wakyn*
> *Till fro under hid heed it be takyn.*'

I have never tried this myself, but what I can say is that being in my clinic when the dehydrators are filled with Agrimony is a very relaxing experience and one that is much commented on by patients and visitors.

Suggestion for the home apothecary

Healing ointment

Take the following:

- » *1 part dried Agrimony aerial parts*
- » *1 part dried Calendula flowers*
- » *1 part dried Comfrey leaves*
- » *1 part dried Lavender flowers*

Add to a slow cooker and cover with mild and light olive oil, warming it very gently over a few days, in the way described for Horse Chestnut. Once the oil is ready, strain it, and measure the volume. Rewarm it gently in a double boiler, adding 1 g of beeswax for each 7 ml of infused oil. Pour the oil and melted wax mixture into a jug, and immediately fill clean dry jars with it. Wait for the ointment to set before picking the jars up to lid them.

This ointment is a staple in my clinic as well as in my home medicine chest. It is perfect for cuts, scrapes, burns, itchy rashes, blisters, sunburn, spots, insect bites, and stings. It is also very effective for bruising or painful swollen smaller joints such as bunions. It even works for warts.

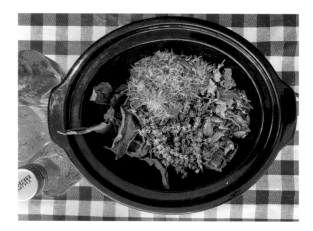

Angelica 🌿 *Angelica archangelica*

'Angelica warms the body and helps us connect to the divine.'

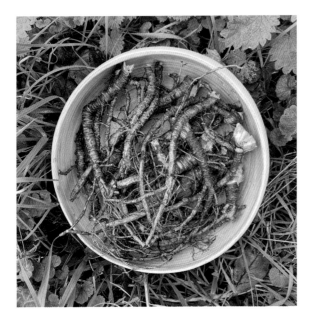

Angelica is a beautiful plant, associated with the warmth and energy of the sun. It holds us and supports us in a great many health circumstances. It enlivens all systems of the body and helps us to balance the spiritual and material realms. This means that it can be a really good herb for people who find it difficult to connect with 'the bigger picture' and accept the interconnectedness of life. The modern name, 'Angelica', is said to have been adopted because the medicinal qualities of the plant were revealed to a monk by an angel who showed him that it was a cure for the plague.

Medicinal parts
- Leaves
- Seeds
- Stems
- Roots

Physiological actions

Summary
- Bitter
- Cholagogue
- Carminative
- Antispasmodic
- Diuretic
- Antimicrobial
- Circulatory stimulant
- Expectorant
- Emmenagogue
- Diaphoretic

Physiological virtues

Angelica is a warming digestive support and cholagogue, especially valuable because most herbal digestive stimulants are cooling. It can increase the appetite, which can be helpful when it is reduced due to disordered digestion. Angelica is also worth considering as a support when a patient's relationship with food and eating is difficult. It relieves nausea and is carminative, easing griping, bloating, and indigestion. It is also generally antispasmodic, reducing habitual muscle tension and easing menstrual cramps.

It is a diuretic, encouraging better elimination through the kidneys, and, since it is directly antimicrobial, it also acts as a urinary antiseptic.

Angelica enlivens the circulation in general, warming chronically cold hands and feet. It is a specific for Buerger's disease (when the arteries of the hands and feet become inflamed, narrowed, and prone to clots) and Raynaud's disease (when there are intermittent spasms of the small arteries, which cause reduced flow to the end arterioles, most often in the fingers).

It can be an especially good choice for cold patients with a tendency to anaemia. It is also anti-inflammatory, well worth considering when there is inflammation that is accompanied by poor circulation, such as in gout or some cases of arthritis. Its circulatory supportive action can also be helpful for patients who complain of foggy thinking.

As well as supporting digestion and circulation and reducing muscular tension, Angelica has a notably positive action on the respiratory system. It is a very good expectorant when taken internally as tea or tincture. The leaves can also be made into a chest compress that helps patients breathe more easily when there is inflammation and congestion in the respiratory tract. Angelica is diaphoretic too, helping to encourage sweating and reducing fever.

You can take fresh or dried Angelica leaf tea as a tonic, or you can take the root in the form of a decoction or tincture. It should be prescribed with care for patients with diabetes, since it tends to increase the level of sugar in the urine. It can stimulate menstruation, so do not take this herb if you are pregnant. Angelica can provoke photosensitivity in some people.

Topically, a fomentation of Angelica root decoction – or an infusion of the leaves – can resolve bruises and encourage the healing of leg ulcers or burns. It is also considered helpful for inflammations of the skin or scalp. Apply to the affected area three times a day. A foot bath can help resolve athlete's foot, or you can dust the powdered dried root onto the feet after washing. The leaves can also be added to the bath as a general health-promoting and relaxing treatment.

Energetics

Angelica is hot, sweet and bitter. It is expansive. It is a herb to consider when a patient seems contracted in themselves and lacking a healthy balance between groundedness and spirituality. It is worth noting here that this balance will be different for each person. Practitioners should not impose their own views about this balance onto their patients; however, if patients themselves mention this as an issue for them, Angelica will support the process of rebalancing.

An old Norse name for Angelica is *Hvann-njoli* (hollow stalk), and it is these hollow stalks that are considered to form a bridge between the groundedness of the earth and the expansiveness and freedom of our soaring spirits. If you need further convincing, just contemplate Angelica's large, fragrant root system anchoring its very tall aerial parts that soar upwards and produce starburst-shaped flowers and seed heads.

When we connect with Angelica, whether that is through ingesting it, applying it topically or even just contemplating it, we receive this message of spiritual and material balance at a deep level, even if we do not consciously realize it. Angelica is an absolutely beautiful, wise, and generous plant being.

In Tibetan medicine

The species of Angelica that is included in the Tibetan pharmacopoeia is *Angelica glauca*. In Tibetan it is called *Ca ba yung ba* [ཙ་བ་གཡུང་བ།]. It has a hot, bitter, and sweet taste, with a sweet post-digestive taste and a warming and heavy potency. This plant is quite unusual in that it is a warming bitter. These virtues are very useful when addressing digestive insufficiency in patients with an energetically cold presentation, for example patients with an excess of *Pekén*. The texts describe Angelica's ability to reduce the Air and Water elements and to increase Fire. They say that it opens the body vessels, restores kidney heat, and acts as a diuretic. It also increases digestive heat and cures stomach disorders. It treats anaemia, debility, fluid retention in the joints, first-stage dropsy, and *rLung* disorders in general. It relieves congestion due to colds or hay fever.

In my dispensary

I regularly meet new patients who tell me that they find their embodiment an encumbrance. They would prefer to concentrate solely on a spiritual life, and they are frustrated by their body's 'inability to be well'. I explain that to be well, we need to take care of and respect our body. In these cases, I most probably include Angelica in their mix too.

On the flip side of that, I also meet patients who find themselves living on a completely worldly and materialistic plane, worrying about their means and their status and feeling more and more anxious about their body and the way that it is aging. There comes a point when people begin to realize that there is more to life than all of this, but the grip of material-based thought patterns can make change very difficult. It is hard to be truly well if we do not balance body, mind, and spirit, and I find that patients instinctively understand this when it is pointed out to them. What that balance means to each of us will be very different, but the thing that we all hold in common is that it is far healthier to have awareness of a 'bigger picture' beyond our worldly and materialistic concerns. When I meet patients who are trying to connect with something beyond the 'daily grind' but are finding it tough, I consider adding Angelica to their prescription. This seems to pave the way for more expansive thought and positive change. It is lovely to see how people's deep suffering falls away as they become more balanced.

'Janie' was 60 years old and had a high-pressure job at which she excelled. She came to see me for support with energy levels and some residual menopausal symptoms. She had some digestive insufficiency and did not have a regular eating pattern. She also found that she was adversely affected by the stress she was under at work.

In recent years she had felt strongly drawn to explore esoteric subjects in her spare time. She wanted to deepen her relationship with energetic and spiritual aspects of healing and personal development, but found it really hard to find the stillness to do this within her habitually busy schedule. She wanted to pursue lots of different fascinating avenues of study and did not feel that she had the time or stillness to see each one through. She told me that she yearned to connect more deeply with her spiritual side, and I wrote 'Angelica' in the margin of her notes.

I prescribed a calming prescription of nervines and digestion-supporting herbs, including Angelica. After a couple of months of treatment her digestion was much better, and her menopausal symptoms had become a thing of the past. She told me that she had begun to spend quiet, contemplative time and was no longer filling her days with busy-ness and unnecessarily long 'to-do lists'. She was keeping a daily gratitude journal and recording her dreams, and overall she was feeling much more settled and comfortable with exploring spiritual aspects in her life. As a result of this she said that she felt better than she had felt for very many years.

Historical applications

Paracelsus referenced Angelica's antimicrobial action when he described it as a '*marvellous medicine*' during the Milan plague epidemic in 1510.

Parkinson places Angelica as the most important medicinal plant of all in his *Paradise in Sole*, which was published in 1629.

Culpeper wrote: '*It resists poison by defending and comforting the heart, blood and spirits. It does the like against the plague and all epidemical diseases. It helps pleurisy as also all other diseases of the lungs and breast.*'

In fact, most of the old writers praise Angelica very highly as a herb to protect against contagion and to purify the blood.

Gerard said it '*cureth the bitings of mad dogs and all other venomous beasts*'.

Maud Grieve describes abundant fields of Angelica, grown on moist soils around London, for the stems to be candied. I would love to see abundant fields of Angelica growing here again, but perhaps for medicine, rather than candy.

The British Flora Medica (1838) reports that '*Laplanders considered this plant as one of the most important productions of the soil.*' Apparently, it was prescribed for a severe colic, something to which they were prone.

Magical

Angelica has a long history of being associated with protection. In the language of flowers, it is believed to symbolize inspiration, ecstasy, and magic. Laplanders used to crown their poets with Angelica leaves and flowers in order to inspire them.

Suggestion for the home apothecary

Angelica leaf bath

Take two handfuls of fresh Angelica leaves, crush them a little, and add them to your bath. This will enliven and stimulate the circulation

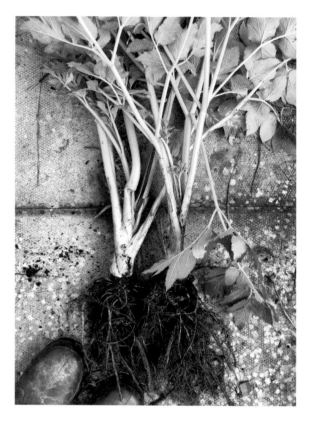

and act as a general tonic. It can be a good thing to try when you have been harvesting Angelica roots. Do not do this if you are pregnant. Remember that, in some people, Angelica can cause photosensitivity, so bear this in mind the first time you try an Angelica bath.

Artichoke 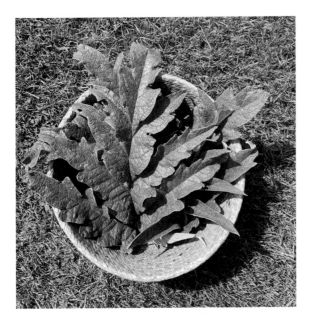 *Cynara scolymus*

'Artichoke supports liver function and reduces blood lipids.'

Artichoke is best known for its edible flower buds and beautiful huge flowers, but the leaves are a valuable and readily available bitter medicine.

Medicinal parts

▹ Leaves

Physiological actions

Summary

▹ Bitter
▹ Cholagogue
▹ Blood sugar balancer
▹ Antihypercholesterolaemic

Physiological virtues

Artichoke is a significant bitter, the levels of the bitter compounds in the leaves being highest just before the plant flowers. Artichoke leaves make a good digestive tonic, stimulating the liver and gallbladder and helping to resolve jaundice and hepatitis. They also have a directly rejuvenating and protective effect on the liver, similar to that of Milk Thistle (*Silybum marianum*).

It helps to stabilize blood sugar levels and therefore can be a helpful herb in the treatment of patients with diabetes. It also reduces blood lipids, perhaps through its ability to help reverse fatty degeneration of the liver. It is a good choice to consider when treating patients with a tendency to form gallstones, its efficacy probably being linked to its ability to normalize cholesterol metabolism. I also suggest considering Artichoke for patients with atherosclerosis.

Energetics

Artichoke is strongly bitter. It tones us and restore us, giving us more zest for life. We all need bitterness in our lives, so that we can truly value and appreciate the moments of sweetness, without craving them. This applies whether we are considering it in a food context or an emotional one.

In Tibetan medicine

Artichoke leaf has a bitter taste and is cooling in potency. It is good in cases of bronchitis, chronic lung disorders, constipation, diabetes, and lymphatic congestion. It is a tonic, a rejuvenative, and an aphrodisiac.

In my dispensary

I prescribe Artichoke as tincture, capsules, and tea, depending on the circumstances of the case. I often choose it when there is hyper-cholesterolaemia. I also encourage patients to supplement their diet with Artichoke hearts in these cases. Regular consumption of Artichoke tones the system and reduces blood lipids, but other factors, for example stress and inflammation, will need to be addressed too, according to the individual case.

I make an Artichoke bitters blend that can be a helpful adjunct to treatment in a range of cases.

Historical applications

Globe Artichokes were cultivated by the Romans, and it is likely that they were first introduced to England during the Roman occupation. They were mostly grown for food, but Dioscorides suggested applying mashed Artichoke root to the underarm area in order to sweeten body odours. When the Romans left, the habit of eating Artichokes must have left with them. Artichokes disappeared until they were re-introduced in 1548.

Culpeper describes how Artichokes not only provoke lust, but they also '*stay the involuntary course of natural seed in man which is commonly called nocturnal pollutions*'.

Suggestion for the home apothecary

Artichoke leaf bitters

This is a great tincture blend to support a sluggish digestion. If you do not have all of the herbal ingredients, just add what you can. It is important that they are all dried, though, otherwise you would need a stronger alcohol percentage to ensure a good shelf life.

» *5 parts dried Artichoke leaves*
» *2 parts dried Karela*
» *4 parts Fennel seed*
» *5 parts dried Dandelion root*
» *2 parts dried Vervain leaf*
» *2 parts dried Orange peel*
» *2 parts dried Ginger*
» *2 parts dried Angelica root*
» *2 parts Cacao nibs*

Place the herbs in a jar and cover completely with 45% ABV alcohol. Leave in a cool, dark place for four weeks, then strain, press, and bottle. Take 5 ml in a little warm water daily in order to boost a sluggish digestion. You can also take a few drops before each meal if you feel you need extra support.

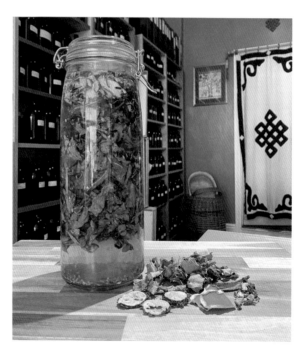

Ashwagandha 🌿 *Withania somnifera*

'Ashwagandha nourishes us deeply. It helps to counteract deficiency and to withstand stresses, both physiological and emotional.'

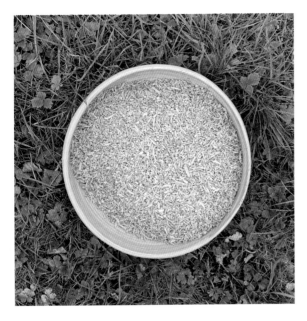

Ashwagandha is also known as 'Indian Ginseng' because of its nourishing and supportive virtues. It is an adaptogen, helping our bodies to deal more effectively with a wide range of stressors, whether they are environmental, behavioural, or emotional. Its name in Hindi, *asgandh*, means 'like a horse'. You could be forgiven for assuming that this is due to its pronounced musky odour, but it also refers to its strengthening, tonifying, and aphrodisiac properties.

Medicinal parts
  ▷ Roots

The leaves are sometimes made into topical preparations, but they should not be ingested. In India the berries are chewed as a tonic.

Physiological actions

Summary
  ▷ Adaptogen
  ▷ Tonic
  ▷ Sedative
  ▷ Hypotensive
  ▷ Anti-inflammatory
  ▷ Immune system amphoteric

Physiological virtues

Ashwagandha is primarily an adaptogen, but also a tonic and a sedative. As an adaptogen it is very supportive for people experiencing physiological or emotional stress. I think of it for people trapped into a cycle of overwork and poor eating habits, as well as those going through harsh allopathic treatment regimes or recovering from chronic illness. The intention here is to support the patient through a particular challenge, rather than to prop up an unsustainable lifestyle choice. Ashwagandha reduces anxiety, fatigue, and cloudy thinking. It is much easier to make constructive changes to our life when we have the clarity and calmness to see the areas where small changes will make a big difference.

Ashwagandha is very rich in bio-available iron, so it is excellent to treat iron deficiency anaemia. It nourishes and invigorates the body, improving libido and reducing the greying of hair, for example. Traditionally, it is often prescribed to the elderly as a tonic to help maintain a good quality of life. Modern research has highlighted the root's ability to support memory and learning. It is thought that it plays a role in protecting nerve cells. This is of great interest in diseases such as Alzheimer's and dementia.

Ashwagandha's ability to act as a general tonic makes it a good choice for patients suffering from nervous exhaustion or long-term stress. It is also excellent as a support to athletes going through an especially rigorous training schedule. In Ayurveda it is considered a *rasayana*, taken to prolong life and promote sexual potency.

It contains alkaloids that lower blood pressure and reduce the heart rate. It also calms us energetically through its grounding and nourishing nature. I say more on this below, when I write about how it is considered in Tibetan medicine. As its specific name, *somnifera*, suggests, Ashwagandha promotes restful sleep. This effect is due not to an immediate sedative action, but to its ability to promote an overall sense of clarity and calm. In fact, if you are drawn to Ashwagandha as a sleep support, I would advise taking it early in the day, rather than last thing at night.

Ashwagandha is a natural anti-inflammatory. It contains steroidal lactones called withanolides, which are similar in structure to our naturally produced steroid hormones and have an anti-inflammatory action. This makes Ashwagandha a good choice when supporting patients with chronic inflammatory diseases such as lupus and rheumatoid arthritis. It balances many aspects of our endocrine system, reducing our cortisol levels, healing our adrenals, and acting as a tonic to the thyroid, helping to re-regulate it, especially when it is under-functioning.

It is also very helpful for the immune system. It is an immune amphoteric, boosting the immune system when it has become weak and calming it when it is over-reactive. These qualities make Ashwagandha a great herb for patients suffering with chronic fatigue immune deficiency syndrome and autoimmune conditions such as rheumatoid arthritis or Sjögren's syndrome. It also plays a very positive role in cancer support. This is due not only to its ability to support the immune system but also because its withanolides have been found to inhibit the growth of cancer cells. This is why I include Ashwagandha in my Fu Zheng blends designed to support patients going through cancer treatment.

In Western herbal practice, Ashwagandha root is most often prescribed as capsules, tincture, or aqueous decoction. In Ayurveda it is traditionally prepared with milk or ghee. The leaves are occasionally prescribed as an anthelmintic. I have done some 'personal practical research' on tea made from the leaves, and I should warn you that they are significantly purgative and gripe-inducing. This may be why you sometimes read of Ashwagandha being taken in some traditions as an abortifacient, whereas, in the vast majority of sources, it is considered completely safe during pregnancy. I believe that this apparent contradiction could well be because the former refers to taking the leaf and the latter to ingesting the root.

Ashwagandha does have topical applications. The powdered root can be made into a poultice and applied to bed sores, boils, and glandular swellings, as can the chopped leaves.

I am a huge fan of Ashwagandha, but it is not the herb for everyone. Take care if you are sensitive to the Nightshade family. Also, like other adaptogens, it is best avoided if you are suffering from an acute infection.

There is widespread tendency for people to take adaptogens, like Ashwagandha, long-term. Sometimes this is fully justified, but at other times it has become a way of propping up an unsustainable lifestyle. If you have been taking

Ashwagandha for a long time, please do not forget about the importance of striving to find balance in lifestyle, diet, and mental attitude. If you have already achieved a well-balanced lifestyle and diet, then Ashwagandha will be much more effective, and you will reap the benefits.

Taste and energetics
Ashwagandha is sweet, bitter, and astringent.

In Tibetan medicine
Ashwagandha is known as *Ashagandha* [ཨ་ཤ་གྷ]. It has a sweet-to-hot taste, with a sweet post-digestive taste. Its potency is warm, dry, and light. It restores kidney heat and strength, and it boosts the physical strength of the body. It reduces accumulations of serous fluid and treats generalized oedema. It reduces inflammation of joints and prevents abnormal calcification. It promotes virility. It is a nourishing, grounding, and slightly warming herb. This, by its very nature, means that it counteracts the airiness of excess *rLung* and therefore has a calming influence when this is needed.

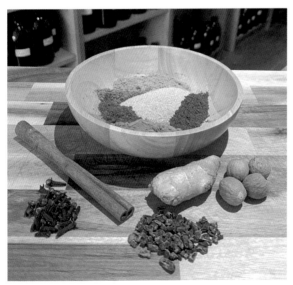

In my dispensary
I frequently prescribe Ashwagandha in tincture, capsule, and decoction form. In tincture form it is most often added to personalized tincture blends. When I prescribe it in capsule form, it can be a simple or in a blood-building blend. As a Fu Zheng decoction, it is mixed in equal parts with *Codonopsis pilosula* (Codonopsis), *Asparagus racemosus* (Shatavari), *Astragalus membranaceus* (Astragalus) and *Lycium barbarum* (Goji). (See also Goji for more details.)

Historical applications
Although in the West it can seem that Ashwagandha is something quite 'new', it is actually a very long-standing and greatly valued herbal medicine. For example, its virtues were described in Sumerian texts written in 1000 BC, and, in the first century AD, Dioscorides recommended Ashwagandha as a tonic. Fragments of Ashwagandha have been found with other medicinal herbs at ancient Egyptian sites.

Suggestion for the home apothecary
Ashwagandha blend

Blend herbal powders as follows, then store in an airtight jar:
> » *2 parts Ashwagandha powder*
> » *1 part Turmeric powder (with 1% Black Pepper)*
> » *1 part Ginger powder*
> » *1 part raw Cacao powder*
> » *½ part Cinnamon powder*
> » *¼ part ground Cloves*
> » *¼ part ground Nutmeg*

Gently heat a mug of milk or non-dairy milk. Stir in 2 tsp of the Ashwagandha powder blend and sweeten to taste. Enjoy.

Bay 🍃 *Laurus nobilis*

'A symbol of triumph, Bay helps us to overcome obstacles and to move forward.'

Bay has a large range of helpful medicinal virtues, as well as a very rich and symbolic magical history. Despite this, it is widely thought of as 'just' a culinary herb. Bay is also known as 'Sweet Bay' or 'Bay Laurel'. Beware: the ornamental plant, *Prunus laurocerasus,* which is known as 'Laurel', is poisonous. Do not confuse it with medicinal Bay.

Medicinal parts
- Leaves

Physiological actions

Summary
- Carminative
- Antispasmodic
- Analgesic
- Diaphoretic
- Emmenagogue
- Antiseptic
- Stimulant
- Astringent

Physiological virtues

Bay leaves are aromatic, containing approximately 3% volatile oil. They improve the appetite and relieve wind and indigestion, being traditionally added to heavy, fatty foods in order to aid digestion. Drinking an infusion of Bay warms and tones the stomach.

The leaves are helpful to ease the symptoms of coughs and colds, and their diaphoretic action reduces fever. They are stimulating, with a particular action on the uterus, bringing on delayed menses and relieving menstrual cramping. They can also warm and tonify the bladder.

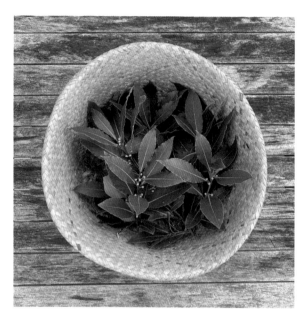

Bay leaves are antispasmodic and analgesic. A bath infused with them can ease period pains or pain in the bowels due to trapped wind. A poultice or fomentation made with Bay leaves is a good first-aid treatment to relieve wasp and bee stings. As an added bonus, Bay is a potent antiseptic. Bay-infused oil can be applied topically to ease joint pains and cramps and was, in old times, prescribed to alleviate palsy and numbness in all parts. Be aware that a minority of people are sensitive to Bay applied topically, whether it is a preparation made with the whole herb or a commercially extracted essential oil. I should mention here that in general I much prefer working with whole herbs, for many reasons, sustainability being one of them.

Avoid medicinal doses of Bay, either internally or in topical treatments, if pregnant.

Energetics

Bay is astringent and warming.

In my dispensary

In my clinic I am especially fond of topical applications of Bay. I often suggest that patients turn to Bay leaves in a bath or footbath, since they are a herb that many people have easy access to. I also make a balm to relieve tension headaches.

Historical applications

Culpeper described Bay leaves as drying and astringent, but the bark of the root has the particular property of '*opening obstructions of the liver, spleen, and other inward parts which bring dropsy, jaundice etc.*'. He also said that the berries were prescribed to speed labour in women. Apparently '*seven berries given to a woman in sore travail of childbirth do cause a speedy delivery*', but he cautions that they should '*not be given to a woman before her time lest they procure abortion or cause labour too soon*'.

Magical

Bay has a rich and symbolic magical history. The leaves symbolize commemoration, both in this life and beyond it. In Ancient Rome, during December, garlands of Bay leaves were made to celebrate the festival of Saturnalia. In Ancient Greece the Bay tree is dedicated to Apollo and is associated with purification and victory. Legend has it that Apollo washed himself after killing the dragon Python in the valley of temples in Delphi and then entered Delphi, a purified victor crowned with Bay.

The Delphic Oracle used to chew Bay leaves before reading oracles. Even nowadays placing a Bay leaf under your pillow is considered to encourage prescient dreams. It does have narcotic properties, so that may help.

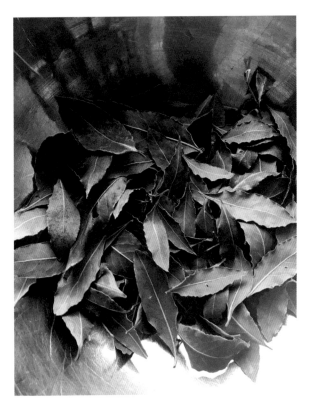

Bay is a traditionally protective herb. Keeping a Bay leaf in your mouth was considered to guard against misfortunes, and wearing a garland of Bay on your head would protect you against lightning strikes. Culpeper said that it: '*resisters witchcraft very potently, as also all the evils old Saturn can do to the body of a man . . . neither witch nor devil, thunder or lightning, will hurt a man in a place where the Bay-tree is*'.

Bay has long been associated with triumph and wisdom. Newly qualified doctors used to be crowned with Bay, a gesture known as '*bacca laureus*', which lives on in the words 'baccalaureate' and 'bachelor' to describe university degrees.

If you have a Bay tree in your herb garden, look after it. If it suddenly fails to thrive, it is said that imminent misfortune is on its way to the household.

Suggestions for the home apothecary

Temple balm

Make an infused oil with Bay leaves in mild and light olive oil. Once it is ready, set it into an ointment (or balm) in jars using a ratio of 1 g beeswax to 7 ml infused oil. (See Plantain for instructions.) Apply the balm to the temples and the back of the neck to ease a tension headache.

Dried bay leaves for tension and pain-relieving baths

If you have a plentiful source of Bay in the garden, you can probably rely on fresh leaves for bathing, but if you do not and are offered some Bay leaves, it is perfectly possible to dry them for year-round medicinal bathing.

Pick the leaves from the branches and spread on trays or hang the branches upside down in an airy place away from direct light and dust. They dry and store easily.

You can add three handfuls of leaves directly to your hot bath and soak in it for 20 minutes. Alternatively, make a strong decoction, adding two handfuls to 1. litre of water and bringing to a very gentle simmer for 5 minutes. Take it off the heat and leave lidded for 20 minutes before adding it to your bath water. Alternatively, you could also make an infused oil from the dried leaves for more localized application.

Birch 🌿 *Betula pendula/B. pubescens*

'Birch sweeps away the old and prepares for the new.'

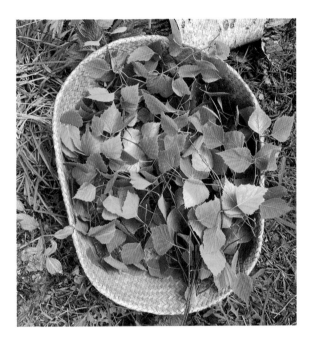

The name 'Birch' is thought to come from the Sanskrit *Bhurga*, which means 'tree on which the bark is used for writing'. European cultures know it as *Beithe* or 'Our Lady of the Woods', and it is considered to represent new beginnings. It is a pioneer tree, the first to colonize new ground, and it nurtures the soil for those that follow. Its branches are traditionally used to create besom brooms that sweep away dirt and obstacles in preparation for new ventures. Medicinally, it cleanses our bodies of old toxins, helping to clear and prepare us for a new phase in our lives.

Medicinal parts
- Leaves
- Buds
- Bark

Physiological actions

Summary
- Diuretic
- Astringent
- Anti-inflammatory
- Antiseptic
- Analgesic

Physiological virtues

Birch leaves are most often thought of as a kidney-supportive remedy. They are diuretic, containing flavonoids and essential oils that gently increase the production of urine without causing stress to the kidneys. They are rich in potassium, so do not deplete the body of this important mineral. Birch leaf tea has long been prescribed to treat cystitis, gout, rheumatism, oedema, and kidney stones. It slows down the formation of kidney stones, perhaps in part due to the high Vitamin C content of the leaves, which increases the secretion of uric acid. Birch leaves can be very helpful for skin conditions due to their ability to support healthy elimination of toxins.

The flavonoids in Birch encourage a more vibrant blood flow in 'harder-to-reach' areas, such as the scalp, making the leaves a traditional remedy to consider in cases of hair loss, dandruff, or skin conditions on the scalp.

The bark and buds of Birch are aromatic and resinous, containing methyl salicylic acid; they are prescribed for inflammatory conditions, urinary tract disorders, psoriasis, and eczema. Decoctions of the bark are astringent and anti-inflammatory, traditionally prescribed for arthritis and gout as well as intermittent fevers. The buds contain a volatile oil, one of the constituents of which is betulin, a substance that has been shown to have promising anti-tumour activity.

Birch tar oil is made by distilling the bark or leaves; it makes a good antiseptic topical treatment. It also has analgesic properties and has some similarities to Wintergreen oil. Birch leaves infused into oil are also traditionally massaged into the body to relieve aching muscles. The infused oil also stimulates the circulation and lymphatic system, making it popular as a cellulite-reducing treatment. The fresh bark can also be applied as a pain-relieving topical treatment. Place the moist internal side against the skin.

Many people like to drink the sap in springtime, but I do not do this. I am influenced by the experience of my tutor, Barbara, who once extracted sap from the Birch tree in her garden and then was then filled with regret when she sensed the tree's displeasure. She tipped the sap back onto the ground at the base of the tree and made her apology. She felt that it had been too invasive and exploitative when the leaves, bark, and buds were offered freely. This is, of course, her own experience, and perhaps her tapping technique was not suitable. Birch trees in different locations and habitats may be more amenable to tapping, especially if it is carried out skilfully.

Energetics

Birch is bitter and astringent. It is all about clearing out the old and making way for the new. If we are clogged with toxins, we do not have the vibrancy and motivation to step confidently into a new phase of our life. Birch cleanses our system and fills us with a new sense of purpose.

In the Celtic tree *Ogham*, Birch, known as *Beithe*, represents new beginnings. It could be birth, rebirth, or a journey, either physical or spiritual. *Beithe* invites us to leave behind old patterns, to lose our sense of fixed expectations or fears, and to get rid of unhelpful associations. When we draw the *Beithe* stave and contemplate it, we know that all will be well. We welcome change. We are stepping forward to fulfil our destiny.

In Tibetan medicine

The species of Betula in the Tibetan pharmacopoeia is *Betula albosinensis*. It is known as *Tregpa shing* [ཁྲེག་པ་ཤིང་]. The small branches are collected in spring and cut into pieces and dried. It has a sweet-to-astringent taste with a sweet post-digestive taste and a cooling potency. It is considered to cure combined disorders of *Tripa* and *rLung*.

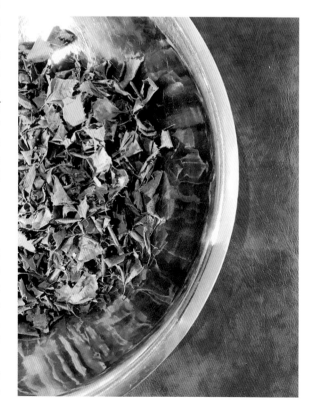

In my dispensary

I mostly prescribe Birch leaves in kidney-supporting teas for my patients. I choose the young bright green spring growth, and they add a lovely cleansing and fragrant note to the herbal tea blends.

Historical applications

Hildegard of Bingen considered Birch to be warming in action and, in her work, *Physica*, described applying the roots to places where '*worms had burrowed into the skin*'.

Magical

In the west of England, crosses made out of Birch were hung over cottage doorways as a way of protecting the house from the possibility of enchantment. It is a tree considered to be able to avert evil and bad luck, as well as being specifically disliked by fairies. Birch twigs were traditionally used to exorcise evil spirits by striking those who are possessed. Cradles were once made of Birch so that the babies sleeping in them would be protected. In Russia a red ribbon was hung around the stem of a Birch tree to get rid of the influence of the evil eye. A personal protective or healing amulet can be made by writing words onto a piece of Birch bark.

Suggestion for the home apothecary

Birch leaf tea

Pick fresh Birch leaves in spring and dry them for tea infusions throughout the year, as needed. Add to a mixed blend as a general support, or drink two cups a day as a simple if more specific Birch support, as needed.

Black Root/Culver's Root   Leptandra virginica

Black Root is also known as 'Culver's Root' after Dr Culver, an eighteenth-century physician who promoted the use of this plant as medicine at that time. It is a potent bitter, removing 'viscid mucus' from the gut. It is wonderful in small doses to help restore a tired and overloaded digestive tract.

It seems to have fallen out of fashion these days, as not many herbal practitioners work with it. Perhaps this is because it is a powerful purgative and needs to be prescribed with care, but also perhaps the knowledge of how best to work with it is no longer being passed on as widely. As demand for this herb has waned, most herbal suppliers now no longer stock it, and this, in turn, means that fewer practitioners want to learn about its virtues. This is a shame, as it is an amazingly effective and valuable medicine that should not be lost from our *materia medica*. I consider it a very important herb in my herb garden, and I prescribe it often.

Medicinal part
▷ Roots

Roots should be dried and preferably aged for 12 months, the fresh root being too harsh in action. If fresh roots are ingested, side effects include vomiting and blood in the stool.

Physiological actions

Summary
▷ Cholagogue
▷ Laxative
▷ Diaphoretic
▷ Emetic

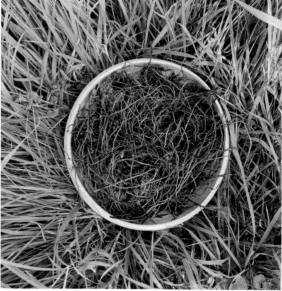

Physiological virtues

Black Root is a cholagogue. It is especially good in cases of chronic constipation associated with chronic insufficiency of bile. One of the reasons that I love it so much for this is that it supports the body holistically and does not create dependency. It helps the body to get rid of a build-up of old hardened mucous lining the bowel without reducing the tone of the bowel.

Think of it for patients who have been suffering with a sluggish bowel for many years and are displaying signs of a build-up of toxicity. They may be experiencing joint pains, lowered immunity, low mood, oedema, poor sleep, and low energy levels as well as chronic named disease states. As it helps to produce a softer and easier stool, it may also be helpful in the treatment of patients with anal prolapse and haemorrhoids.

It can also be a good choice to include in a blend for patients suffering with gallbladder and liver insufficiency, including cases of jaundice and hepatitis, as well as some skin diseases where reduced liver function is a factor.

It is diaphoretic and was in the past prescribed for typhus and 'bilious fevers', its efficacy probably being partly due its action in inducing sweating. It is also considered helpful in treating pleurisy, but I do not have personal experience of prescribing it in this way.

It is usually prescribed at low doses and combined in a prescription with other herbs such as Dandelion root. It has emetic properties: high doses can cause nausea, vomiting, and diarrhoea. It should not be prescribed in pregnancy or while breastfeeding and must be avoided with children.

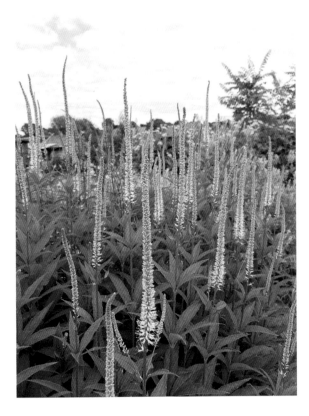

Energetics

Black Root is bitter and cooling. In clearing viscid mucus from the gut, it helps people let go of old hardened attitudes and emotional baggage. Many patients mention a sense of renewal and 'cleanliness' when they have been taking it in their blend.

In my dispensary

I usually prescribe this at a low level in a pair with Fringe Tree bark (*Chionanthus virginica*). I include it either in personalized tincture blends or within a bowel-supporting capsule formula. It would normally not be more than 5% of any blend or formula, with another 5% being Fringe Tree bark. The habitually constipated patient will report an immediate improvement in the ability to pass a stool, and those who have always had a 'sticky' stool will announce that the stickiness is gone, often adding that they had never realized what passing a healthy stool felt like.

The following is a typical case of where Black Root is very helpful. 'Rosemary' was 70 years old and had suffered with chronic constipation, regularly going for several days without having a bowel movement. When she did have one, her stool was like rabbit droppings. She tried very hard to have a healthy diet, drinking plenty of water and eating a lot of superfoods and supplements which she added to a smoothie daily. She mentioned that she avoided wheat in the afternoons as she always suffered with bloating after she ate it. She also told me that she carried a lot of tension in her body and often did not sleep well.

I recommended that she took a break from gluten and dairy and I suggested that she also reduced caffeine as she was in the habit of having several cappuccinos and espressos each day. I prescribed a general calming and relaxing tincture blend which included Skullcap,

Cramp Bark, Ashwagandha and Wild Oat. I also prescribed two capsules daily of my general bowel-supporting blend which includes Black Root alongside herbs such as Dandelion root, Rhubarb root, *Cascara sagrada,* and various carminatives and demulcents.

Within three weeks her bowels were much better, and she was having a bowel movement every other day. She had also noticed an improvement in her sleep. After another four weeks she was having a bowel movement most days, which was quite momentous for her, and her sleep continued to improve. A year later she had a consistent regular bowel and good sleep, no longer needing any herbal support. She told me that she continues to stick to the dietary and lifestyle recommendations that I made as she notices an immediate adverse impact if she goes back to her old ways. She said it was well worth while being more careful about her diet, and she was absolutely delighted with the improvement. She was feeling fabulous.

Historical applications

Black Root is a medicine considered primarily a laxative and emetic by many indigenous Americans. It was believed to cure typhus and bilious fevers, chills and seizures. The Seneca Indians induced vomiting by drinking a tea made from the dried root. As well as this, the Seneca and Ojibwa cleaned scrofula (tuberculous) sores with the mashed root, and the Cherokee chewed the plant to relieve the symptoms of colic. The Meskwaki chose it to assist women in labour, and the Chippewa considered it as a blood cleanser. The Chippewa name is *wi'sûgidji'bĭ,* which means '*bitter root*'.

It was adopted into the European herbal pharmacopoeia primarily as a cholagogue and laxative.

Magical

In early settler folklore it was said to be often found with 'evil' medicines, so that a sorcerer may undo his work. It was also found in war bundles, used to purify people, animals, medicine, and weapons. In certain indigenous American rituals, the fresh root was taken to induce vomiting as part of purification rites. The Menomini specifically used the plant for purification after being 'defiled' by being touched by a bereaved person.

Bogbean   Menyanthes trifoliata

'Bogbean is a herb for deep-seated chronic conditions associated with weakness and debility.'

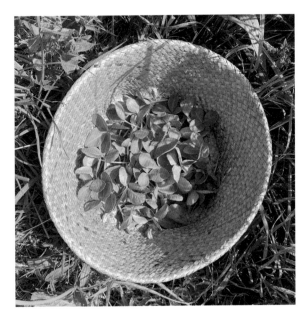

Bogbean is a member of the Gentian family, which, as its name suggests, grows wild in spongy bogs, marshes, and shallow water throughout Europe. Since it is scarce in the South of England and I do not have room to create a pond in my garden, I grow it in a large ceramic pot with the drainage holes stopped up. A healthy established plant produces enough to supply what I need for my clinic in terms of tincture. If I had a lot of patients requiring Bogbean in tea form, I would need to increase production significantly. However, Bogbean is so very bitter, a little goes a long way, and I am most unlikely to prescribe a large volume of it in tea form.

The generic name, 'Menyanthes', is derived from the Greek words for 'month' and 'flower'. The eighteenth-century naturalist, Carolus Linnaeus chose it because it is usually in flower for at least a month each year. The specific name, 'trifoliata', refers to its trifoliate leaves, reminiscent of a garden bean, hence its common name.

The flowers are absolutely beautiful. An unknown historical source – mentioned by Maud Grieve in her *A Modern Herbal* (1931) – described its inflorescence as a '*bush of feather-like floures of a white colour, dasht ouer slightly with a wash of light carnation*'.

Medicinal parts

▷ Leaves
▷ Flowers

Physiological actions

Summary

▷ Bitter
▷ Cholagogue
▷ Alterative
▷ Purgative
▷ Tonic

Physiological virtues

Bogbean is a very bitter herb, helpful for stimulating the digestion in general and liver function in particular. It is traditionally prescribed to alleviate rheumatism and gout.

A tea made from the leaves mixed with Wormwood, Centaury, or Sage was prescribed for a sluggish liver. It stimulates the appetite and can help to alleviate bloating and abdominal discomfort. It can also be helpful to help support healthy weight gain in underweight patients. Be warned, it is purgative and in large doses can cause abdominal pain. Avoid for patients with inflammatory conditions of the digestive tract, such as colitis, IBS, and ulcers.

It is traditionally considered to be tonic, cathartic, and very helpful for rheumatoid arthritis and gout, as well as skin diseases. It is especially indicated when patients show lack of vitality and weight loss associated with these conditions.

As a topical treatment it can be applied to reduce glandular swellings.

Energetics
Bogbean is bitter.

In Tibetan medicine
As far as I know, this species is not part of the Tibetan pharmacopoeia. However, we can make some extrapolations as to how it could be prescribed within a Tibetan medicinal framework. It is strongly bitter and cooling, so is especially suited to situations where there is raised *Tripa*.

In my dispensary
I see Bogbean as a herb for deep-seated chronic conditions associated with weakness and debility. It helps the body to clear away toxins when it has been worn down by long-standing obstacles to that process. In these cases, it is important to introduce lifestyle changes slowly and steadily, so that it is not too overwhelming for the

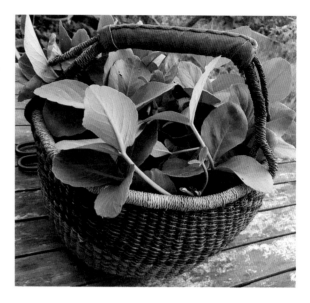

patient. Lifestyle and dietary changes will be necessary to support the process of healing.

Historical applications
Bogbean was once prescribed to treat scurvy, since it is a digestive tonic that is rich in Vitamin C. Its name in German, *Scharbock*, is derived from the Latin word *scorbutus*, which is the former medical term for scurvy. The juice of the fresh leaves, mixed with whey, was said to cure gout. Due to its bitterness, it was sometimes used instead of hops, for brewing beer.

Magical
Bogbean's cleansing properties can help clear obstacles and remove clutter and debris from the psychic sphere.

Boneset ❦ *Eupatorium perfoliatum*

'A specific for colds and influenza accompanied by aching muscles and bones.'

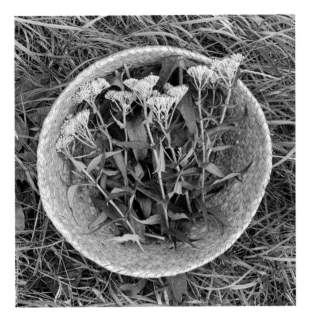

Eupatorium perfoliatum is also known as 'Thoroughwort', 'Feverwort', or 'Agueweed'. Its generic name was chosen because of Mithridates Eupator, the ruler of Pontus in old Asia Minor, who lived from 135–63 BC. He was very interested in herbal medicines and specifically tried to become immune to poisons for his own safety.

Boneset is a very popular diaphoretic, fever herb, and tonic in the United States but it is not so commonly prescribed in the United Kingdom. As its name suggests, it is also prescribed to help strengthen ligaments and speed the healing of bone fractures. It contains pyrrolizidine alkaloids, so, on the basis of the precautionary principle, it is best avoided if there is liver disease. I aim to choose this herb for short-term treatments such as for the duration of an acute illness or for speeding bone healing after a break.

Medicinal parts
▷ Aerial parts

Aerial parts should be harvested at the time of flowering.

Physiological actions

Summary

▷ Diaphoretic
▷ Tonic
▷ Expectorant
▷ Bitter
▷ Cholagogue
▷ Aperient
▷ Emetic

Physiological virtues

Maud Grieve states that Boneset acts slowly and persistently with its greatest power being '*manifested upon the stomach, liver, bowels and uterus*'. It is probably best known these days for its capacity to treat catarrh, colds, influenza, and fever. It lowers fevers effectively due to its diaphoretic and peripheral vasodilatory actions. It is also expectorant and supports the immune response. Its expectorant action makes it suitable in cases of acute bronchitis and pneumonia.

Timely dosing at the onset of an attack of influenza or fever can be extremely effective at minimizing the symptoms and duration of the illness. In these cases, administer the Boneset as a decoction or as a tincture in hot water. You can also consider it for eruptive illnesses like chickenpox and measles. If internal prescribing is difficult, it can be prescribed topically in the form of a body wash or foot bath. Fomentations of the cooled tepid decoction can be wrapped around the wrists and ankles to help reduce the fever. Change them frequently at first, whenever the cloths warm up.

When taken cold, small doses act as a tonic. Boneset is a very good all-round support to the bodily systems, especially when there are frequent infections or a tendency to chronic joint or muscle pain. It encourages the digestion and is a cholagogue, stimulating bile production and acting as a mild aperient. This means it can be helpful to encourage the bowels to move when there has been sluggishness. It is also a vermifuge. Be warned: it is an emetic, and too much of it will cause nausea.

Energetics
Boneset has a bitter and hot taste with a light and dry quality.

In my dispensary
I have grown Boneset on a small scale for many years. I most often prescribe it as a small proportion of an individual tincture blend as a tonic ingredient, especially in general nervine or respiratory blends. It is of course very helpful for patients who ask for help at the onset of fever or influenza.

Historical applications
In the nineteenth century, Boneset was probably the most frequently prescribed herb in the United States. It was the herb of choice for fevers, including break bone (dengue) fever, influenza, coughs, headaches, and rheumatism. It was widely respected as a plant that would cause profuse perspiration and also loosen the bowels. For this, it was typically prepared as a strong hot infusion. A cold infusion was considered more of a tonic. The leaves were also applied as a poultice to help mend broken bones.

Boneset is bitter to the taste, and so, for treating children, was traditionally made into a syrup with Ginger and Anise as a cough remedy.

Magical
The Chippewa people made a deer-summoning whistle from the root fibres combined with Milkweed. Boneset is also associated with protection and exorcism. It is said to ward off evil spirits. If you feel the need, make an infusion and sprinkle it about the house to drive away evil.

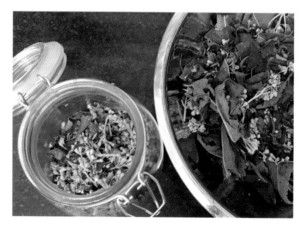

Borage 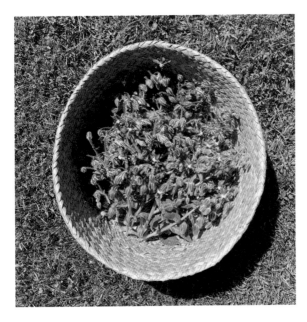 *Borago officinalis*

'I Borage always bring courage.'

As a herbal medicine, Borage is diuretic, antitussive, and anti-inflammatory, and it helps to promote lactation. Most interesting, perhaps, is its action in supporting the adrenal cortex. So many patients these days have exhausted adrenals or are withdrawing gradually from steroid treatment and need adrenal support. The addition of a little Borage to their prescription can be very helpful.

I absolutely love Borage, but I do not prescribe it liberally. Unfortunately, it is another herb that has fallen out of favour due to the fact that it contains a very low level (0.01%) of pyrrolizidine alkaloids. I view it as a herb for occasional short-term prescribing in specific circumstances.

Medicinal parts
- Aerial parts
- Seeds

Aerial parts are harvested during flowering; oil is prepared from the seeds.

Physiological actions

Summary
- Anti-inflammatory
- Antitussive
- Diuretic
- Galactagogue

Physiological virtues
Borage contains mucilage and can be a soothing influence for sore and inflamed skin. The leaves are diuretic, and the flowers are diaphoretic. Traditionally Borage leaves and flowers are considered anti-inflammatory and a galactagogue as well as helpful to alleviate depression. Borage is antitussive and can be a good first-aid choice for dry, irritated coughs, especially if the patient is feeling very low in mood. The leaves and flowers promote the regeneration of the adrenal cortex so can play a part in promoting the recovery from adrenal burnout or supporting patients withdrawing from long-term steroid treatment. Due to the theoretical toxicity of its pyrrolizidine alkaloid content, it is suggested that Borage is taken only at a low dose over a short period, say 6 weeks..

Borage oil contains gamma linolenic acid, so can be a good alternative to Evening Primrose oil. It can be helpful in cases of eczema as well as to protect the cardiovascular system from inflammation.

Energetics
Borage is cool, moist, and slightly sweet. It has long been associated with courage. In the first

century AD, Pliny the Elder [Gaius Plinius Secundus], in his *Naturalis Historia,* referred to it as '*Euphrosinum*' because of its euphoric effect. '*Ego Borago gaudia semper ago*' ['I Borage always bring courage'].

In my dispensary

Sometimes I have a patient for whom life seems to have become a challenge, and they are exhausted by it. Their adrenals are exhausted, and they do not have the energy to move forward with confidence. They need Borage, but I tend to prescribe it in very small doses, often just a few drops or at a very low level within a tailor-made formula. It is wonderful to see the patient blossoming again as their system gradually relaxes and their zest for life is rekindled.

Historical applications

Gerard wrote: '*Those of our time do use the floures in sallads, to exhilarate and make the mind glad. There be also many things made of them, used for the comfort of the heart, to drive away sorrow, & increase the joy of the minde. . . The leaves and floures of Borrage put into wine make men and women glad and merry, driving away all sadnesse, dulnesse, and melancholy, as Dioscorides and Pliny affirme.*'

Francis Bacon said: '*The leaf of Burrage hath an excellent spirit to repress the vapour of dusky melancholie.*'

Magical

Borage is also known as 'Burrage' or 'Herb of gladness'.

Drinking an infusion of Borage is said to help develop one's psychic powers. If you carry the fresh flowers, it will strengthen your courage.

Suggestion for the home apothecary

Borage-flower ice cubes

Make these ice cubes to 'exhilarate and make the mind glad'.

Pick Borage flowers and freeze into ice cubes, placing one in each cube. Add to summer drinks and enjoy.

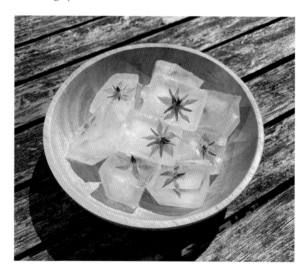

Burdock   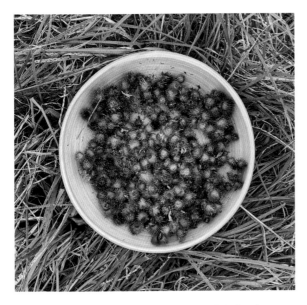   *Arctium lappa*

'Burdock is a stimulating blood purifier especially indicated in dry skin conditions.'

Burdock is an impressive biennial hedgerow plant spending its first year developing enormous, almost wearable leaves; in its second year it throws up impressive flower stalks, which eventually produce a crop of barbed, clinging burrs or seed heads. These burrs were once used to fasten clothing, giving rise to some of its country names: 'Beggar's Buttons' and 'Batchelor's Buttons', for example. It was also called 'Butter Dock' because the leaves were used to wrap butter and 'Gypsy Rhubarb' or 'Snakes Rhubarb' due to the appearance of its stems. The temperance drink, Dandelion and Burdock, used to be a popular healthful bitter tonic. These days it is usually a sweetened and artificially flavoured shadow of the original recipe.

Medicinal parts
- Roots
- Leaves
- Seeds

Physiological actions

Summary
- Alterative
- Bitter
- Circulatory stimulant
- Sudorific
- Diuretic
- Antimicrobial

Physiological virtues

Burdock root is an alterative, supporting elimination of metabolic waste products from the body, especially via the liver and the kidneys. It can help to 'clean' the blood and take the pressure off an overburdened skin. It is quite oily in nature so is specific for skin conditions characterized by soreness, dryness, and flakiness. Consider it when there is dry, scaly eczema or psoriasis, for example. It is a stimulating herb and can be rather 'pushy', so do not be too enthusiastic with it until you know how your patient is going to react to it. They will not thank you for a huge skin flare-up.

The leaves are milder in action than the root. They are a gentle digestive stimulant and a hypoglycaemic agent. A tea of fresh leaves is often easier to obtain than digging up the roots, and for general support it can be a good option.

The seeds have a definite oily quality, and this is quite noticeable when you are picking them. The oiliness is a very helpful energetic consideration when treating patients prone to dryness. When ingested as medicine, they are stimulating and diffusive, creating a tingling sensation in the mouth similar to that produced by good-quality extractions of Echinacea root. Be warned though, never try them straight from the plant. The barbs will attach themselves firmly to your tongue. It is best to make a decoction or a tincture or to separate the barbs from the seeds in a food processor. The seeds are 'faster-acting' than the roots or the leaves, moving heat to the periphery, reducing fever, encouraging sweating, and bringing out the rash in viral illnesses such as measles and chickenpox. It is interesting to note that while the seeds support increased sweating, they can also help to reduce it when it is excessive. It seems that they have an amphoteric action, bringing elimination from the skin into healthful balance, perhaps through supporting the lymphatic system. I always consider Burdock when a patient complains either of excessive sweating or that they never sweat, or that they have a skin issue that manifests in the armpits or other sweat-gland-rich areas.

While the root and leaves are often thought of as acting primarily on the liver, the seeds are considered to have a primary action on the urinary system. They are diuretic, removing calculus and reducing oedema. They are also very good as a support to an inflamed prostate. In China they are prescribed for colds, dry coughs, and sore throats.

Burdock's virtues are not limited just to the skin. It is an excellent herb to consider for gout and other inflammatory joint conditions. It seems to not only clean the blood but also to encourage the blood supply to 'harder-to-reach areas' – for example, the big toe in gout or the deep interior of large joints in arthritis. This blood-cleaning and stimulating action may also help to explain Burdock's traditional association with reversing hair loss either when taken internally or when applied as a wash.

All parts of Burdock can be applied topically as a poultice for skin sores, leg ulcers, and infections. A cooled decoction can be helpful as a wash for acne as well as for fungal skin infections such as ringworm and athlete's foot. It has directly antimicrobial and antifungal properties.

Burdock has a long history of being considered an anti-cancer treatment; it was mentioned by Hildegard of Bingen and it is an ingredient in a traditional First Nations cleansing formula (the proper name and the original herbal ingredients I am afraid I do not know). Canadian nurse Rene M. Caisse, who promoted it from the 1920s through the 1970s, said that she was originally passed the formula by one of her Ontario patients. She 'renamed' it as 'Essiac'. These days, Essiac is usually based on Burdock root, Turkey Rhubarb root, Sheep's Sorrel, and Slippery Elm bark. Rene Caisse must have made some herbal substitutions, as Burdock, Turkey Rhubarb, and Sheep's Sorrel are not indigenous to the land we now call North America. Either way, the 'renamed' formula became popular among Europeans and their descendants as a cancer cure – a claim that has now been widely discredited by the powers that be. Research by non-herbalists has revealed 'no direct activity' against cancer. When considering this, we should bear in mind that the whole issue of making claims about natural cancer treatments is a minefield these days. I feel that, while no one herbal treatment or formula can be a 'cure' on its own, we should not disregard the potential for healing that can be stimulated in a body with good pathways of elimination, reduced inflammation, and an enlivened immune system. I think that Essiac can be a helpful support to certain patients, and I regularly prescribe the formula in various health presentations. I would love to know its lineage, original name, and formula, so that I can properly credit those who taught its benefits to the Europeans.

Energetics

Burdock root is bitter, sweet, and oily. The leaves are bitter, cooling, and astringent; the seeds are bitter, astringent, and fast-acting.

In Tibetan medicine

Burdock is known as *Byi dzin* [བྱི་འཛིན་]. The medicinal parts are the root and the fruit. It has a hot and astringent taste, with a bitter post-digestive taste. It is both warming and cooling in power. Although this latter seems contradictory, I would say that it is warming in the short term and cooling over a longer period of treatment. *Byi dzin* dissolves stones, heals tumours, cleanses channels, ripens the pimples of a disease called 'sib bi', and cures '*rLung* fevers'. It is also considered good for neurological problems.

In my dispensary

Burdock comes to my mind whenever I see patients with a dry, flaky skin condition but I team it with other herbs according to the unique circumstances of the case. I favour the root for internal prescribing and make an infused oil with the leaves, which is applied topically to alleviate itchiness and discomfort. As an internal medicine, Burdock is rather powerful, so I always work slowly and steadily with new patients. I think it is counterproductive to create a dramatic and worrying healing crisis. The proportions of Burdock in a prescription can be increased gradually over a few months, if needed. I have noticed that when prescribed for skin conditions, the improvements often start from the very top and bottom of the body – that is, the scalp and the feet. I put this down to its stimulating effects as well as its blood-cleaning action. The following is a good example of a case requiring Burdock.

'Sally' was 42 years old and came to see me because she had had a long-term problem with psoriasis in her scalp. She had tried all sorts of different topical treatments and had worked her way through multiple different shampoos and conditioners. She had also followed various exclusion diets and had installed a water softener system in their house. Sadly, all of this was to no avail. The itchy and flaky psoriasis remained all over her scalp.

I felt that she could make a few dietary adjustments, mostly to keep her blood sugar more stable, and I prescribed herbs, in the form of a tincture, to support her nervous system, her digestion, and her elimination pathways. She was pretty fit and healthy apart from her scalp, but she had always had a rather low blood pressure. I wondered if this reduced the effective blood supply to the skin on her scalp. I prescribed Hawthorn to see if this would gently help things, and I included Burdock, starting at a low level and increasing it gradually, ending up after a few months with it making up a quarter of her blend. I will admit that this is a rather high level for my usual prescribing, but it suited her well, and over the next 12 months the patch of psoriasis shrank steadily, and the dryness and itchiness reduced. The skin on her scalp became completely clear, apart from one little patch behind one of her ears, which occasionally flared up when she was stressed. The other herbs in her mix were Skullcap, Hawthorn berry, and Cleavers.

This case illustrates Burdock's action in normalizing sweating: 'Liam' was a dancer in his 30s who came to me for help with anxiety and lack of focus. His main prescription was a Tibetan medicinal blend to calm and ground him. After the first month of treatment he felt much calmer and more focused, but he mentioned that for most of his life he had sweated profusely, even when not exercising. He said it as an aside and explained that he was used to it. I had already been thinking about introducing an element of digestive support into his treatment, so, armed with this specific indication, I chose to prescribe drop doses of Burdock tincture alongside his main prescription. Within four weeks the excessive sweating disappeared completely.

Historical applications

Plinius (Pliny the Elder) named it '*Lappa*' which means to 'hold onto' while Dioscorides knew this plant as '*Arcteion*', the Greek for 'Bear Plant'. Dioscorides suggested a decoction of the root and seeds as a toothache cure '*if it be holden awhile in the mouth*'.

In the Middle Ages it was prepared in wine and prescribed to treat leprosy. Henry VIII took it for syphilis, and while it did not cure him, it was said to have improved it. Perhaps it also helped to treat his gout.

Culpeper writes a great deal about Burdock, recommending the leaves bruised with egg white as an application for burns, and the seeds as a treatment for urinary calculus. He also describes applying the leaf and seed to the body in order to '*draw the womb which way you please*'. Apparently, Burdock was applied to the crown of the head to treat prolapse, to the soles of the feet to treat menstrual cramping, or to the navel to help prevent miscarriage.

John Pechey, in his '*Compleat Herbal of Physical Plants* (1694), wrote that its virtues were '*Drying, Pulmonick, Diuretick, Diaphoretick Cleansing, and somewhat astringent.*'

Gerard wrote that the young stalks, peeled and eaten raw with salt and pepper, or boiled in meat broth, are pleasant to eat, and increase seed and '*stir up lust*'.

Parkinson included the following account of Burdock's medicinal qualities: '*The Burre leaves are cooling, and drying moderately, and discussth withal as Galen saith, whereby it is good to heale old Ulcers and sores.*' . . . '*A dramme of the rootes taken with Pine kernels, doth helpe them that spit foul mattery and bloody flegme.*' . . . '*The juyce of the leaves taken with hony provoketh urine, and remedieth the pains of the bladder.*' . . . '*The seede being drunke with wine, forty days together doth wonderfully helpe the Sciatica. . . . It is much commended to breake the stone, and cause it to be expelled by Urine, and is often used with other seedes and things for that purpose.*'

Magical

Burdock is associated with protection and healing. The dried herb can be sewn into sachets and placed around the home to ward off negativity. You could also add it to protection incense and protection spells. Burdock roots were gathered during the waning Moon, dried, and then cut into small pieces, strung on a red thread, and worn for protection. The leaves of the Burdock laid on the soles of the feet were said to cure gout.

Suggestion for the home apothecary

Burdock-leaf infusion for indigestion

Make an infusion with Burdock leaves and take a wineglassful dose before meals.

For leg ulcers and for itchy skin you can make an infused oil, or steam a fresh leaf and apply as a warm poultice.

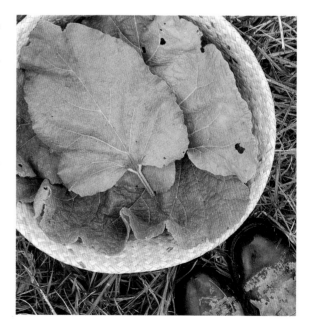

California Poppy 🌿 *Eschscholzia californica*

'Calms churning thoughts, improves mental focus and aids restful sleep.'

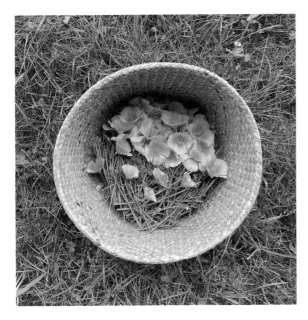

California Poppy is an annual bitter nervine that grows to 60 cm in height and bears beautiful orange poppy-like flowers in the summer. It has a long history of being taken as a pain-reliever and sedative. It is the state flower of California.

Medicinal parts
> Aerial parts

Physiological actions

Summary

> Nervine
> Antispasmodic
> Sedative
> Anodyne

Physiological virtues

First Nation peoples have long recognized California Poppy's pain-relieving properties – for example, chewing it to relieve the pain of toothache. Nowadays, it has become popular in Europe and is often prescribed to promote restful sleep and to calm the tendency to have churning, obsessive, circular thoughts. It is sometimes prescribed for hyperactivity in children. Matthew Wood, herbalist and author of the excellent *The Earthwise Herbal* (2008, 2009), considers it a specific for tinnitus caused by listening to loud music.

Although related to the Opium Poppy, California Poppy has a very different mode of action. Rather than being disorientating, it helps to promote healthy focus and calm, clear thought patterns. It helps to calm obsessive churning thoughts and is especially helpful when these contribute to insomnia. It is gently antispasmodic, sedative, and analgesic and is, in appropriate circumstances, suitable for children.

Think of California Poppy for bedwetting, psychological problems, insomnia, nervous tension, and anxiety. As well as its calming effects, it is said to oxygenate the circulatory system and help the body to absorb Vitamin A.

Do not take in pregnancy.

Energetics
California Poppy is bitter and cooling. It helps to break our obsessive patterns of circular or negative thoughts. We can get into habits of how we think, and it can be difficult to change them. California Poppy will support us in changing this if we choose to reach out to it for help.

In Tibetan medicine
California Poppy is bitter and should therefore be prescribed with caution in those suffering

from an excess of *rLung*. It can be prescribed, but it is recommended that the patient ensures they have increased the rich, oily, and nutritious aspects of their diet and lifestyle, or, if this is not possible, the prescription is balanced by the presence of oily, nourishing, and warming herbs.

In my dispensary

I love this herb for patients who lie awake at night with churning thoughts. I am always careful to work on the premise that the herbal prescription is a temporary solution while the root cause of their problem is addressed. California Poppy can be very effective, but unfortunately this in itself can lead to psychological dependence and an unwillingness of the patient to look again at lifestyle or dietary issues. In the case of patients with a tendency to an excess of the *rLung* in Tibetan medicine, it is important to balance bitter nervines with nourishing and grounding foods, medicines, and behaviours, otherwise long-term reliance on herbs like California Poppy could worsen the underlying imbalance and increase psychological dependence.

This is one of the few herbs that I always tincture from fresh plant; I do not dry any for teas or capsules.

Historical applications

Indigenous Americans chewed the fresh plant in order to alleviate the pain of toothache. They shared their knowledge with early settlers, who learned that this plant was a helpful, mild sedative. It became popular as a herbal remedy for children who found it hard to sleep.

Magical

California Poppy can help to promote intuition and pave the way for prophetic dreams.

Suggestion for the home apothecary

California Poppy tincture

Loosely fill a jar with freshly harvested California Poppy that was surface-dry on harvesting. Cover with at least 50% ABV alcohol and leave in a cool, dark place for 4 weeks. Drain, press, and bottle. Take 2.5–5 ml in hot water before bed as a temporary help for sleeplessness.

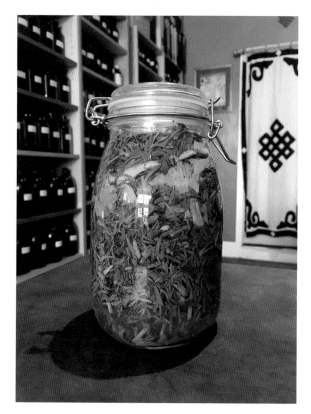

Caraway 🌿 *Carum carvi*

'Caraway is warming, calming and astringent.'

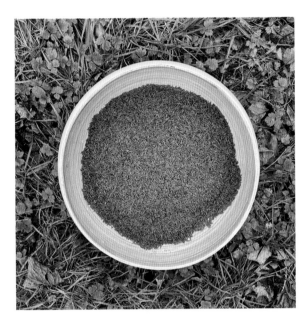

Caraway has a very long medicinal and culinary history. It is a good digestive, astringent, and gentle sedative. It is a very important herb within Tibetan medicine, being calming and grounding. I very often rely on it in my prescriptions for patients suffering from *rLung* disorders.

Medicinal parts
▷ Seeds

Physiological actions

Summary

▷ Carminative
▷ Antispasmodic
▷ Astringent
▷ Sedative
▷ Galactagogue
▷ Analgesic

Physiological virtues

Caraway is a relaxing herb considered to be similar in action to Anise (*Pimpinella anisum*) and Fennel (*Foeniculum vulgare*). It is carminative and antispasmodic, relaxing the intestinal muscles and relieving colic, griping, bloating, and flatulence. You can make a cold overnight infusion using about 30 g of seeds to 570 ml of water and give drop or teaspoonful doses to infants with colic. The dose depends on the age and size of the infant. It is worth noting here that Caraway can help promote more abundant breast milk, so in some cases mother and baby would do well to share the same preparation.

In adults, if excess digestive wind is causing heart arrhythmia, Caraway tea or tincture will solve this. As an added bonus, its nervine action will help to soothe their understandable anxiety at the same time. Caraway seed tea is a good calming drink and has the benefit of being something that can be sourced pretty much wherever you are in the world.

Its antispasmodic action makes Caraway an effective and readily available remedy for period pains. It also has a directly analgesic action. The bruised seeds, pounded with a bit of newly baked bread and moistened with a little spirit, was an old topical remedy for earache. It is a common ingredient in cough medicines, being an expectorant and bronchodilator. It can be helpful for bronchitis and bronchial asthma.

Overall, Caraway's medicinal virtues are so numerous that I consider it an indispensable herb in any dispensary or home apothecary.

Energetics

Caraway has a hot, bitter, and astringent taste, with a potency that is oily and nutritious.

In Tibetan medicine

Caraway, called *Ko nyeu* [ཀོ་སྙེའུ།] has a taste that is bitter, hot, and astringent, with a bitter post-digestive taste. Its potency is equalising and oily. It counteracts raised *rLung*, particularly when it is combined with heat and is manifesting in gastric upset. Its calming and relaxing nature makes it a good choice to help in cases of nervousness and insomnia accompanied by diarrhoea. The *Gyudzhi* reports that it is prescribed for *rLung* fevers, poisoning, and eye diseases. It is light and mild in power, and this makes it suitable for eye diseases and some *Pekén* disorders. It is especially indicated for heart fever and *rLung* disorders affecting the heart. It improves appetite and reduces swelling.

In my dispensary

I very often reach for Caraway when I want a gentle astringent nervine herb that is not bitter in nature. Bitter nervine herbs, such as Skullcap, Mugwort, Vervain, Hops, Wild Lettuce, or California Poppy, may seem calming at first, but on their own they do not properly counteract a *rLung* imbalance and can lead to dependency problems over the longer term. Patients with raised *rLung* need more warming, oily, and nutritious influences in their treatment, whether through diet, medicine, or both. Caraway is therefore a good choice in these circumstances, along with other nourishing nervines like Wild Oat and Ashwagandha.

The following case shows how wonderful Caraway can be when a calming, astringent and carminative herb is called for. 'Leanne' was 60 and had been suffering with ulcerative colitis since she was a young adult. She had a demanding job, which she enjoyed, but she was prone to anxiety and insomnia. She had been given a total colectomy with ileorectal anastomosis while she was in her 20s. The surgery had helped her to cope with the condition, but she still had to be very careful with what she ate. If she ate certain triggering foods, she suffered with very painful trapped wind. She always tried to avoid the things that did not agree with her, but she travelled a lot for her work and found it difficult when she was away from home. Even on a good day her bowel movements were frequent and loose.

To me, her case immediately called out for Caraway, so her personalized tincture blend had that as the main herb. I added Calendula, Agrimony, Wild Oat, and Cleavers, as these were indicated by other details of her case, and I asked her to cut out both dairy and gluten. Three weeks later she reported that her tendency to trapped wind pain had lessened considerably, and she was feeling quite a bit calmer. Her sleep was still not good though. Four weeks after that she reported that she was feeling 'much, much better', saying that her digestion had been more comfortable than she had ever remembered. There was no trapped wind pain, and her bowel movements were firmer and less frequent. She was also feeling calmer and was sleeping more soundly. She continued with the dietary recommendations after finishing her course of herbal medicine and has been able to maintain her improved health without relying on a daily herbal prescription.

Historical applications

Fossilized Caraway seeds have been found at Mesolithic sites, showing that its history as a medicinal herb goes back at least 5,000 years. It became popular as a spice in Europe during the thirteenth century.

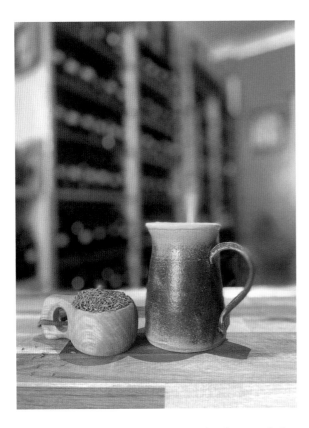

Lyte considered Caraway to be hot and dry in the third degree. He said that Caraway is '*very good and convenient for the stomack and for*

the mouth, it helpeth digestion, and provoketh urine, and it swageth and dissolveth all kinds of windinesse'.

Culpeper wrote that Caraway seed is '*conducive to all cold griefs of the head and stomach . . . and has a moderate quality whereby it breaketh wind, and provoketh urine*'.

Magical

Caraway is associated with protection against theft as well as all manner of evil spirits, entities, and negativity. Any object that contains some Caraway seeds is considered to be theft-proof.

It also encourages fidelity. Chewing the seeds is helpful to gain the love of the one that you desire, and when baked into cakes (or added to cheese), they encourage lust. They also strengthen the memory.

Suggestion for the home apothecary

Caraway-seed tea

Take 1 tsp, heaped, of Caraway seeds and infuse, covered in a mug of hot water, for 10 minutes. Sip slowly while connecting with calming and grounding thoughts.

Cardamom 🌿 *Elettaria cardamomum*

Cardamom warms the digestion and calms the mind. It is a spice that has been traded between East and West for thousands of years, coming to Europe along the old caravan routes. Known as *Elachi* in Hindi and *Sukmel* in Tibetan, it has always been greatly valued.

Medicinal parts

▷ Seeds
▷ Pods

Physiological actions

Summary

▷ Carminative
▷ Digestive stimulant
▷ Antispasmodic
▷ Expectorant
▷ Kidney tonic
▷ Aphrodisiac
▷ Nervine
▷ Anti-inflammatory

Physiological virtues

Cardamom is rich in volatile oils, including camphor, pinene, humulene, caryophyllene, carvone, eucalyptol, terpinene, and sabinene. These make it significantly carminative, as well as being a warming digestive stimulant. It is a good herb to consider when appetite is depleted or when there are blood sugar imbalances. Adding Cardamom to mucus-forming foods such as milk can neutralize these undesirable effects on the body. A Cardamom pod can also be an excellent first-aid treatment for nausea.

It is antispasmodic and is a stimulating expectorant. It has a decongestant action and

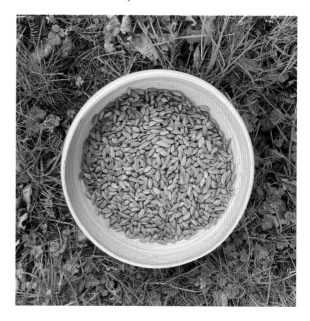

is traditionally prescribed for both acute and chronic respiratory conditions such as bronchitis and asthma. Chewing the seeds can be helpful when you have a sore throat.

Cardamom has a long-standing reputation as an aphrodisiac as well as being a tonic for the urinary and reproductive systems. It can be a good choice of herb when there is oedema, and it is also helpful to treat kidney stones and urinary incontinence.

It can alleviate lethargy and exhaustion and is an excellent general tonic. It is rich in antioxidants and is anti-inflammatory. It is said that it helps neutralize the effects of caffeine when it is added to a cup of coffee, but I have not tried this. Overall, it is a calming and grounding herb, very suitable for those suffering from anxiety and insomnia or from an inability to focus and sit still.

Energetics

Green Cardamom has a hot and bitter taste. It lifts the spirits, calms the mind, and improves memory and concentration.

In Tibetan medicine

Green Cardamom is known as *Sukmel* [སུག་སྨེལ།] in Tibetan. It is a specific for all kidney illnesses caused by cold. It has a hot and sweet taste, with a post-digestive taste that is bitter. It has a potency that is oily, warm, dry, and fast-acting. It is stimulant and carminative. The texts teach that it is helpful in cases of poor circulation, abdominal cramps, gas, indigestion, and malabsorption. It is described as 'binding the openings of the nerves', a pathology that is caused by a cold disease of *Pekén* and *rLung* affecting the kidneys; *Sukmel* reduces *Pekén* and *rLung* but increases *Tripa*.

In my dispensary

I most often prescribe Cardamom in a tincture blend designed to counteract excess *rLung*. Alongside Cardamom, this blend contains a range of *rLung*-reducing herbs and spices, including Cloves, Caraway, Garlic, Nutmeg, Cinnamon.

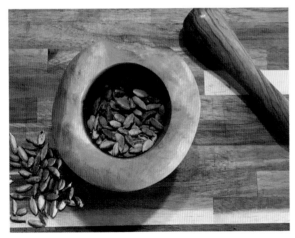

Historical applications

Cardamom has been part of the Tibetan and Ayurvedic *Materia Medica* for thousands of years. By the fourth century BC it was known in Greece and much valued as a medicine, being traded along the caravan routes that ran from the East to the West. It is an ingredient of the ancient Egyptian ointment called '*metopion*', which was both a perfume and a medicine. Cardamom was introduced to Europe by the Romans. It was not recorded as a medicinal plant within Chinese medicine until the eighth century AD, when it was described as being indicated for urinary incontinence.

Magical

Cardamom is associated with lust and love. The ground seeds are added to warmed wine for a quick lust potion. They are also baked into apple pies or added to sachets and incense to attract love.

Suggestion for the home apothecary

Warming spicy chai

This is a great recipe for midwinter when you instinctively feel that you need the influence of warming spices in your life. The Cardamom pods are a key ingredient, but the recipe also contains several other wonderful medicinal warming spices. Adjust the ingredients to your own preference and their availability. Makes two large cups.

> » *2.5 cups water*
> » *6–8 green Cardamom pods*
> » *5–6 whole Black Peppercorns*
> » *1–2 slices fresh Ginger*
> » *3 thin slices fresh Turmeric*
> » *2.5–5 cm of Cinnamon*
> » *4–5 Cloves*
> » *1 Star Anise*

» *½ tsp Caraway seeds*
» *1 Bay leaf*
» *1 cup milk (I use non-dairy milk)*
» *2–3 tsp loose leaf black tea*
» *Honey or unrefined sugar to taste*

Put the water in a saucepan and add the spices. Bring to the boil, turn down the heat, and simmer for 10 minutes. Add the milk, and simmer gently for a couple of minutes. Turn off the heat, add the black tea, and leave that to infuse passively for 2–3 minutes. Strain into two cups and add honey or refined sugar to taste.

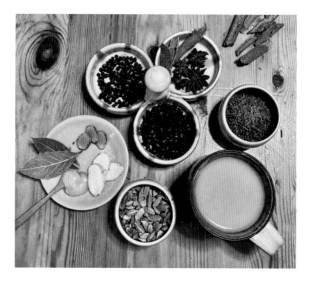

Catmint 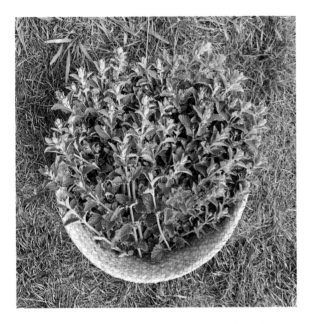 *Nepeta mussinii*

'Catmint is calming as well as stimulating.'

Catmint is a bit of a paradox. It is calming while also being stimulating. It is antispasmodic and carminative while stimulating digestion and encouraging sweating. It is a herb that needs to be protected from our feline friends during the establishment phase. I have always dreamed of establishing a sea of the blue-flowered version under a standard deep pink-flowered Rose in my garden. Alas, where I live, the local cat population is not going to let me. As soon as I try to plant some cuttings, the word spreads, and a succession of felines come and luxuriate in and roll on the plants until they disappear into the soil, never to recover. Apparently, if grown from seed and not disturbed, cats overlook it. Luckily, I am able to grow and cut it at my allotment, so I have access to this lovely medicine.

Medicinal parts
  ▷ Aerial parts

Physiological actions

Summary
  ▷ Nervine
  ▷ Carminative
  ▷ Antispasmodic
  ▷ Diaphoretic
  ▷ Decongestant
  ▷ Antitussive
  ▷ Stimulant

Physiological virtues

Catmint is a nervine, helpful for anxiety, restlessness, and nervousness. It is a good, relaxing diaphoretic, producing perspiration without being heating. It is well indicated for children, but doses should be kept small in those under 12 because as well as being calming, it can be quite stimulating. It is a pleasant herbal tea, but do not underestimate its potency. According to Maud Grieve: '*it is good in restlessness, colic, insanity and nervousness*', but also '*the root when chewed is said to make the most gentle person fierce and quarrelsome*'. As a tea, for older children and adults, it is very calming to the nervous system and promotes restful sleep. It is a good choice for anxiety, tension headaches, and nightmares. Cats go mad for it, so expect your cat to be very interested while you are sipping it.

Catmint's aromatic constituents give it the property of settling an upset stomach and easing colic, flatulence, and diarrhoea. It is also decongestant and a bronchodilator, helpful to relieve coughs, bronchitis, sinusitis, and asthma. Old writers advised a decoction sweetened with honey in order to relieve a cough.

Topical applications of Catmint can be helpful to reduce fevers. Apply fomentations of the infusion to the wrists and ankles or massage the patient with the infused oil.

Energetics

Catmint is hot and astringent.

In Tibetan medicine

In the Tibetan pharmacopoeia *Nepeta mussinii* is considered to be interchangeable medicinally with *Elsholtzia strobilifera* and other Elsholtzias. *Elsholtzia* and *Nepeta* medicine is generally called *Phur mug* [སུར་སྨུག]. *Elsholtzia densa* is called *Ji rug mukpo* [བྱི་རུག་སྨུག་པོ].

The medicinal parts are the leaves, stems, flowers, and fruit. It is usually prepared as a concentrated decoction. It has a hot to astringent and a bitter post-digestive taste. Its potency is cooling as well as warm and rough. It is considered to cure diphtheria, muscle inflammation, muscle cramps in the small intestine caused by microorganisms, epidemic diseases in general and inflammation associated with them, as well as sores, pimples, and swelling.

Please do not confuse the generic name 'Elsholtzia' with the similar sounding 'Eschscholzia', which is the generic name for California Poppy. These two are not related.

In my dispensary

I most often prescribe Catmint in calming tea blends mixed with Wild Oat, Skullcap, and Agrimony. The following is a typical example of where I would choose Catmint.

'Finn' was 5 years old and often complained of tummy aches. He did not always feel hungry and only ate his evening meal perhaps once per week. His parents were very conscious of providing their children with a healthy diet and Finn had excellent wholesome, low-sugar, organically sourced meals. When I took his case, it seemed to me that Finn needed help with his digestive system and that he would benefit from a herbal calming influence. It had become clear that his symptoms had worsened since he started school, and I wondered if he was finding it difficult to adjust to the change in lifestyle. I prescribed a blend of Catmint and Chamomile, which was to be infused and made into natural jelly cubes. He was to take two per day, one in the morning and one in the evening. He loved his special medicinal jelly cubes and told me that his older sister was a bit jealous. Four weeks after starting his herbal medicine, his tummy aches were much less frequent, and his appetite was improving. Later on, his sister came for a checkup and got her own herbal blend for jelly cubes too.

Historical applications

Lyte described it as '*hot and dry in the third degree*'. He said that it: '*prevaileth much against the bitings of venomous beastes . . . and drunken . . . aforehand with wine, preserveth a bodie from all deadly poison, and rhaseth and driveth away all venoumous beastes from that place where as it is either strowen or burned. . . . Dronken with honied water,* [it] *. . . warmeth the body, and cutteth or severeth the grosse humors, and driveth away all cold shiverings, and causeth to sweat. It hath the same power if ye boile it in oile, and annoint all the body therewith.*'

Maud Grieve wrote that Catmint was traditionally combined with Saffron and prescribed for scarlet fever and smallpox.

Magical

Catmint is popular in love sachets (often combined with Rose petals). It is said that if you hold Catmint in your hand until it is warm, then hold someone's hand, they will be your friend forever – as long as you carefully keep the sprig. Pressed Catmint leaves are used as bookmarks in magical texts.

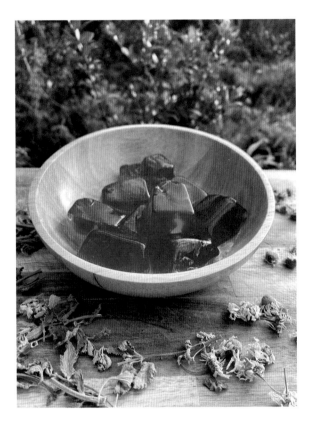

Suggestion for the home apothecary

Catmint and Chamomile jelly cubes

These jelly (or Jello) cubes can be made with any herbal infusion and are much loved by children. All you need to do is to make a herbal infusion, steeping the herbs covered in hot water for 10 minutes. If preparing roots, bark or seeds, you may wish to make a decoction instead, simmering gently for 10 minutes. The volume of water you choose is based on the volume of water required to make a batch of jelly. Strain the herbal tea or decoction, put it back in a pan and bring it to a gentle boil. Use this herbal tea or decoction instead of boiling water when making your jelly. Pour the herbal jelly mixture into an ice cube tray and allow to set. Store in the fridge. Give 1–2 as a medicinal treat daily, depending on the circumstances. I prefer to make these with vegan jelly crystals, the type you can buy from wholefood stores, as they have no gelatine, less sugar, and fewer additives.

Chamomile *Chamaemelum nobile* (Roman)/ *Matricaria recutita* (German)

'Chamomile helps us to digest our emotions and resolves weepiness.'

There are two main types of Chamomile: Roman and German. I consider both Roman and German Chamomiles to be pretty much interchangeable in medicinal practice, so I refer to them both as 'Chamomile'. The name 'Chamaemelum' is derived from the Greek *chamaimelon*, which means Earth Apple. This name alludes to its intensely apple-like scent.

Chamomile has a wide range of very helpful physiological virtues. It has the special quality of helping us to digest our emotions when everything seems too much and all we can do is weep. This makes Chamomile a particularly helpful herb for children but it should not be underestimated as a herb for overwhelm in sensitive and overly stressed adults.

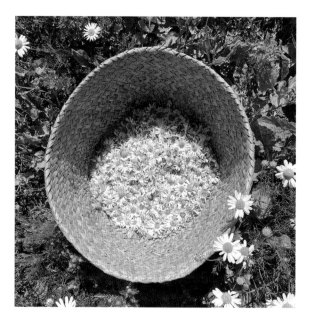

Medicinal parts
▷ Flowers

Physiological actions

Summary

▷ Bitter
▷ Carminative
▷ Sedative
▷ Antispasmodic
▷ Analgesic
▷ Diaphoretic
▷ Diuretic

Physiological virtues

Chamomile supports the liver and digestion. In the Beatrix Potter stories, Peter Rabbit was told to drink it for his indigestion. It is gentle but effective, so is excellent for soothing chil-dren's tummy aches or helping to support a weak digestion in elderly patients. In elders with a loss of appetite and sluggish digestion, it is recommended that a small cup of Chamomile tea is drunk about an hour before the main meal. This will help to stimulate the appetite and encourage better digestion.

Chamomile is relaxing and antispasmodic, helping to relieve griping and nausea. It has a mild analgesic action and sometimes, if taken promptly at the onset of a headache, a dose of Chamomile can avert it. Typically, this works best if the headache is associated with liverishness. Maud Grieve describes Chamomile as being able to cut short an attack of *delirium tremens* if taken in the early stages.

It is a diaphoretic and can be helpful in fever management. In times gone by it was prescribed for intermittent fevers. Another of Chamomile's virtues is that it is a diuretic and tonic. These qualities make it helpful in cases of dropsy, especially when combined with stimulating herbs to support the circulation.

As a topical treatment, Chamomile is anti-inflammatory and soothing, excellent to relieve nappy rash, itchy skin, or sunburn. Maud Grieve describes it being applied as a poultice made of equal parts Chamomile flowers and crushed Poppy seeds to relieve the pain of congested neuralgia and inflammation of the face caused by tooth abscesses.

It is also strongly antiseptic. It is said to be 120 times stronger than sea water for this purpose. This may explain some of the reverence with which it is held in the traditional Nine Herbs Charm.

Regarding Chamomile's specificity with weepiness, it is interesting to note that crying is the only way for the body to excrete stress hormones whole. If they are not excreted whole, they need to be broken down by the liver, and this is quite hard work, especially if there is liver

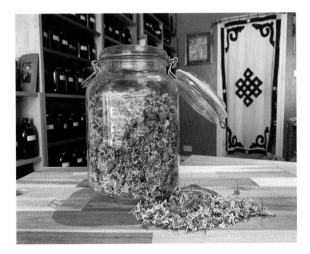

congestion. In these circumstances it makes sense that the body will need to cry more often. Chamomile supports the liver, and it therefore helps it to better break down stress hormones. Perhaps this is the reason that it reduces the urge to cry so often.

Energetics

Chamomile is my herb of choice for people prone to weepiness. The patient is overwhelmed by their suffering and they weep easily because they are unable to digest their emotions. They feel unable to cope with their own suffering and that of the world around them. This overwhelm can lead to a child-like demeanour of just wanting everything to be made better and feeling completely unable to take constructive action for themselves. Chamomile allows us to turn a feeling of helplessness into a feeling of acceptance. It helps us to feel that it is possible to move forward from our overwhelm and despair in a positive way. With Chamomile we find that we can better digest our emotions (as well as our food).

In Tibetan medicine

Despite its sweet fragrance, Chamomile is significantly bitter. This makes it an excellent choice to treat excesses of *Tripa* in sensitive and stressed individuals. Over-prescribing of Chamomile should be avoided for patients with an excess of *rLung*, but a little will be helpful if there is weepiness.

In my dispensary

If there is a tendency to weepiness or if there is a childlike quality, I include Chamomile in prescriptions for patients who already need bitters or nervines. A very helpful attribute of Chamomile is that it is widely available as a herbal tea and is therefore a familiar herb to most. This means that in those who are especially anxious about taking herbal medicine, it poses less of a challenge. In my clinic I have found that there are certain patients who, despite desperately and genuinely wanting help, find themselves very fearful about taking 'new' herbal medicines. Their underlying anxiety can make it difficult for them to engage wholeheartedly in the herbal therapeutic process if unfamiliar herbs are prescribed. The status quo can feel much safer than making changes, especially when there is the fear of an adverse reaction. In these cases, we take things very slowly and steadily in order to work towards the changes required to start the healing process. On many occasions, I have started the treatment of such patients entirely with gentle dietary changes and regular Chamomile tea. It is wonderful to see people begin to feel less fearful and more trusting of herbal medicine.

'Cally' was 32 years old and had been suffering with anxiety since she was at school. She told me that she did not have any 'logical reason' to feel anxious but it was completely dominating her life. She was also very honest about her fears surrounding taking herbal medicine, fearing that she might have a bad reaction to something. When she told me that she suffered with a frequent loose stool and digestive bloating and was prone to feeling weepy, I knew that Chamomile was going to be the best herb to start her on her herbal healing process. I prescribed half a mug of Chamomile tea 30 minutes before each meal and asked her to try to stick to a more regular eating pattern. When I next saw her, she reported that her digestion was much better and her anxiety seemed less. Unusually for her, she had hardly felt weepy at all during the intervening time. She continued to feel less anxious and began to feel more trusting about

the prospect of taking a tailor-made herbal prescription. We moved onto more tailored support and Chamomile continued to support her continued recovery within her personalized blend.

Historical applications

Chamomile has an extremely long medicinal history. Archaeological evidence shows that it was part of life in Neanderthal communities.

Gerard wrote: '*It is of force to digest, slacken, and rarifie…wherefore it is a special helpe against wearisomeness, it easeth and mitigateth paine, it mollifieth and suppleth.*'

Parkinson wrote: '*Camomil is put to divers and sundry users, both for pleasure and profit. Both for the sick and the sound, in bathing to comfort and strengthen the sound and to ease pains in the diseased.*'

Magical

Chamomile is known as 'Maythen' in Anglo-Saxon. It was considered to be one of the nine herbs given to the world by the god Woden. These herbs are combined in a special formula or 'charm' against infection caused by 'worms and flying venom'. It is likely that the charm was a topical treatment applied to wounds. The Lacnunga manuscript which dates from the ninth or tenth century contains our only surviving reference to this charm. As the charm is put together, an address to each of the nine herbs is spoken. This is a translation of the address to Chamomile:

> '*Remember, Chamomile,*
> *what you brought to pass,*
> *what you accomplished,*
> *at Alorford,*
> *that no one should lose their life to disease,*
> *since for him Chamomile was prepared.*'

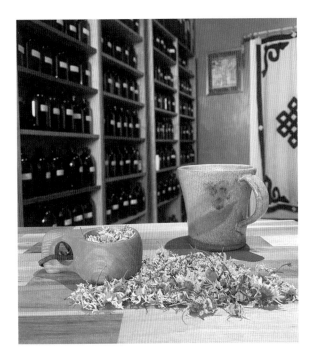

Alorford is a place name which can be translated roughly as Alder Ford. I would love to know what happened there but sadly that information is now lost. It probably refers to a dramatic healing event which was precipitated by treatment with Chamomile.

Suggestion for the home apothecary

Chamomile tea

Keep a stock of dried Chamomile flowers in your home apothecary. Prescribe a cup of Chamomile tea an hour before the main meal for older relatives or those who suffer with a weak digestion.

Chickweed 🍃 *Stellaria media*

'Chickweed soothes inflammation, reduces itching, resolves lumps and promotes tissue repair.'

Chickweed is also known as 'Star Weed' due to its beautiful little white star-like flowers. As its name suggests, it is beloved by hens and other birds. It can vary quite a bit according to where it is growing, but once you get your eye in, you will see it everywhere. Chickweed is a versatile and valuable herb for skin conditions, wounds, and abscesses. It is rich in saponins that can be very helpful to relieve itching.

Medicinal parts
 ▹ Aerial parts

Physiological actions

Summary

 ▹ Demulcent
 ▹ Anti-inflammatory
 ▹ Antipruritic
 ▹ Aperient
 ▹ Expectorant

Physiological virtues

Chickweed is demulcent and refrigerant. It is most popularly prescribed topically as an ointment, juice, poultice, or cream. A poultice made from the fresh leaves can be applied to reduce inflammation, treat slow-healing ulcers, or to help resolve abscesses. Do not waste the boiling water used to prepare it. It makes a good initial wash before applying the poultice.

An ointment or wash of Chickweed juice or infusion is absolutely indispensable for itchy skin conditions, including bites, eczema, allergic reactions, and chickenpox. It also soothes haemorrhoids. Topical applications of Chickweed are traditional to relieve ophthalmia. You

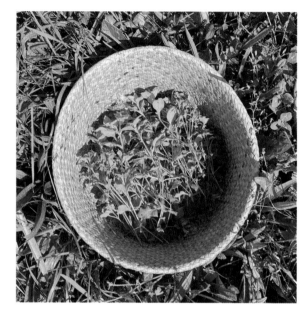

can even add Chickweed infusion to the bath in order to reduce inflammation in the joints and encourage tissue repair.

A decoction made with the fresh plant can act as an aperient, relieving constipation; an infusion made with the dried herb is a good expectorant, relieving coughs and hoarseness. Chickweed's saponins mildly irritate the stomach, and it is believed that this effect transfers to the lungs by a process known as reflex expectoration. This is possibly due to the fact that both lungs and stomach share a common nerve root. Chickweed may also thin the mucus and make it easier for the cilia in the lungs to expel it.

Energetics
Chickweed is sweet, salty, and astringent, cooling, and moistening.

In my dispensary

I prescribe Chickweed internally and topically, as needed by patients. For practical reasons, the main topical application I prescribe is an ointment, although I often encourage patients to gather their own fresh Chickweed as a treatment. I have two stories to tell you about the wonders of Chickweed as a topical application.

The first took place when I had not been in practice for very long, and I was still working from home in West Dorset. A woman in her early 70s arrived for a consultation, accompanied by her husband. She had had a severe allergic reaction to a course of antibiotics that had been prescribed by her GP. I cannot remember now what the problem was that had required the antibiotics, but the main thing that needed to be dealt with was the very severe itching that she was experiencing. She had a raised red rash all over her body. She continually rubbed her arms and legs while she spoke, and all the while her husband gently rubbed her back. I could see that her whole body was filled with tension and suffering, and no matter how hard she was trying not to scratch, the situation was clearly unbearable. I immediately handed her husband a jar of my Chickweed ointment and asked him to help her apply it to all of the areas that were worst affected. Almost immediately, her tension melted away, and her whole body began to relax. 'Goodness that's very effective!' she said. Within minutes the tension had gone, and she looked like a completely different person. With the help of Chickweed, I was able to properly assess her case and formulate a treatment plan for the underlying health issue. By the end of the session, her rash was much less livid. She left with a personalized prescription and a jar of Chickweed ointment.

The second was a patient, also in his 70s, who was experiencing a painful and itchy rash where his prosthetic leg fitted onto his stump. He had been fitted with the prosthesis many years earlier, but in the last couple of years it had started to cause problems. It rubbed and chafed and was very itchy, significantly limiting his ability to remain mobile. His wife, also in her 70s, was pushing him in a wheelchair most of the time. He was not a light man, and she struggled to push him up inclines or to bump the wheelchair up kerbs.

On inspection, it looked as though the skin on the stump had become fragile and inflamed. I was already treating him for other issues, including supporting his circulation, so I hoped that once the inflammation in the area had resolved, the tissue would heal properly and would be more able to withstand the pressure from the prosthesis. I gave him a jar of Chickweed ointment to try, and he reported that the area had stopped itching immediately and had quickly healed up. It seems that, as well as making him much more comfortable, Chickweed had reduced the longstanding inflammation, allowing the prosthesis to fit again. The skin on his stump stayed healthy, and he continued to apply Chickweed every morning as a safeguard. I supplied him with regular jars of ointment for many years, until he died.

Historical applications

Dioscorides wrote that Chickweed: '*may usefully be applied with cornmeal for inflammation of the eyes. The juice may be introduced into the ear in earache.*'

Gerard wrote that '*Little birds in cages (especially Linnets) are refreshed with the lesser Chickweed when they loathe their meat, whereupon it was called of some "Passerina"*'. . . . '*the leaves of Chickweed boyled in water very soft, adding thereto some hog's grease, the powder of Fenugreeke and Linseed, and a few roots of Marsh Mallows, and stamped to the forme of Ctaplasme or pultesse, taketh away the swelling of the legs or any other part . . in a word it comforteth, digesteth, defendeth and suppurateth.'*

Culpeper describes using repeated fresh poultices of Chickweed to the liver area in order to reduce liver inflammation. '*The herb bruised, or the juice applied, with cloths or sponges dipped therein to the region of the liver, and as they dry to have fresh applied, doth wonderfully temper the heat of the liver, and is effectual for all impostumes and swellings whatsoever, for all redness in the face, wheals, pushes, itch or scabs, the juice either simply used, or boiled in hog's grease.'* Fascinatingly, he also mentions the application of Chickweed and Rose leaf ointment to relieve the shrinking and hardening of the sinews: '*It helpeth the sinews when they are shrunk by cramps or otherwise, and extends and makes them pliable again. . . . Boil a handful of Chickweed and a handful of dried red Rose leaves . . . in a quart of Muscadine, until a fourth part is consumed; then put to them a pint of oil of trotters, or sheep's feet; let them boil a good while, still stirring them well which being strained, anoint the grieved part therewith warm against the fire, rubbing it well with your hand, and bind, also some of the herb to the place if you choose.'*

Magical

Chickweed is associated with fidelity and love. Carry it in order to attract or retain love.

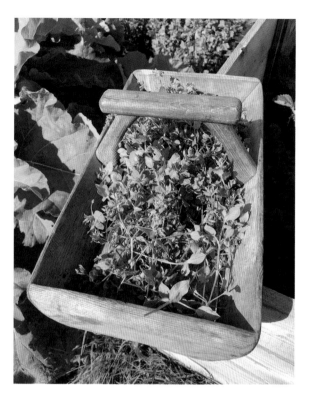

Suggestion for the home apothecary

Chickweed poultice for bites and itchy skin

Gather fresh Chickweed. Chop a handful and apply directly to the affected area, holding the herb in place with a clean muslin cloth. You can also dry some herb for out-of-season applications.

Chilli 🌶 *Capsicum frutescens/C. annuum*

'Chilli is the King of Heat.'

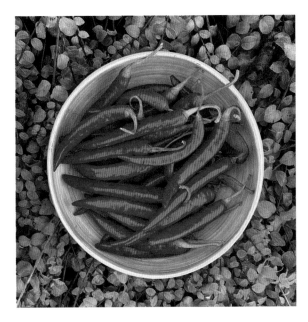

Chilli is indigenous to Mexico and Northern South America. It is a tonic to the whole body, increasing blood flow to the surface as well as the deep organs, tonifying the nervous system, and increasing the appetite. It was described by Gerard as 'extreme hot and dry, even in the fourth degree.' Whenever I read that, I somehow have an image of Gerard's reaction after nibbling a little bit of Chilli for the first time.

Medicinal parts
- Fruit

Physiological actions

Summary
- Circulatory stimulant
- Diaphoretic
- Expectorant
- Carminative
- Digestive stimulant
- Laxative
- Analgesic
- Antiseptic
- Vulnerary

Physiological virtues

Chilli is a powerful stimulant herb, encouraging blood circulation, especially to the periphery; but it also helps to enliven circulation to the major organs of the body. One of my tutors described how Chilli had saved his wife's life after she had suffered a heart attack. He acted quickly, calling an ambulance and then immediately administered a teaspoon of neat Chilli tincture before commencing CPR (cardio-pulmonary-resuscitation). The ambulance arrived within a just a few minutes, and the paramedics found her conscious, and with a regular heartbeat. With a combination of allopathic emergency healthcare and good herbal support from her husband, she went on to make a full recovery.

On a less dramatic note, Chilli is a really good medicine for those who have a chronically sluggish circulation and a cold constitution. It increases blood flow to the skin and can be helpful both to stimulate sweating and to encourage better temperature regulation. It is also an excellent digestive herb, being carminative and relieving wind and colic. It stimulates better secretion of digestive juices, and it improves the appetite. Doses for these health conditions are obviously much lower than in the first example.

Chilli is an expectorant and is worth considering for prescriptions to help with catarrh and sinus issues. It is a key ingredient of Fire Cider.

It was a pillar of eclectic herbal prescribing in which stimulating and relaxing herbs were combined. Chilli and *Lobelia inflata* are a pair that work very well together: the Lobelia relaxes the tissues and the Chilli enlivens the circulation to them. It is also worth noting that Chilli causes sweating and Lobelia is an emetic, both actions being promoted by the eclectics as cleansing and healing strategies.

Topical treatments, such as infused oils, compresses, and ointments are a great way of stimulating the circulation in those who are unable to tolerate too much Chilli orally. It is a popular ingredient in creams and ointments designed to help relieve cold hands and feet. For obvious reasons it is important to apply only to unbroken skin. If using a compress, do not leave it in place for too long, as it could cause blistering. Chilli contains capsaicin, which desensitizes nerve endings and acts as an analgesic. This means that topical Chilli can be helpful for neuralgia, back pain, headaches, and arthritic pain, especially when these manifestations of pain are associated with poor blood flow to the affected area. It is an excellent treatment for unbroken chilblains.

Chilli is antiseptic, so, if applied to a wound, it will disinfect it; but there are other antiseptic herbs that feel less 'intense' when applied, so you may want to bear that in mind. Its antimicrobial action is effective to treat infections of the digestive tract, and it can even kill certain stomach nematodes. It is surprisingly helpful for some manifestations of diarrhoea. Eating spicy food can be a very great idea when travelling if you are not used to the local 'bugs', but you will need to be guided by your own system. It is also worth remembering that a pinch of Chilli powder in water is an excellent readily available first-aid gargle for the onset of a sore throat.

Energetics

Chilli is hot and a little sweet. It helps to encourage movement where there is stagnation, whether that is in the body or the mind or, as is most often the case, both.

In Tibetan medicine

Cayenne Pepper is called *Tsitraka* [ཚི་ཏྲ་ཀ] in Tibetan. It has a taste that is hot and a post-digestive taste that is bitter. Its potency is rough, warm, and light. It is strongly warming and is known as 'The King of Heat'. It treats shifting oedema, colonic growths, micro-organism diseases, and leprosy. Chilli brings the element of Fire to the system, counteracting excesses of Earth and Water.

In my dispensary

As the active ingredients of Chilli are oil-soluble, you need a very high alcohol content and therefore minimal water content if you are making a tincture. I use 90% ABV alcohol to make mine. Luckily a little goes a long way. I include a little Chilli in many of my prescriptions as a carrier or 'medicine horse' in order to help the medicine get to where it is needed in the body. The rate of inclusion is perhaps only 5 ml in a 300 ml bottle.

Historical applications

Lloyd and Felter's *King's American Dispensatory* (1905) suggests Cayenne tincture mixed with Orange peel tincture for tackling alcoholism and delirium tremens.

Magical

Chillies are associated with breaking hexes and encouraging fidelity in a relationship. If you suspect that your love is tempted to be unfaithful, take two dried Chillies, cross them and tie them with a red thread and place this beneath

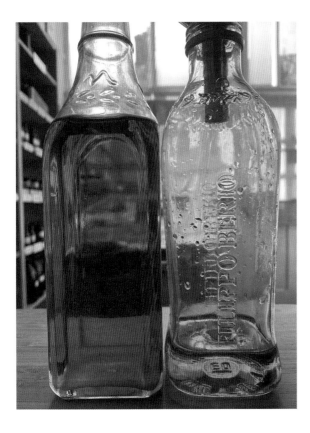

your pillow. It is said that this will keep your love from straying.

Suggestions for the home apothecary

Chilli infusion

Make an infusion by adding ½ tsp of dried Chilli (or a whole fresh Chilli) to a cup of boiling water. Take 1 tbsp of this base infusion, dilute that in a cup of hot water, and sip it to ease shock, depression, cold hands and feet, or to ease the symptoms of colds. You can also gargle with this mix to help sore throats. Two or three drops of the undiluted base infusion can be taken neat to stimulate the digestion.

Chilli-infused oil

Slice fresh Chillies, add to a jar and cover with olive oil. Leave for four weeks, then strain, filter, and bottle, taking care to leave the aqueous layer at the bottom of the jar when decanting. Apply to cold hands and feet, chilblains, or painful joints.

Cinnamon 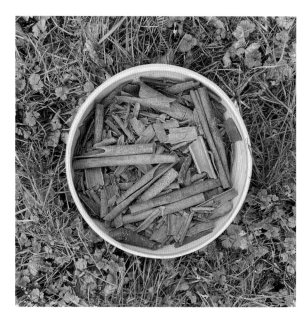 *Cinnamomum verum/C. zeylanicum*

'Cinnamon is warming and calming, counteracting feebleness and laxity.'

There are various species of Cinnamon, but generally *Cinnamomum verum* and *Cinnamomum zeylanicum* are the species chosen for medicine in the West. Cinnamon has a very wide range of medicinal virtues, having a helpful supportive action on the digestive, nervous, respiratory, circulatory, urinary, and reproductive systems. It also acts as an antimicrobial and antiviral. It is warming and comforting, as well as being delicious.

Medicinal part

▷ Bark

Physiological actions

Summary

▷ Circulatory stimulant
▷ Diaphoretic
▷ Astringent
▷ Antibacterial
▷ Antifungal
▷ Antiviral
▷ Blood sugar balancing
▷ Nervine
▷ Antispasmodic
▷ Antidepressant
▷ Expectorant
▷ Diuretic

Physiological virtues

Cinnamon is a warming and stimulating herb and, as such, can be a good choice to support people with a cold constitution. It especially warms and relaxes the uterus. Consider it for patients who have painful congested menses with large clots.

It has antibacterial, antifungal, and antiviral properties, making it a good first aid herb if you are away from home, since you can nearly always get access to some if you need it. It is quite astringent in nature, due to its tannins, so it is excellent for diarrhoea while travelling. On the flip side, if you are someone with a tendency to constipation and are in the habit of adding a generous spoonful of Cinnamon powder to your porridge every morning, you will be making it much worse. Ease off on the Cinnamon and enjoy the difference.

The essential oil of Cinnamon is very irritating if taken internally. Beware of herbal tea products that contain essential oil of Cinnamon to boost the flavour of their inferior-quality herbs. If you have a sensitive digestion and you drink that sort of tea regularly, it could be causing significant inflammatory gut problems, and, ironically, this could lead to a loose stool. Change your tea choice, and you will be amazed. As a side note I do not recommend drinking any herbal tea that has essential oils added, and I never recommend taking essential oils internally.

Cinnamon helps to balance the blood sugar, so if you have insulin resistance or Type II diabetes, choosing good-quality Cinnamon tea – or decocting your own – can be a good idea. Please check with your practitioner first, though. I certainly like to consider Cinnamon in formulae that I make up for patients with blood sugar imbalances, but I am careful to adjust the amounts and balance it with other herbs if, for example, the patient is prone to a sluggish bowel.

Cinnamon is a nervine, helping to promote relaxation and a sense of grounded calm. It is analgesic, antispasmodic, and antidepressant. In Tibetan medicine it is an important calming herb.

It is also an expectorant, a diaphoretic, and a diuretic kidney tonic. Overall, Cinnamon is a veritable medicine chest.

Energetics
Cinnamon is sweet, hot, astringent. It is comforting and warming, bringing a sense of grounding and security to us when we take it. It helps us to resist the urge to eat high glycaemic index sugary snacks which will destabilize our mood and upset our blood sugar balance.

In Tibetan medicine
In Tibetan Cinnamon it is known as *Shingtsha* [ཤིང་ཚ] (which literally means 'Hot Wood'). Its taste qualities are hot, sweet, astringent and salty. Its post-digestive taste is bitter and its potency is oily, warming and light. It is considered to counteract cold disorders of the stomach and liver. Its astringency makes it helpful in cases of cold diarrhoea as well as in cases of cough, asthma, pus in the lungs, toothache and nerve pain. It reduces *rLung* and *Pekén* while increasing *Tripa*.

I should like to add one note of caution when prescribing Cinnamon according to elemental principles. In theory, Cinnamon counteracts *rLung* but its significant astringency could worsen an existing tendency to constipation. *rLung* disorders are often accompanied by a tendency to constipation so in these cases, the inclusion of Cinnamon within a prescription should not be too heavy handed.

In my dispensary
Cinnamon is a hugely valuable herb in my dispensary. It is helpful in a wide range of circumstances, but I most often reach for it when treating anxious patients who feel the cold and suffer with a loose stool and congested, painful periods. It is also one of the herbs in my *rLung* tincture mix.

Historical applications
Cinnamon was one of the first traded spices in the ancient world, and ancient Egyptians used Cinnamon as part of their embalming rituals. There are many references to it (as the Hebrew name *Kannamon*), in the Bible in Psalms, Proverbs, Ezekiel, and Revelations. It was regarded as a suitable gift for Monarchs and for Gods. It is said that the Roman Emperor Nero ordered a year's supply of Cinnamon to be burnt after he murdered his wife, as a sign of remorse.

In the first century AD, Pliny the Elder wrote that the equivalent weight of 350 grams of Cinnamon was equal in value to over the equivalent of 5 kg of silver. This made Cinnamon about fifteen times the value of silver at that time.

In the Middle Ages, Cinnamon was considered to be primarily a remedy to treat cold and throat ailments, such as coughing, hoarseness, and sore throats.

Gerard was very enthusiastic about Cinnamon: '*To write as the worthinesse of the subject requireth, would ask more time than we have to bestow upon any one plant.*'

He did manage to encapsulate some of the main virtues of Cinnamon: '*Dioscorides writeth, that Cinnamon hath power to warme, and is of thinne parts, it is also drie and astringent, it provoketh urine, cleareth the eies, and maketh sweet breath. The decoction bringeth down the menses, prevaileth against the bitings of venoumous beasts, the inflammation of the intestines and reines. The distilled water hereof is profitable to many, and for divers infirmities, it comforteth the weake, cold and feeble stomacke, easeth the paines and frettings of the guts and intrailes proceeding of cold causes, it amendeth the evill colour of the face, maketh sweet breath, and giveth a most pleasant taste unti divers sorts of meats, and maketh the same not only more pleasant, but also more wholesome for any bodies of what constitution soever they be, notwithstanding the binding qualitie.*'

Magical

Cinnamon is associated with spirituality, success, and healing. It is also thought to help to increase psychic sensitivity and to confer protection. It is particularly grounding and therefore helps us to have a more stable mind, from which other benefits flow. Burn it as an incense or make it into amulets or sachets.

Suggestion for the home apothecary

Hildegard spice biscuits

Hildegard of Bingen wrote that if these spice biscuits are eaten regularly, they will bring joy and positivity.

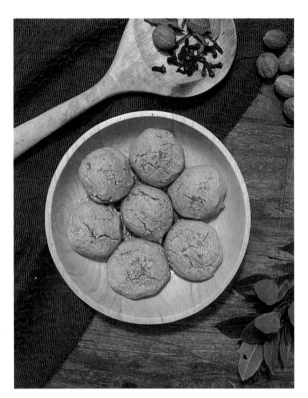

» ¾ cup butter or coconut oil
» 1 cup brown sugar
» 1 egg
» 1 tsp baking powder
» ¼ tsp salt
» 1½ cups flour
» 1 tsp ground Cinnamon
» 1 tsp ground Nutmeg
» ½ tsp ground Cloves

Soften the butter and then cream it with the brown sugar. Beat in the egg. Sift the dry ingredients. Add half the dry ingredients and mix. Add the other half and mix thoroughly, until it forms a dough. You may need to adjust the proportions if working with gluten-free flours. Chill the dough to make it easier to work. Form into walnut-sized balls, place on greased and floured cookie sheet, and bake for 12–15 minutes at 175°C (until the edges are golden brown).

Citrus fruits 🍋 *Citrus aurantium/C. limonum/C. aurantiifolia*

'Citrus stimulates our digestion and increases our inner wealth.'

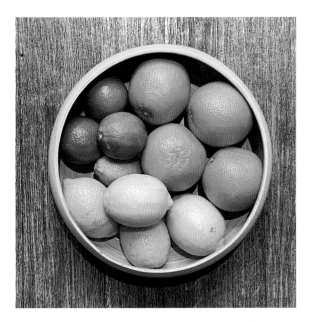

Citrus peel is a valued herbal medicine because of its bitter and antioxidant-rich qualities. Bitterness stimulates the digestion, encouraging better assimilation of nutrients, and immune-boosting antioxidants help to support our immune systems and safeguard us against infections. This, in turn, increases our inner health and wealth. In Sanskrit, Orange is *Nagaranga* and Lemon or Lime is *Nimbuka* or *Chura*.

Medicinal parts
▷ Peel
▷ Fruit
▷ Blossom

Physiological actions
Summary
▷ Bitter
▷ Carminative
▷ Cardiovascular tonic
▷ Diaphoretic
▷ Diuretic
▷ Anti-inflammatory
▷ Nervine

Physiological virtues

Citrus rind is packed with antioxidants and bioflavonoids. It can help to support the integrity of the blood vessels and contribute to the prevention of circulatory disorders such as varicose veins and easy bruising. It is also considered to help prevent the build-up of arteriosclerosis.

It is naturally bitter and acts as a digestive stimulant, encouraging better secretion of bile but also supporting pancreatic function. Including Citrus in the diet encourages a healthy appetite, improved digestion, and better absorption of minerals, particularly iron. It is a diaphoretic and diuretic, and it helps to reduce arthritis, gout, and rheumatism.

Lemon is a familiar home remedy in cold and influenza remedies. It has a high Vitamin C content, improving our resistance to infections, and is antiseptic and antimicrobial. Although it is acidic upon ingestion, once digested, it has an alkalizing effect on the body. It is a very good anti-inflammatory astringent and is worth considering topically in cases of sunburn. It is also a very well-known option as a gargle for sore throats, gingivitis, and mouth ulcers. Drinking Lemon juice can stop a severe and persistent attack of hiccoughs.

In traditional Chinese medicine, whole unripe Bitter Orange, called *Zhi shi*, can help to support the digestion, relieving bloating and flatulence as well as alleviating constipation. It is also a calming nervine, helpful for insomnia and shock. The ripe dried fruit, known as *Zhi ke*, is an excellent digestive support. Both are also considered helpful for prolapse.

The dried rind of ripe Satsumas, known as *Chen pi*, is prescribed as an expectorant when there is thin, watery phlegm. The green unripe rind, *Qing pi*, is a qi tonic, which supports the digestion.

The fresh juice of Limes (*Citrus aurantiifolia*) is a popular medicinal ingredient in south-east Asia and Guyana, especially as a treatment for diarrhoea. An infusion of the leaves is said to relieve a bilious headache.

Orange blossom is a wonderful sedative nervine. I will never forget the gorgeous fragrance coming from the Orange orchards while visiting in Cyprus in springtime – definitely a magical and relaxing experience.

Energetics

Bitter Orange (*Citrus aurantium*) is sour, bitter and cooling; Satsuma (*Citrus reticulata*) is warm and bitter.

Citrus supports us in numerous ways, improving digestion and elimination and improving all sorts of health conditions. The traditional association of Citrus fruits with good fortune and wealth is well deserved. Citrus supports better digestion and assimilation and therefore helps us to increase our 'inner wealth'.

In my dispensary

Many patients struggle with sluggish digestion and find it difficult to maintain healthy iron levels. While there can be many reasons for this, in most cases it can be very helpful to support digestion and absorption alongside targeted treatments to tackle other underlying causes. I often suggest that they drink hot water with a slice of Lemon to support their herbal treatment for sluggish digestion or low iron levels.

I want to share a story here about the power of Citrus, even though this was a case for which I cannot claim any direct involvement. I once met a lovely lady at a social gathering. She was perhaps in her late 60s and had been suffering for many years with Type II diabetes. She had apparently been quite overweight, although when I met her, she was not. When she discovered that I was a medical herbalist, she generously shared her experience with the healing power of Lemons. A year or so previously, her health had been deteriorating, and she had been advised by her spiritual teacher to juice a whole Lemon, flesh, rind, and pips, and to drink this mixture daily. She did this without fail for a year; she lost two stone, enlivened her digestive system, and improved her insulin sensitivity, eventually curing herself from Type II diabetes. She was continuing with her daily juiced fresh whole Lemon and remained vibrant and well.

Historical applications

Oranges originated in China, and by the Middle Ages were popular among Arab physicians. They were mentioned in Arabian medicinal texts long before they were known to Europeans. Once they found out about Citrus fruits, Europeans came to prize them very highly in order to counteract scurvy. English ships were required by law to carry enough Lemons to allow every seaman to have an ounce daily after being at sea for more than ten days.

Lemon juice was considered a good first-aid herb to counteract opium poisoning. Drinking an infusion of Orange peel was considered to guard against later drunkenness.

In folk tradition, Orange blossom was included in bridal bouquets: not only would they have smelled gorgeous, but perhaps they were helpful to calm any anxieties in either the bride or the groom.

Magical

Citrus fruits have a rich history of being associated with winter festivities. They represent the sun and warmth and have come to be part of winter solstice celebrations to remind us of the return of the light. There is a Christmas tradition that Santa leaves an Orange, Satsuma, or Clementine in the toe of the stockings that he fills with presents. This is because folklore has it that he would leave small gifts of gold, symbolised as round golden balls. Citrus fruits make an ideal substitute for gold, especially as they represent wealth and good fortune. They are given as gifts to celebrate the Chinese New Year and are enjoyed in Russian New Year's celebrations for the same reasons.

Citrus fruits are magically associated with love. The dried peel is added to love sachets, and Orange blossom added to bath water is considered to make the bather irresistible to the one they wish to attract. You can also perform a divination with Orange seeds. As you eat an Orange, think of a question that can be answered by either yes or no. After you have eaten it, count the pips. And even number indicates 'no', an odd number indicates 'yes'.

Suggestions for the home apothecary

Citrus digestive tonic

This tonic is a delicious addition to the home medicine chest. I suggest that you take 1 tsp of the tonic diluted in hot water if you are feeling bloated or have indigestion. You can also take a little about half an hour before meal-times if you are suffering from a poor appetite. If you have a sluggish digestive system, try a once-a-day dose over the course of four weeks in order to liven things up. For very elderly patients, reduce the dose to half.

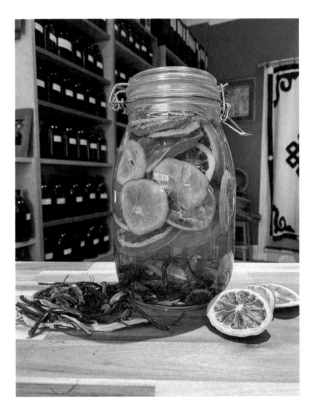

Loosely fill a jar with dried Orange and Lemon slices and add 1 tbsp, heaped, of chopped dried Dandelion root, 1 tbsp of dried Dock root, 1 tbsp of dried Ashwagandha root, and a few slices of fresh Ginger root. Cover the herbs completely with vodka that is at least 40% ABV (alcohol by volume). If your country labels alcohol in terms of 'proof', this is at least 80% proof. Leave the tonic in the dark for four weeks before draining, pressing, and bottling. If you wish to avoid alcohol, you can use cider vinegar instead of vodka as the menstruum.

Citrus peel headache treatment

Pound fresh Citrus peel into a paste with a little water and apply to forehead to cool a headache caused by heat.

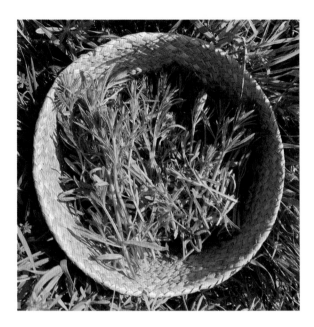
'Cleavers moves water. It encourages the flow of lymph and stimulates the kidneys.'

Cleavers is a wonderful lymphatic tonic. If you observe its natural growth habit, you will see that it is a specialist at transporting water over long distances. In my locality, Cleavers often grows with its roots in damp ditches, its succulent pre-seeding stems reaching over 2 metres long when climbing up the neighbouring hedge. These stems are pliable and soft. Cleavers does not waste its energy on stem-strengthening structures. It focuses on the efficient transportation of water and relies on other plants for its support.

The folk names for Cleavers include 'Sticky Willy', 'Goose Grass', 'Catch Weed', and 'Beggar Lice', due to its clingy bristly foliage and persistent sticky seeds. When I was first in practice, I often used to give talks. I remember speaking at a Women's Institute, where an elderly lady told me how she and her school friends had called it 'Sweet Hearts'. She described how, at play time, the 'done thing' was to pick pieces of it and throw it at the boys. I could not help but wonder about the number of new romances that had started in that way.

Cleavers is related to the Bedstraws, Madder, and, perhaps surprisingly, Coffee. The seeds can be gathered and lightly roasted as a Coffee substitute.

Medicinal parts

> Aerial parts

These should be gathered before the plant begins to seed.

Physiological actions

Summary

> Lymphatic tonic
> Diuretic
> Aperient

Physiological virtues

Cleavers is a lymphatic tonic, considered to be a drying herb according to the Galenic tradition. This is because it is so effective at moving water through the lymphatic system and out of the kidneys. Patients who suffer from swollen glands, lymphoedema, tender breasts, skin breakouts, or repeated bouts of tonsillitis are most probably suffering from an overloaded lymphatic system. It is essential to look at diet and lifestyle to get to the root cause, for example cutting out rich fatty foods and improving water intake, but, while the necessary changes are being made, Cleavers is an excellent support to the lymphatic system.

If you are taking Cleavers in the spring as a seasonal cleanse, you will need to ensure that you maintain good water intake, as it could be drying. This is one of the reasons why, for a cleanse, a cold overnight infusion of fresh young Cleavers in water is usually preferable to a quick dose of tincture. However, as part of a tailor-made tincture blend for ongoing herbal treatment, a tincture is perfect. As ever, if tinctures are not suitable, Cleavers can be added to a tea blend and drunk hot.

Cleavers mostly encourages excretion of toxins via the kidneys, but it also has a mild laxative effect. Some people find that a spring cleanse with Cleavers can be a bit too stimulating in this regard.

Cleavers is also one of the first herbs to consider for skin conditions such as acne, eczema, and psoriasis. Its diuretic action also means that it can be a good herb in cases of urinary infections, gravel, and urinary system stones.

Energetics

Cleavers is slightly bitter and hot. Since, according to Tibetan medicine, the inner workings of our bodies directly affect our experience of the world around us, a clogged and over-loaded lymphatic system is very often accompanied by a sense of 'being stuck' and feeling stagnant. We may find ourselves surrounded by clutter – physically and emotionally – and not have the energy and motivation to sort it out. Taking Cleavers brings new energy and motivation to clear out the old stuff. Many of my patients have told me that they not only felt a new lease of life, but they also completely de-cluttered their houses when they began to take Cleavers.

In Tibetan medicine

Cleavers is called *Sang tsee karpo* [ཟངས་རྩི་དཀར་པོ།]. As well as being slightly bitter and hot, it has a cool and rough potency. It treats *Tripa* disorders, yellowing of the sclera due to jaundice, bone fracture and rupture of blood vessels, and

it stops haemorrhage. It also increases sperm count. *Sang tsee karpo* can exacerbate *rLung*, so those with a tendency to airiness – anxiety, insomnia, mood swings, blood sugar instability, for example – would do well to resist the urge to drinks large amounts of cold overnight Cleavers infusion each spring.

In my dispensary

I often prescribe Cleavers for patients who present with oedema, indicated by tooth indentations on their tongue and a sense of being stuck and exhausted. They tend to have poor circulation and find that they gain weight easily and struggle to lose it. They may tell me about premenstrual mood changes, cyclical breast tenderness with a worrying tendency to lumpiness, as well as painful periods. Very often I discover that they are eating a diet quite high in mucus-forming foods, especially dairy products and refined carbohydrates. This can happen gradually after first becoming a parent, as that is when we often change our eating habits to make life easier. Other times it can be part of the initial adjustment phase after giving up meat. Once the patient's diet is cleaned up and they take a course of herbal medicine, they generally start to feel much better very quickly. I love seeing patients with a new zest for life and a new confidence in their bodies.

This is an example where Cleavers helped to resolve severe symptoms associated with lymphatic congestion: 'Georgina' was 19 years old and had frequent episodes of tonsillitis, as well as constantly swollen cervical glands. She also had eczema and IBS and felt exhausted much of the time. After going through her case in detail, I advised her to completely cut out dairy, and I prescribed a tailor-made tincture blend with Cleavers as the main herb, supported by Plantain leaf, Marshmallow leaf, Phytolacca root, Chamomile flowers, and Peach leaf. She improved steadily on the new regime. Her swollen glands resolved, her tonsillitis ceased, and her eczema reduced, although she still experienced flare-ups every so often. Her IBS symptoms also became much better over time. She did find it really tough to give up dairy completely, especially when going out with her friends. She decided to opt for having occasional dairy when she went out, feeling that a bit of discomfort was a price worth paying to be able to hang out with her friends.

Historical applications

Cleavers had the reputation of helping the body to deal with tumours, perhaps due to its ability to clear the lymphatic system and stimulate the immune system. An ointment was applied topically to ulcerated areas, and the juice was drunk to support the healing process.

In the days when freckles were frowned upon, a simple infusion of Cleavers was applied to reduce freckles and relieve sunburn.

According to Maud Grieve, an infusion drunk later in the day can be helpful in cases of insomnia – a somewhat surprising virtue given the fact that it is related to Coffee, but perhaps less so when you consider how effective homeopathic '*Coffea*' can be for insomnia.

Gerard wrote that '*Clivers*' was a marvellous remedy '*for the bites of snakes, spiders and all venomous creatures.*' He quoted Pliny, who said that '*A pottage made of Cleavers, a little mutton and oatmeal is good to cause lankness and keep from fatnesse.*'

According to Culpeper, Cleavers is a remedy for earache.

Magical

Magically, Cleavers represents tenacity. This may be in relationships, commitment, or protection.

One of the names of Cleavers has been Christianised as 'Our Lady's Bedstraw', since it was said that it was used as bedding at the birth of Christ. This name may have come about to make acceptable an old German pagan custom of putting a handful of Cleavers into the birthing bed in order to ensure an easy birth and a plentiful supply of milk. Or perhaps it is the other way around. You can choose.

Suggestion for the home apothecary

Cold overnight Cleavers infusion

Harvest a small handful of Cleavers in early spring, when the shoots are small and delicate and smell a little of Vanilla. Chop it and leave it to infuse in cold water overnight. Strain and drink in the morning. Continue for 3–4 weeks. As the season progresses, your gathered Cleavers becomes more mature and stronger, and you will be better accustomed to its cleansing effects.

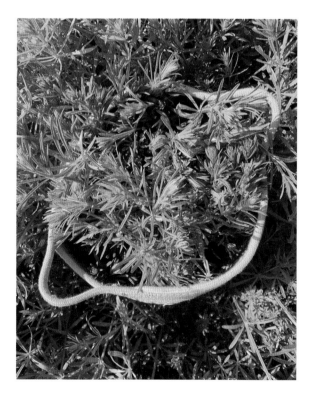

Clove Syzygium aromaticum/Eugenia caryophyllata

'Cloves are the most stimulating and calming of all the aromatics.'

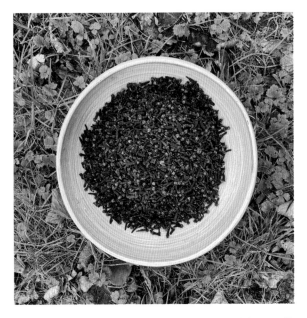

Cloves are a familiar spice and a valuable medicine that has been part of mankind's medicine chest for at least 3,000 years. The name 'Clove' comes from the Latin word *clavus*, which means 'nail'. Many years ago, I was fortunate enough to visit the island of Zanzibar. I will never forget the scent of Cloves in the air as I stepped out of the light aircraft onto the airport tarmac. Cloves are still a very important crop there.

Medicinal part
- Flower calyx

While often referred to as the 'flower bud', strictly speaking, the medicinal part of Cloves is the flower calyx after the petals have fallen. They should be harvested before ripening, since at that time the aromatic properties are at their height. At the time of harvest, each calyx has an embryo seed developing at its tip. These calyces look a bit like nails, hence the name.

Physiological actions

Summary
- Aromatic
- Stimulant
- Expectorant
- Analgesic
- Antiemetic
- Diaphoretic
- Emmenagogue
- Galactagogue
- Aphrodisiac
- Vermifuge

Physiological virtues

Cloves are the most stimulating and calming of all the aromatics. They support the circulation and enliven the systems of the body. They can be helpful in cases of hypotension, but if blood pressure is high, they should be taken with caution. They can ease nausea, flatulence, and dyspepsia, as well as stimulating the appetite when it is failing. They are also strongly antiseptic and act as a stimulating expectorant, which makes them an excellent remedy for congested conditions of the respiratory tract, especially when there is active infection present. Consider Cloves for patients with colds, coughs, and asthma. They are diaphoretic, encouraging sweating if there is a latent fever, but they are to be avoided if there is high fever present. They have analgesic properties and are very well known as a home remedy for toothache. An infused oil of Cloves is also a good pain-relieving treatment for wider aches and pains, such as backaches or joint pain. It can also be a lovely, enlivening massage oil.

Cloves can stimulate the uterus and are therefore worth considering when there is congestion and sluggishness in this area – clotted and painful menses, for example. Obviously, that means that they should be avoided in medicinal doses during pregnancy. Cloves also have a galactagogue action, so can help to stimulate lactation once the baby is born. They are also helpful for the reproductive system in males. They are traditionally considered to be an aphrodisiac herb, promoting a healthy libido and treating erectile dysfunction or premature ejaculation.

On top of all of these wonderful medicinal virtues, they are significantly antimicrobial and antifungal. A decoction of Cloves can, for example, be a good topical treatment for athlete's foot. They can help to calm outbreaks of Candida, although the root cause of Candida overgrowth needs to be addressed for lasting relief. Cloves are also antiparasitic and are a good option to include in a prescription for patients with intestinal worms, especially roundworms. When we see how helpful they are against various infections and infestations, it is perhaps not surprising that Cloves are traditionally associated with protecting us from plagues and epidemics.

Energetics
Cloves are hot and dry, and a bit bitter. Cloves are warming, so they should be prescribed with caution to patients with a fiery constitution or a feverish presentation. They are, however, a very good medicine to help calm excess *rLung*. A weak Clove infusion sipped throughout the day is a very good support in the first (shock) stages of bereavement.

In Tibetan medicine
Cloves are known as *Lishi* [ལི་ཤི༌] in Tibetan. They have a taste that is astringent, hot, and bitter, with a post-digestive taste that is bitter. The potency is oily and stable, as well as smooth and warming. Cloves are considered to be superlative medicine to support the life channel,

curing 'life-channel disorder' and cold disorders of *rLung*. Cloves are especially effective against respiratory diseases. They have a bitter, pungent taste and a warming effect on the body. They will help to ripen a fever when a patient is suffering from a lingering respiratory infection that does not seem to reach a resolution. They are pain-relieving, and they calm coughing, congestion, colds, and sinus problems.

In my dispensary
In my clinic I mostly work with Cloves within Tibetan medicinal formulae, such as *Manu Zhi Thang*. They are excellent to support people suffering from the onset of respiratory illnesses or who lack the immune system vibrancy to resolve a lingering cold. They are also a very good option as part of a prescription to treat intestinal parasites. When prescribing herbs for worm infestations, I find that a blend of herbs is often much more effective and palatable than just one single vermifuge herb.

Sometimes I recommend 'Clove tea' for people with a cold constitution who are suffering with anxiety, shock, or recent bereavement. Just infuse a couple of Cloves in a mug of hot water and take small sips throughout the day.

Historical applications
In the third century BC in China, Cloves were known as '*bird's tongue*' or *hi-sho-hiang*. Officers of the court were required to place Cloves in their mouths before audiences with the sovereign in order to ensure that their breath was fresh. As a medicine, Cloves were recognized as a stimulant, an antiseptic, and a tonic. They were applied topically to treat scorpion stings, toothaches, and cracked nipples.

When they found their way to India a few hundred years later, Cloves became very popular within Ayurveda, and from there found their way into the Tibetan pharmacopoeia.

Pliny the Elder described Cloves in his *Natural History* of AD 70, saying that they were imported to the West for the sake of their scent. In the sixth century AD, Byzantine physician Alexander of Tralles recommended Cloves for seasickness, gout, and to restore a weak appetite.

Magical

Cloves attract prosperity and drive away hostile or negative forces. They are burned as an incense in order to purify the home and prevent others from spreading gossip about you.

It is said that if carried as an amulet, they bring comfort to the bereaved.

Suggestion for the home apothecary

Garam masala

Making small batches of freshly ground garam masala is a fantastic way of getting the health-promoting and tonic effects of various spices, including Cloves.
You will need:

- » *2 tbsp Cloves*
- » *¼ cup Coriander seeds*
- » *2 tbsp Cardamom pods*
- » *2 tbsp Peppercorns*
- » *1 tbsp Fennel seeds*
- » *3–4 Star anise*
- » *10 cm Cinnamon sticks*
- » *half of a Nutmeg*
- » *2 dried Bay leaves*

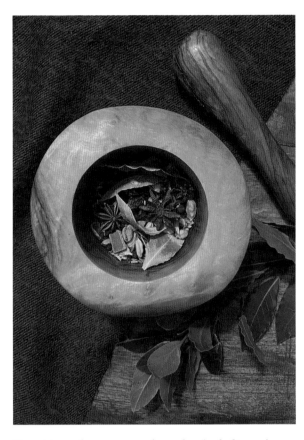

Roast in a dry pan, cool, and grind. Store in an airtight jar in a dark place or use a recycled dark jar. I have a whole kitchen spice rack based on classic dark glass jars with yellow lids, the type that used to contain yeast extract. Once you have your garam masala, you will want to add it to lots of dishes.

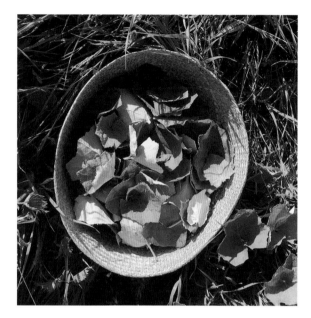
'Coltsfoot is Nature's best herb for the lungs and her most eminent thoracic.'

Coltsfoot's Latin binomial means 'Cough dispeller' and 'like White Poplar' – a reference to the white underside and the shape of the leaves. Its country name is 'Son Before Father', due to the fact that the flowers appear in the spring before the leaves. The most common name, 'Coltsfoot', arises because of the shape of the leaf. It is also known as 'Coughwort', and 'Foal's Foot'. In Russian, its name is 'Mother and Step-Mother', and in Finnish it is called 'Widow's Leaf'.

It is a fabulous cough remedy and a demulcent respiratory tonic: 'Nature's most eminent thoracic'.

Medicinal parts
▷ Leaves
▷ Flowers

Physiological actions

Summary

▷ Expectorant
▷ Demulcent
▷ Antispasmodic
▷ Antitussive

Physiological virtues

Despite Coltsfoot's huge value as a respiratory supportive herb, it has rather fallen from grace for prolonged internal prescribing – rather than inhalation – due to theoretical concerns over its unsaturated pyrrolizidine alkaloid content. Unsaturated pyrrolizidine alkaloids can be converted to toxic pyrroles in the liver, and these can, in theory, be hepato-toxic in large or prolonged doses. There have been recorded cases of fatalities, which have occurred when people have consumed large quantities of unsaturated pyrrolizidine alkaloids in, for example, famine or drought situations. Research is still ongoing and opinions evolving. In my practice, I have considerably reduced my prescribing of Coltsfoot until there is more clarity over the issue. However, given that Coltsfoot is such an incredibly effective respiratory support, I feel that for patients with no liver problems it is safe to use for short periods, such as when suffering from an acute episode of influenza or a cough.

As I write these words, it is no longer possible to source Coltsfoot through normal herbal wholesale channels. If we want to maintain access to its medicine, we have to grow or gather it ourselves. This brings up an important point about the herb supply chain and how vulnerable our traditional prescribing practices are if we rely on it. There is a constant risk of more and more herbs being reclassified as 'potentially toxic' once they are examined and considered on the basis of individual constituents rather than the whole plant. If we have access to our own plants, we can decide for ourselves whether or not we will work with them. If we can no longer source them, that decision has been made for us by people who have no real herbal connection or lineage.

Coltsfoot reduces inflammation, relaxes spasms, soothes irritation, expels mucus, and stimulates the immune system. It is especially good when combined with Horehound (*Marrubium vulgare*) and Mullein (*Verbascum thapsus*) for dry, irritating coughs, and, with Wild Cherry bark (*Prunus avium* or *P. serotina*) and Thyme (*Thymus vulgaris*), for spasmodic coughs.

I hope that as herbalists we will be able to safely prescribe Coltsfoot for generations to come.

Energetics
Coltsfoot is pungent, sweet, neutral, moist.

In my dispensary
'Mary' was in her late 70s and had recently had a frightening episode where she could not

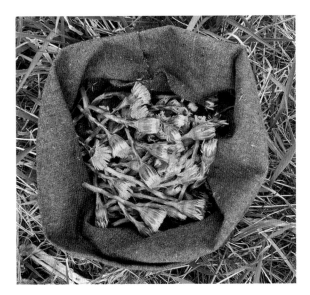

breathe. She had spent some time in hospital, and it was thought that it was adult-onset asthma triggered by a pollen allergy. She had been prescribed two inhalers but still felt very wheezy and had a persistent cough. She was nervous and wanted more support.

I prescribed a respiratory blend temporarily while her general levels of inflammation and reactivity were addressed holistically. The blend contained Coltsfoot as well as Thyme, Horehound, Honeysuckle, Elecampane, Lobelia, Chilli, and Bloodroot. She immediately felt that she could breathe more easily, was able to sleep better, and felt less tense. She had the original respiratory supportive blend for four weeks, after which the Coltsfoot was removed from the mix. She gradually reduced her dosage over the next eight weeks and remains well without a respiratory blend.

Historical applications
Dioscorides and Galen recommended smoking the leaves as a treatment for a cough. Pliny recommended that the smoke was swallowed rather than inhaled. It was also commonly prescribed as an aqueous decoction for asthma.

Gerard wrote: '*A decoction made of the greene leaves and roots, or else a syrrup thereof, is good for the cough that proceedeth of a thin rheume. The green leaves of Fole-foot pound with hony, do cure and heale inflammations. . . . The fume of the dried leaves taken through a funnel or tunnel, burned upon coles, effectually helpeth those that are troubled with shortness of breath, and fetch their winde thicke and often. Being taken in the manner as they take Tobaco, it mightily prevaileth against the diseases aforesaid.*'

Magical
Coltsfoot is magically associated with peace and tranquillity. It can be sewn into sachets to promote a sense of calm and a feeling of being able to breathe freely.

Comfrey 🦫 *Symphytum officinale*

'Comfrey is the supreme healer of connective tissue but beware of trapping in dirt and infection if treating deep wounds.'

Comfrey is a supreme healer of skin, connective tissue, and bone. The name 'Comfrey' is derived from the words *con firma*, which mean 'made firm'; the generic name 'Symphytum' comes from the Greek 'to unite'. Its country name is 'Knitbone', with good reason. Its roots look like bones and joints, and they exude slimy mucilage, which gives away its healing demulcent properties. Comfrey is a herb that has fallen from grace for long-term internal prescribing, due to the presence of pyrrolizidine alkaloids. These compounds can cause veno-occlusive disease in the liver if taken at high doses over a long period, or even at lower doses by particularly vulnerable patients. We still do not know exactly which cases prove to be more vulnerable than others, so we need to err on the side of caution. These days, Comfrey is mostly reserved for topical applications or short-term internal prescribing of the leaf in suitable cases.

Medicinal parts
- Leaves
- Flowers
- Roots

Physiological actions

Summary
- Vulnerary
- Demulcent
- Anti-inflammatory
- Bone and ligament healer
- Expectorant
- Astringent

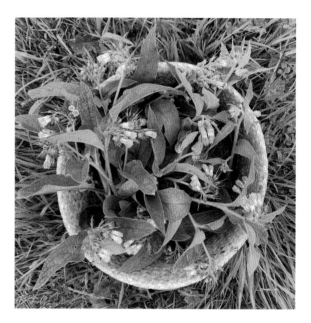

Physiological virtues

Comfrey is demulcent, mildly astringent, and expectorant. It contains more mucilage than Marshmallow root and used to be the go to herb for inflammation of the digestive tract. Before the pyrrolizidine alkaloid issue came under investigation, Comfrey was a very valuable remedy for diarrhoea and dysentery. In these cases, patients were prescribed a wineglassful dose of the root decoction, to be drunk frequently. It was also a very valuable remedy for respiratory troubles, such as consumption and whooping cough, soothing inflammation and resolving bleeding from the lungs. The root was preferred to the leaves for this. Additionally, it was very effective to resolve bleeding from the digestive tract, including ulcers and bleeding haemorrhoids, as well as treating urinary-tract inflammation and haematuria.

Comfrey's ability to assist with the alignment and healing of broken bones is thought to be linked to its potent anti-inflammatory action around the break. By reducing the inflammation, the bones are better able to become aligned and knit back together. These days, apart from 6-week internal courses of the leaf in the case of broken bones or ligament injuries, Comfrey tends to be reserved for topical prescription. The leaves make an excellent fomentation for sprains, inflammation, and bruises, including arthritis and gout. Where there are abscesses or infected cuts, a poultice can be applied to promote suppuration. Comfrey can be an especially good healing support for eczema, acne, psoriasis, and burns, working well as a wash or an ointment. Swift application of Comfrey cream or ointment to a burn is extremely effective and has to be experienced to be believed. It can reduce the appearance of scars too. It helps to disperse and resolve bruising, so is a good first aid treatment for bruises, another of its country names being 'Bruisewort'. It also makes a good poultice to treat varicose ulcers and a compress to soothe varicose veins.

One of Comfrey's active constituents is a compound called allantoin, which is a cell proliferant, hence its efficiency at supporting wound-healing. As a side note, this substance is also secreted by maggots, one of the reasons that maggot therapy can be very effective in suppurative infections. Beware of applying Comfrey to a deep and potentially dirty wound though: there is a risk that Comfrey will heal the surface layers too quickly and trap the dirt inside. My tutor, Barbara, was a very keen advocate of the traditional ways of working with Comfrey, and she used to tell us a story about applying the fresh leaves to a deep puncture wound caused by a garden fork. Apparently, it healed up beautifully, with no infection. I should add that she did also treat the patient internally with anti-infectives.

As an infusion, Comfrey leaves make a good gargle for inflammation of the oral mucous membranes.

Energetics

Comfrey is sweet, astringent, and bitter. It knits together wounds in the fabric of our being. It is heavy and supportive, yet it can encourage growth and change.

In my dispensary

I love Comfrey as an external treatment for inflammation, burns, and sprains. I make a healing ointment with a blend of Comfrey leaves, Calendula flowers, Agrimony leaves, and Lavender flowers, and it has become an oft-prescribed topical product. Not every patient is in a position to source and prepare fresh Comfrey poultices, and I have found application of the ointment to be excellent for inflamed joints and gout, as well as skin problems.

This is a case where Comfrey leaf poultices made a significant difference in a bad case of gout. 'Jeremy' was in his early 50s, and, despite an active lifestyle and a very healthy diet, he was prone to gout in his hands and elbows, areas where he had suffered injuries in a road traffic accident. Unusually for a gout sufferer, his lower legs and feet were rarely affected. Every so often the joints in his arms would become very swollen and painful, and he had to take strong allopathic pain relief. When I first met him, one of his elbows was very swollen and had recently had an infection, for which he had needed antibiotics. During the consultation I discovered that Jeremy's circulation was not good, and he had a tendency to Raynaud's syndrome. He had to drive long distances for his work and was in the habit of driving with the windows down, regardless of the time of the year.

We agreed that he should reduce caffeine intake and hydrate more consistently. I also suggested that he should try to keep his hands and upper arms warmer while driving: I felt that driving with the windows down was probably contributing to the poor circulation in his hands and elbows. As well as a circulation-supporting and gout-reducing internal blend – containing Yarrow, Celery seed, and Burdock among others – we decided on Comfrey leaf poultices applied to the affected areas twice a day. Four weeks later he reported that the swelling had come down very quickly and he was no longer taking any allopathic medication. He still suffered quite a bit of joint stiffness in his arms though. A further four weeks later he reported full movement in both elbows and said that his hands no longer felt cold.

Historical applications

Gerard, writing about Comfrey in his *Generall Historie of Plants*, said: '*The slimie substance of the roots made in a posset of ale, be given to cure pains in the back suffered by wrestlers and immoderate wenchers.*'

Comfrey was not just for men's aches and pains. Young women, about to be married, would take Comfrey baths as a way of repairing their hymens in order to '*restore their virginity*'.

Culpeper wrote: '*The root, being outwardly applied, helpeth fresh wounds or cuts immediately, being bruised and laid thereunto; and is especial good for ruptures and broken bones; yea, it is said to be so powerful to consolidate and knit together, that if they are boiled with dissevered pieces of flesh in a pot, it will join them together again.*'

Magical

Worn as an amulet, Comfrey is associated with safety during travel. It is also chosen for money spells due to its association with proliferation and abundance.

Suggestion for the home apothecary

Comfrey poultice for sprains, swollen joints, or broken bones

If the bone is in plaster, apply the poultice above and below the cast. It if is a small bone that remains unset, apply to the area. Finely chop or blend equal parts of fresh root and leaves. Spread the resulting sticky and slimy paste onto a piece of clean muslin, and lay it onto the area to be treated. Cover with another piece of muslin, so it is contained like a sandwich. Apply a fresh poultice daily.

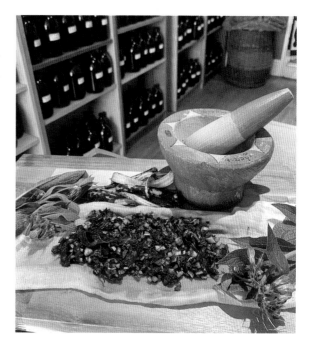

Couch Grass   *Elymus repens*

'Couch balances sweetness with cleansing.'

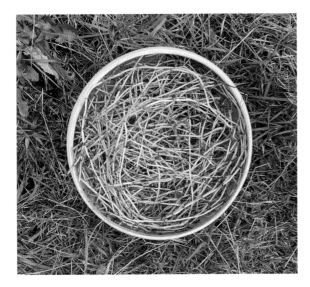

To most gardeners, Couch Grass (*Elymus repens,* formerly *Agropyron repens*) is the bane of their lives, a weed to be eradicated at all costs. The reason for this is that it spreads throughout cultivated beds by means of long spreading underground rhizomes and surface stolons. When weeding it out, every little piece of rhizome and stolon needs to be removed, as the tiniest fragment will develop into a new plant.

To me, Couch is a valuable and precious medicine. It is also an exuberant plant that needs to be confined to keep it from taking over the herb garden. I used to grow a crop of it each year in a barrel of compost. Harvesting is easy, just tip out the barrel onto a tarpaulin, remove the stolons, and then replace the compost for next year's crop.

Medicinal parts
- Rhizomes
- Stolons

Physiological actions

Summary
- Diuretic
- Antiseptic
- Demulcent
- Anti-inflammatory
- Expectorant

Physiological virtues

Couch is a valuable urinary system antiseptic and demulcent diuretic, providing a soothing action on hot, irritated urinary passages while encouraging increased production of urine. It is also anti-inflammatory and antimicrobial – a helpful herb in many conditions, including cystitis, dysuria, haematuria, irritable bladder, prostatitis, urethritis, benign prostatic hyperplasia, oedema, and incontinence. It soothes the urinary passages and eases discomfort, as well as assisting with the passage of urinary gravel. It is an old remedy for hypercholesterolaemia, arthritis, and gout.

Couch also brings its antimicrobial and demulcent qualities to the respiratory system, being expectorant and decongestant. It is sometimes prescribed for irritating coughs and bronchitis.

Energetics

Couch has a sweet taste: the roots taste a little like Liquorice. My tutor Ifanca used to say that when people are prone to urinary infections and inflammations, it was important to discover what was irritating them in their life. We should ask: 'What are they trying to get rid of?' I used to be quite sceptical about this link, but over the years I have noticed that patients prone to repeated cystitis do much better when they have, for example, resolved their difficult relationship, cleared the air with a relative, or left the job that they found frustrating. It is certainly something to bear in mind. I feel that Couch can be helpful in smoothing the way for us to make life changes more skilfully.

In Tibetan medicine

The sweetness of Couch helps to reduce heated inflammatory states seen in certain excess *Tripa* presentations, such as urinary system infections. It is worth noting that its sweet and nourishing nature is a natural balance to *rLung*, so, when a very anxious person with an excess of *rLung* has long-term urinary-tract inflammation, it may be preferable to include more Couch Grass (sweet) and Celery seed (oily) than, say, Pellitory-of-the-Wall (astringent and salty) and Buchu (bitter, astringent, and warming) in their prescription. It is not to say that the latter two herbs cannot be prescribed at all, it is just that we can produce better results by being aware of the elemental balance and adjusting herb choices where possible. Also, I should point out that, if suitable herbs are not available, one can balance the herbs chosen by asking the patient to make appropriate lifestyle and dietary adjustments, such as eating regularly and choosing warming and nutritious foods.

In my dispensary

The following case is a good example of Couch as a readily available first-aid treatment for a urinary-tract infection. 'Gerry' was a keen gardener in his mid-70s, with a beautifully kept garden. He was very keen on natural approaches to health and drank a large pot of 'garden herbal tea' daily. His wife had died about seven years previously, and after this he had struggled to find the motivation to take care of himself, telling me that he sometimes no longer saw the point.

He had developed high blood pressure after his wife died and was taking allopathic hypotensive drugs, but wanted to come off them. We worked together on a personalized herbal and lifestyle plan, and over the next few months his blood pressure came down steadily. He felt able to gradually reduce his medication, with the support of his doctor. At that point he was signed off from my clinic, and I thought that I would not see him again.

A year later he telephoned me, saying that he had developed a painful urinary infection and urgently wanted some herbal tea to help shift it. He had tried the usual self-help approaches of drinking plenty of water and Cranberry juice, but it was not going away, and he wanted to avoid antibiotics. I asked about his prostate in order to gauge whether he was likely to be suffering from urinary retention, but nothing seemed to have changed since I had last seen him. He had telephoned when I was just shutting up my shop for the weekend, so I asked him if he had Couch Grass anywhere in his garden. I half expected him to say he did not, since he always gave the impression that his garden was immaculate, but he said yes, of course. I told him to dig up some couch rhizomes, wash them, and make a strong cup of tea with them. He was to drink two large cups a day over the weekend. If things had not improved after that, he was to come in and collect some of my kidney supportive tea blend. He did as I recommended and reported back after the weekend to say that the Couch had resolved the infection quickly and efficiently. He said that he had not realized how useful it was, and from now on he would always make sure he had some in his garden.

Historical applications

Gerard wrote that '*Although the Couch-grasse be an unwelcome guest to fields and gardens, yet his physicke virtues do recompense those hurts: for it openeth the stoppings of the liver and reins without any manifest heat.'*

Magical

To attract a lover, put Couch Grass root in a sachet and hide it under the bed of the person you wish to attract.

Suggestion for the home apothecary

Couch Grass infusion for cystitis

Harvest some fresh Couch Grass rhizomes, and wash them thoroughly. Take a small handful, and chop into small pieces. Put into a teapot or jug, and pour over 570 ml/1 pint of water. Allow to infuse for 10–15 minutes. Drink two cups per day if suffering from a urinary system infection.

For year-round supplies, dry some and store in an airtight container.

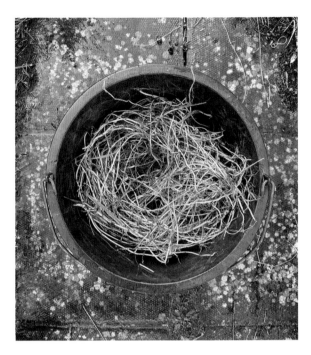

'Cowslip, or Palsy Wort, is specific for respiratory congestion accompanied by repetitive tics or compulsive behaviour patterns.'

The name 'Cowslip' comes from 'Cow-slop' in old English, referring to its tendency to grow in pastures where there are plenty of cow pats. The yellow flowers look a bit like a bunch of keys, originally being called 'Freya's Keys' and being dedicated to the goddess Freya, the virgin of the key. Later it was Christianized by being named 'St Peter's Keys' or 'Our Lady's Keys'. Its other names are 'Palsywort,' 'Paralytica', and 'Arthritica', names that refer to its medicinal actions.

These days Cowslips are too scarce to wild harvest. If you want Cowslips as medicine, you need to establish a colony in your herb garden. Medicinally it is generally considered to be interchangeable with Primrose (*Primula vulgaris*), but I like to work with Cowslips, and I grow them at my allotment.

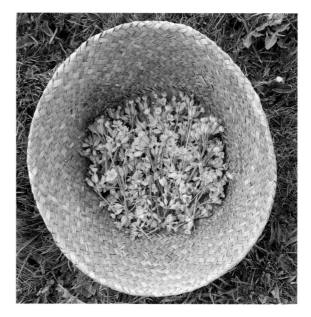

Medicinal parts
▷ Roots
▷ Flowers

Traditionally, roots are best, although flowers are a good and more sustainable substitute.

Physiological actions

Summary
▷ Sedative
▷ Antispasmodic
▷ Expectorant
▷ Antitussive
▷ Anti-inflammatory

Physiological virtues

Cowslips are sedative and antispasmodic. Cowslip tea is a good remedy for nervous tension and headaches, as well as sleeplessness. The roots contain saponins and are high in anti-inflammatory and pain-relieving salicylates. This is probably why Cowslip was known as 'Arthritica'. These days, most herbalists work with the flowers, and think of Cowslip mostly as a gentle sedative and cough reliever. They are indeed very good to treat dry respiratory infections where the lungs are congested with hardened phlegm. Cowslips thin the mucus, helping with the process of expectoration, and they soothe tickly coughs. They are also a mild diuretic and are anti-inflammatory.

Old sources are a rich seam of information about different, perhaps more exciting, medicinal properties of Cowslip. It is reported as having a special affinity for nerves and the brain. Maud Grieve, in her *A Modern Herbal*, mentions that '*in earlier times*' it was used in all paralytic or spasmodic ailments, being known as 'Palsy Wort' or 'Herba Paralysis'.

In my dispensary

In my dispensary I have Cowslip flowers as a tincture and dried whole flowers for infusions. I absolutely love Cowslip for children who have long-standing respiratory congestion, accompanied with nervous tics. The following two cases, one where Cowslip formed part of an infusion and one where Cowslip tincture was prescribed in drop doses, are typical examples of how Cowslip's virtues are helpful in my practice.

'Anthony' was 7 years old when I first met him. He alternated between being withdrawn and being impulsively active, and he had a very poor attention span. He also had a periodic involuntary tic, which had been steadily worsening over the last year. Anthony had a strong tendency to respiratory congestion, especially at night. He suffered from allergies, and had very dark circles under his eyes. His tongue had a thick yellowish coating.

Anthony's mum was very worried, because his tic was worsening, and he was becoming prone to angry outbursts as well as periods of intense withdrawal. She had sought an allopathic assessment, and the specialists had suggested that Anthony's problem could be related to a rare form of attention deficit disorder linked to a personality disorder. Understandably, Anthony's mum did not want to accept this. She told me that Anthony had always struggled to acknowledge his feelings, preferring to say that everything was fine when she asked him if he was alright. She was aware that he was feeling unsettled due to her recent divorce from Anthony's father. Anthony was finding it quite unsettling to move between his parents' homes and to adapt to different routines, house 'rules',

and meal choices. Anthony liked things to be predictable and stable.

We went through his case history, including his dietary patterns. It was clear to me that he most likely had a significant dairy intolerance, so we agreed that as far as possible Anthony was going to cut out dairy. I also prescribed a nice calming tea blend in order to relax him, help improve his hydration, and support his digestion. The tea contained Cowslip, Rose, Calendula, Cleavers, and Skullcap. He was to drink two cups a day.

When Anthony returned for his first follow-up four weeks later, the dark circles under his eyes had completely gone, and he looked much more vibrant. His eyes were shining, and he was more engaged. He was excited to see me and to show me that his tongue was now clear. His mum told me that he was a different child, his congestion was lessening, the tic was much reduced, and his behaviour was becoming more settled. After a couple more months of herbal treatment, his tic was completely gone, and his allergies were greatly lessened.

In Anthony's mix, the Cleavers and Calendula were intended to help clear his lymphatic system, and the Rose, Skullcap, and Cowslip were to help release tension, allowing him to start digesting his emotions. The Calendula, Skullcap, and Rose would also gently support his digestion physically, by virtue of their bitterness. I chose the Cowslip in his tea blend specifically because of the tic, and I believe that it played a very significant role in its disappearance.

'Will', 9 years old, was pretty active and healthy most of the time, but suffered with episodes of severe breathing difficulties at night. Each time it happened, he required emergency admission to hospital and high doses of steroids. It was not clear what was causing the episodes, but his parents were pursuing every possible avenue to understand and treat this very worrying issue. The episodes were happening on average once a month.

Will had a lot of energy and found it quite difficult to settle down at bedtime. He had a lingering phlegmy unproductive cough and often suffered with coughs and colds. He also had some repetitive behaviours, such as throat clearing and humming. I suspected dairy intolerance and asked Will to cut it out completely. He was a very intelligent and determined young man and immediately took on board my advice and adapted to his new way of eating. One month later the cough had changed in character, and the repetitive throat clearing had lessened. He was also settling down and going to sleep more easily. During that first month, he had suffered with one episode of breathing issues, but it was milder than usual, and he did not require hospitalization. At this stage I prescribed Cowslip tincture as a simple, 5 drops to be taken twice a day in a drink. Over the next four weeks his cough became much more productive, he had no more breathing difficulties at night, and all of his repetitive behaviours completely ceased. He felt much more ready for bed in the evening and settled down to sleep more easily.

Historical applications

Hildegard of Bingen recommended applying a warm compress of Cowslips over the heart while sleeping, in order to cure melancholia. This is a really fascinating idea, which I have yet to try in my practice.

The mediaeval *Regimen Sanitatis Salernitanum* recorded Cowslip as a cure for palsy or paralysis. Geoffrey Grigson, writing about Cowslip in his *The Englishman's Flora*, suggests that this association had come about due to the trembling or nodding of the flower heads.

Warren R. Dawson's *A Leech Book of the Fifteenth Century* reported that Cowslip and Lavender should be boiled together in ale for: '*tremblelynge hand and handis a slepe*'.

Gerard referred to the treatment of '*the phrensie*' with Cowslips as follows: '*A practitioner of London who was famous for curing the phrensie, after he had performed his cure by the due observation of Physicke, accustomed every yeare in the moneth of May to dyet his patients after this manner: take the leaves and floures of Primrose, boile them a little in fountaine water, and in some rose and Betony waters, adding thereto sugar, pepper, salt and butter which being strained, he gave them to drinke thereof first and last.*' He also wrote about their properties as expectorants, phlegm clearers, and pain relievers: '*the Antients have named them "Verbasculi", that is to say, small Mulleins . . . the roots of Primrose stamped and strained, and the juice sniffed into the nose with a quill or such like, purgeth the brain, and qualifieth the pain of the megrim.*' Regarding Cowslip as an external healing treatment he wrote: '*An unguent made with the juice of Cowslips and oile of Linseed, cureth all scaldings or burnings with fire, water, or otherwise.*'

Parkinson also referred to the ability of Cowslips to ease headaches and joint pain: '*They are eaten in Tansies and Sallets, by those beyond Sea, and are accounted very profitable for paines in the head, and are accounted the best for that purpose next unto Betony, they are excellent good against any joynt aches as the palsie and to ease the pains of the sinews.*'

Magical

A bit of Cowslip placed underneath the door mat at the entrance to a house is said to discourage visitors if you want to be alone. Tradition has it that a bunch of Cowslips worn or held in the hand will help you to find hidden treasure. Cowslips are also associated with restoring or preserving youth.

Cramp Bark 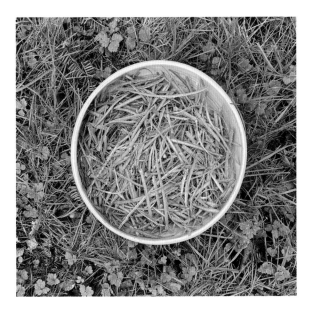 *Viburnum opulus*

'Cramp Bark is the master of letting go.'

Cramp Bark is the master of helping us to 'let go'. While taking this herb, we find it easier to let go of tension, stress, and, above all, our own rigidity. Its names are 'Cramp Bark', 'Guelder Rose', 'High Cranberry', or, in Russian, *Kalina*. It is a beautiful shrub of unspoilt hedgerows and damp woodlands. Where I live, it is becoming scarcer in the wild, but nowadays it is widely planted in wildlife-friendly landscaping around new developments. It is closely related to *Viburnum prunifolium*, which tends to be favoured in the United States.

Medicinal parts
- Bark
- Berries

The bark is harvested in early spring from coppiced stems or pruned branches. Some people make medicines and condiments from the berries too, but I do not. The berries are said to require cooking in order to neutralize their toxicity. Russian folk medicine includes knowledge of working with decoctions of the flowers.

Physiological actions

Summary
- Antispasmodic
- Nervine
- Sedative
- Analgesic
- Astringent

Physiological virtues

This herb is an excellent antispasmodic, working effectively on either smooth muscle or skeletal muscle. It is also a nervine herb that works on many different levels. It is sedative, pain-relieving, and a little astringent.

Cramp Bark contains hydroquinones, including arbutin, coumarins, scopoletin, tannins, resin, and the alkyl carboxylic acid, valeric acid, which is also found in Valerian. When you scrape a little fresh bark from a stem of Cramp Bark, you can smell the valeric acid. It smells like Valerian.

It is helpful in prescriptions for patients suffering with cramps, spasms, chronic tension, or asthma. It offers itself up to support those experiencing severe period pain, or the painful gripes associated with IBS. It is worth considering for constipation associated with an inability to relax, although in these cases care should be taken as it contains tannins that can also exacerbate constipation. Through relaxing muscles of the bile duct or ureters, it can assist with the passage of gallstones or kidney stones. It can also help to relax the smooth muscle of the circulatory system, improving peripheral circulation and therefore reducing hypertension. When children wet the bed due to tension or anxiety, Cramp Bark can be helpful. It is also a valuable first aid treatment to allay threatened miscarriage.

It relaxes skeletal muscles and plays a useful role in relieving back pain when it is exacerbated by associated muscle spasm. It also relieves the pain of arthritis when there is muscle spasm surrounding an affected joint. In these examples it is often prescribed topically as an oil or liniment rub.

Maud Grieve says: '*It has been employed with benefit in all nervous complaints and debility and used with success in cramps and spasms of all kinds.*'

The Maskwaki people of North America saw Cramp Bark as being primarily an antispasmodic, while the Penobscot people chose it to treat swollen glands and mumps.

Russian folk medicine recommends infusing the berries in brandy as the best home medicine for ulcers. A topical application is also made by pounding the berries and applying them to the ulcer in the fold of a cotton cloth. A decoction of the flowers is prescribed for coughs, colds, fever sclerosis, tuberculosis of the lungs, and stomach sickness.

Energetics

Cramp bark is bitter and astringent. On an emotional level, it can help us let go of unhelpful patterns and feel more at ease in our bodies, minds, and spirits. There is a natural tendency to become more fixed in our ways as responsibilities mount up and we learn 'what works for us'. When life becomes challenging or uncertain, we seek the security of regular patterns and tend to adopt fixed responses to situations, but if we are unwell or unhappy, change is not only good, it is essential.

In Tibetan medicine

Cramp Bark has an astringent, bitter, and aromatic quality. Although its taste would not immediately indicate it as a primary choice for *rLung* imbalances, its action is specific at a deep level, since it helps us to let go. *rLung* is ultimately exacerbated by a tendency to grasping and attachment, so the inclusion of Cramp Bark in the prescription can be very helpful.

In my dispensary

Cramp Bark is the first herb to which I turn when an antispasmodic influence is needed. I include it in personalized prescriptions where tension, or unwillingness to change, is a factor. It is also a key ingredient in my circulation-supporting capsule blend. It is no good prescribing circulatory stimulants if the system is too tense to accommodate a more vibrant blood flow. Cramp Bark relaxes the smooth muscles of the circulatory system and allows better flow.

Cramp Bark is, of course, excellent for period pain. I lose count of the number female patients in their late teens and 20s who present with severe dysmenorrhea. Their cramping pain is so intense that they are completely unable to function on at least two days out of each cycle. They have to stop everything and spend the time doubled up in the foetal position, feeling worn out and hopeless. This is always a miserable and heart-rending state of affairs to hear about, but fortunately there is a great deal that can be done to help through holistic herbal medicine. I always seek to address the underlying cause, and this usually requires a change to the diet and lifestyle, as well as supporting the circulation to the uterine area and boosting liver health. I prescribe a daily herbal blend that is formulated for the unique circumstances of each patient.

Let us take 'Imogen'. She was a 21-year-old student suffering from severe period pains. She experienced so much pain during her period that she was completely unable to function. During her consultation we went through her lifestyle and diet, and I suggested some changes, mostly around eating more regularly and reducing sugary snacks. Her periods were not unduly heavy, but the pain was intense, so I prescribed a 'period mix' based on Cramp Bark tincture to help with managing symptoms during the period until the main treatment had time to take effect. She was to take 5 ml in hot water up to four times a day during the most painful days of her period. She also had a main daily tincture mix that supported her circulatory system and digestion, in particular liver function. After the first month of treatment, she said that it was amazing to have had a much more bearable period, reporting that 'the period mix you gave me is absolutely miraculous!' After a couple more months of treatment she was virtually pain-free during her period and no longer needed to rely on the Cramp Bark so heavily. She no longer dreaded her period and felt that she had 'got her life back'.

Apart from living up to its name, Cramp Bark works on more subtle levels. The following story is a nice illustration of that.

'Jayne' came to me for support in lowering her blood pressure. She was on hypotensive allopathic medication, but even so, her blood pressure and her weight had been creeping up over the last few years. She was in her 70s and was one of those people who seemed especially set in her ways. She liked to stick to a familiar routine in terms of eating and day-to-day activities. When describing her diet, she had explained that on each day of the week she and her husband always had a particular meal. This cycle of a 7-day recurring menu and their eating habits in general seemed pretty rigid. I could see that Jayne was greatly attracted to discipline and routine. She had been a staunch member of the Girl Guide movement when she

was younger and, although no doubt this would have involved quite a lot of adventures, it was clear that she had also enjoyed the disciplined framework that it had offered.

I felt that this was a patient who needed to make some significant changes and become less rigid, both physiologically and in her habitual tendencies. She was quite horrified at first when I suggested that she made changes to her diet and lifestyle. Drinking less black tea and more water were probably the most challenging ones for her. I also prescribed a more varied diet, with more vegetables and less sugar, and I asked her to go for a walk every day, preferably in a natural environment. To support her ability to make these changes, I added Cramp Bark to her tailor-made prescription.

Jayne surprised herself and did very well with implementing the changes that I had suggested. Over the next few months her blood pressure and her weight began to reduce, and she felt much better in herself. When she attended for her follow-up appointments, I could see that she had improved energy levels and more zest for life. I recognized the particular influence of Cramp Bark when, out of the blue, she told me that she had decided to book an experience day at a motor-racing circuit because she had always wanted to become a racing driver when she was younger, and she wanted to have a go at it.

In this case, while Cramp Bark had definitely helped to support Jayne physiologically by reducing long-term tension and rigidity in her circulatory system, it had also helped her on an energetic and emotional level by encouraging her to let go of her own rather rigid attitudes to life and her lifestyle.

Historical applications

Geoffrey Chaucer suggested eating the berries: '*The Gaitre-Beries are among the plants that "shal be for your hele"*' to '*picke hem right as they grow and ete hem in'*. He did not caution against eating them raw – perhaps folk in the fourteenth century had stronger stomachs than we have.

Suggestion for the home apothecary

Cramp Bark decoction or tincture for period pain

To make the decoction, add 15 g of dried bark to 750 ml of cold water. Bring to the boil and gently simmer for about 20 minutes until the volume is reduced to 500 ml. Drink half a cupful every 3 hours. The preparation can be refrigerated and stored for 48 hours.

To make a tincture, fill one third of a clean jar with dried Cramp Bark, and then pour over enough 50% ABV vodka to fill the jar. Leave it for four weeks in the dark, then strain, press (or squeeze), and bottle. Take 2.5 ml in a little hot water as needed, up to five times per day. A tincture will keep for many years in a dark bottle on the shelf.

You can also make an infused oil with the bark as a topical application to relieve period pain when massaged into affected areas.

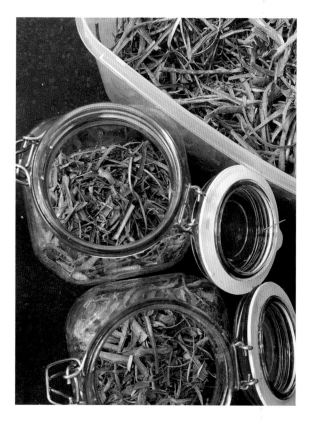

Daisy ❦ *Bellis perennis*

'Daisy is our native Bruisewort. It is also an expectorant which opens the chest and encourages lightness of spirit.'

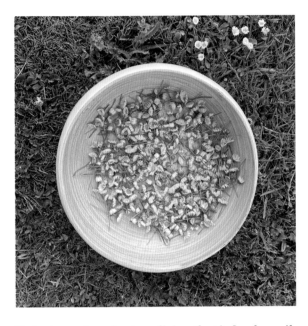

Daisy is an abundant medicine that is freely available throughout most of the year. We should make the most of it. One its country names is 'Bruisewort', and it is our native version of Arnica. These days Daisy has rather fallen out of fashion in the world of herbal medicine. Perhaps it is too common, too available, and therefore taken for granted. Physiologically, it is vulnerary and expectorant, while energetically it is playful and joyful. It encourages a lightness of spirit in us, helping us to open our chest if we have been feeling contracted and weighed down by life's challenges. In fact, Culpeper writes that Daisy *'cures wounds made in the hollowness of the breast'*.

Medicinal parts
- Flowers
- Leaves

Physiological actions

Summary
- Astringent
- Vulnerary
- Expectorant
- Antitussive
- Anti-inflammatory

Physiological virtues

Daisy's vulnerary and astringent virtues make it good to treat all sorts of wounds and burns. It is an excellent treatment to help resolve bruising, and, unlike Arnica, it is safe to apply where the skin is broken. Daisy is also especially indicated for slow-healing wounds, such as infected leg ulcers. You can combine internal and topical applications.

It is a good anti-inflammatory. It is traditionally prescribed for mucous colitis. Christopher Hedley taught that it is a herb to consider for chronic inflammation where there is angiogenesis.

Daisy contains saponins that act as an expectorant and antitussive, which makes it a good medicine to help with expectoration and to relieve coughs. The mechanism of action is thought to be reflex expectoration, a process where the saponins are slightly irritating to the stomach, and this stimulates the respiratory system due to a shared nerve root. Moderate doses should not cause any gastric problems, but excessive intake could cause nausea and stomach upset. Make a 10-minute infused tea, and drink it three times a day. Be guided by your own system. If you start to feel nauseous, you need to lower your dose.

Energetics

Daisy is astringent and cooling. It is associated with playfulness and joyfulness. I take this into account when choosing it for patients suffering with respiratory or catarrhal issues. Patients who are weighed down by life often develop a constriction of the chest, perhaps as a subconscious way of guarding their heart area. If the situation persists, it can impact respiratory health and balance. By encouraging a lightness of spirit and an opening of the chest area, Daisy can assist with deeper breathing and more efficient expectoration in more ways than just through the physical action of its constituents. It is considered to be a specific for loneliness in children.

In my dispensary

I have practiced martial arts for many years and, in the past, I tended to be a bit blasé about the minor bruises that are a regular hazard of training. Nowadays, if I do get a bruise, I treat it. Daisy ointment is helpful in more serious cases of bruising too. A patient of mine fell off a ladder, and another was trampled by a cow. In both cases Daisy ointment helped to resolve the bruising surprisingly quickly and considerably eased their discomfort.

I regularly add Daisy tincture to expectorant and anticatarrhal prescriptions, especially when those respiratory challenges seem to be accompanied by a loss of joyfulness and playfulness in the patient's life.

Historical applications

Culpeper wrote of Daisies: '*A decoction made of them, and drank, helpeth to cure wounds made in the hollowness of the breast. The same also cureth all ulcers and pustules in the mouth or tongue, or in the secret parts.*' He went on to describe that a fomentation of Daisies mixed with Agrimony was good to relieve sciatica, gout, and palsy, and that an ointment of Daisies could help wounds that are '*kept long from healing*'.

Gerard said: '*The Daisies do mitigate all kinde of paines, but especially in the joints, and gout, if they be stamped with new butter unsalted, and applied upon the pained place: but they worke more effectually if Mallowes be added thereto. The juice of the leaves and roots snift up into the nostrils, purgeth the head mightily, and helpeth the megrim. The leaves stamped take away bruises and swellings proceeding of some stroke, if they be stamped and laid thereon; whereupon it was called in old time Bruisewort. The juice put into the eis cleareth them, and taketh away the watering of them. The decoction of the field Daisie (which is best for physicks use) made in water and drunke, is good against agues.*'

Magical

Daisies are associated with lust and love. It is said that whoever picks the first Daisy of the season will be possessed of 'a spirit of coquetry' beyond any control. Attract love by wearing a Daisy and sleep with a Daisy root beneath the pillow to draw an absent lover back to you.

Suggestion for the home apothecary

Daisy-infused oil for bruises

Take fresh Daisies picked on a dry day, or dried Daisies, loosely filling a jar with them. Pour over mild and light olive oil until the herb is thoroughly covered. Start by placing the jar in a gentle warm water bath or place on a sunny windowsill. If you are making this with fresh Daisies, cover the jar with a temporary muslin 'lid' so that any moisture in the flowers can evaporate. Once the oil has had a few hours of warmth, leave it in a cool, dark place for four weeks, checking regularly to make sure that the flowers are still submerged. When the oil is ready, strain it and filter it into bottles. If you have made it with fresh Daisies, you will have to decant the oil very carefully to leave the small layer of watery fraction behind in the infusing container.

Once you have your infused oil, you can make an ointment by setting the oil with beeswax or a vegan setting agent. I choose 1 g of beeswax to each 7 ml of infused oil. Measure the volume of oil, then warm it gently in a double boiler, add the required amount of beeswax, and stir until it has melted. Immediately pour the oil and melted beeswax mixture into clean dry jars. Allow the ointment to set before picking up the jars to lid them.

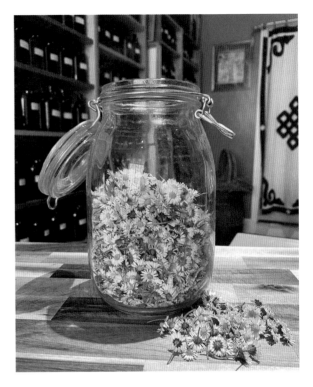

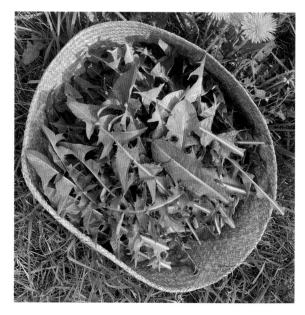
'Dandelion enhances the metabolism and clears away toxins.'

Dandelion's common name stems from the shape of its leaves. They remind us of lion's teeth – *dent de lion* in French. It is also known as *Pis en lit* because of its diuretic properties. The various parts of Dandelion are considered to have different medicinal properties, making this herb a medicine chest all on its own. It clears away toxins by supporting the action of the liver, bowel, and kidneys.

Medicinal parts

- Roots
- Leaves
- Flowers
- Seed heads

Physiological actions

Summary

- Bitter
- Diuretic
- Alterative
- Aperient
- Blood sugar balancer/hypoglycaemic
- Cholagogue
- Anti-inflammatory

Physiological virtues

Dandelion leaf is a wonderful diuretic, with significant advantages over allopathic diuretics such as bendroflumethiazide. These drugs are widely prescribed for hypertension and other conditions where enhanced diuresis can be helpful. Unfortunately, they can potentially lead to potassium losses from the body, and this is the reason that health-care providers monitor their patients carefully while they are taking them. Dandelion leaf is very high in potassium,

supplying more to the body than is removed by increased diuresis. This quality makes Dandelion especially helpful in cases of cardiac-related oedema or dropsy (caused by left heart failure) when patients are taking the drug digoxin or the whole herb, Foxglove. These treatments can cause irritability of the heart muscle when potassium levels are low, but as Dandelion safeguards potassium levels, it makes the treatment much safer. All traditional remedies for dropsy included both Dandelion and Foxglove. Dandelion leaf is also well indicated for oedema, especially when there is a tendency to ankle swelling. It flushes out the urinary system and can help to resolve urinary calculus.

The leaves are bitter, but there is a more pronounced bitterness in the roots. These are the plant part chosen by herbalists when digestive stimulation and bitterness are the primary herbal actions that are sought. The roots improve the appetite, encourage the secretion and the release of bile, reduce blood sugar levels, and are aperient, encouraging a healthier and more regular bowel habit. They support the gallbladder and are a good choice to prevent and even dissolve gallstones, as well as to treat jaundice. Be careful, though, if you have a large gallstone. Dandelion could potentially encourage it to move somewhere where it will cause much more trouble and pain.

It is worth bearing in mind that roots harvested in the spring have a higher level of bitterness, while roots harvested in the autumn have more inulin, which enhances their prebiotic qualities.

Dandelion is a herbal alterative, steadily removing toxins from the body via the liver and the kidneys. Its cleansing and stimulating properties make it helpful to resolve long-standing chronic conditions such as arthritis or skin conditions. In these cases, it can be a good strategy to encourage patients to consume 2–3 Dandelion leaves a day during every spring and then again in the autumn. An infusion can be taken instead if fresh leaves are not available.

Dandelion is probably the first herb to consider when people are suffering from illnesses derived from exposure to pollutants. Think of it for patients who work with chemicals, including people who have to work with paints, herbicides, or cleaning products.

It can help to resolve chronic deep-seated sinus infections as well as infected root canals. In this latter scenario, it encourages recalcification if bone loss has been occurring. It also has a reputation for being helpful in resolving cancerous tumours and is a good support in cases of viral hepatitis. Since Dandelion is a nourishing herb as well as a cleansing one, it is a very good choice for those who are convalescing after a long illness.

The flowers are anti-inflammatory, and an infused oil makes a lovely topical treatment for muscle aches and joint pain, especially where tension is a contributory factor. The fresh sap is a traditional topical application to treat warts.

As it is a diuretic, Dandelion should be taken with care by those who suffer with hypotension, since it could further lower their blood pressure. It is safe in moderate doses during pregnancy and lactation, but extreme 'detox' regimes are not advised.

Energetics

Dandelion is bitter, sweet, and cooling.

A few years ago I discovered that it is possible to work with the energetic aspects of Dandelion to help patients find balance amidst the bewildering highs and lows of bipolar disorder. Dandelion manifests a bright, sunny, fiery flower that is balanced by an ethereal, dreamy, cooling seed head. I make separate preparations from the flowers and the seed heads (I personally choose to make tinctures). These are prescribed in drop doses (usually 5 drops a day), depending on how the patient is feeling. The sunny flower preparation is taken during low, depressed phases, and the cooling 'moon' seed head preparation is taken during high, manic phases. If the patient feels balanced, they can take equal parts of each. On a physiological level, Dandelion has long been known to be helpful in depression, probably through its ability to support liver cleansing and to free up sluggish bowel function, but this 'Sun and Moon' treatment is much more subtle and more energetic in nature and is a very valuable awareness-building tool.

Patients who have tried it have reported that it has enabled them to be more mindful of trying to follow helpful behaviour and dietary patterns during each episode. They tell me that taking it daily helps them to become more aware of the shifts in their condition before these develop into full 'highs' or 'lows'. As doses are extremely small, any changes to the rate at which the liver breaks down allopathic medication are minimal, making this strategy safe for those relying on carefully balanced doses of prescription drugs.

I am very happy to report that one of my patients is now managing well and completely 'drug-free' on this regime after over thirty years of relying on allopathic medication. Several others have told me how helpful the preparations are for them to manage their condition.

In Tibetan medicine

Taraxacum tibetanum is the Dandelion species within the Tibetan pharmacopoeia. It is known as *Khur mong* [ཁུར་མོང་]. It has a bitter-to-sweet taste, a bitter post-digestive taste, and a cooling potency. It is prescribed for hot disorders of *rLung*, *Pekén mukpo* (brown phlegm), and chronic fever. It cures *Tripa* and stomach disorders and relieves cramp attacks due to poisoning. It cures poisoning caused by precious stones and metals. *Khur mong* restores lost appetite and is the best herb for curing a blood-*Tripa* disorder. The roots are included in formulae for liver and gallbladder support as well as congested lymph nodes. They are also considered specific for healing ruptured nerves, while the leaves and flowers are considered to help mend broken bones.

In my dispensary

I work with Dandelion in tinctures, teas, and capsules. I make a separate tincture of roots, leaves, flowers, and seed heads, although these two latter preparations are only prescribed in tiny drop doses so only small volumes are needed. I powder the roots to include in my bowel-supporting capsule blend, and the powder of the leaves forms part of both my blood-building and my kidney-supporting capsule blends. The leaves are included in personalized teas, as needed.

The following case illustrates the value of Dandelion root – along with other bitters and carminatives – alongside lifestyle changes to address chronic constipation. 'Josie' was 64 years old and suffered with painful oral lichen planus. She had been prescribed a steroid mouthwash, but it had not improved things. She explained that she could hardly eat anything at the moment due to the intense discomfort in her mouth, but that she was very happy with her current weight and did not want to gain any. She described herself as a 'long-term dieter'. She was stressed and weepy, and her bowels were very irregular, with a bowel movement only every second or third day. They had apparently been like this for some time. I felt that encouraging her bowels to be more regular was absolutely essential to make headway with the oral lichen planus, and I started out by recommending that she hydrated better and reduced her intake of caffeine. I prescribed a dilute mouthwash based on Myrrh and Calendula tinctures, with which she was to swill and gargle twice a day. To start with it was diluted at a rate of 6 drops in 20 ml of water. She also had two of my Dandelion-root-based bowel-supporting capsules daily after supper. Within the first couple of weeks her oral lichen planus started to reduce, but her bowels were taking their time to respond. I increased the dose of the capsules to two in the evening and two in the morning, emphasizing the need to keep water intake up. The bowels began to steadily improve, and the lichen-planus-affected area gradually shrank. She soon began to be able to tolerate a wider range of foods and kept on with the dietary and lifestyle improvements; six months after her first appointment her oral lichen planus was completely resolved, and her bowels were regular for the first time in years. She felt a lot better in herself on many levels, including her emotional stability.

Historical applications

In the thirteenth century, the Physicians of Myddfai included Dandelion in their pharmacopoeia, describing its effectiveness in treating jaundice. This constitutes the earliest record of Dandelion as a medicine in the West.

Four centuries later Culpeper heaped much praise on Dandelion: '*Whoever is drawing towards a consumption, or an evil disposition of the whole body called cachexia, by the use hereof for some time together, shall find wonderful help.*' (Cachexia is the wasting of the body due to a severe chronic condition.)

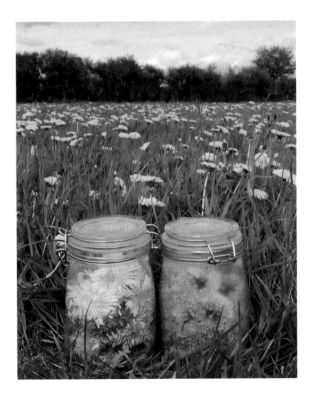

Gerard did not write about Dandelion's '*vertues*', but he did write a lovely description of its flower: '*Upon every stalk standeth a floure greater than that of Succorie, but double, and thick set together, of colour yellow, and sweet in smell which is turned into a downy blowball that is carried away with the wind.*'

Magical

Dandelion is associated with divination and the calling of spirits. Place a steaming cup of Dandelion root decoction next to your bed in order to make use of this quality. This is also said to enhance psychic sensitivity.

The seed heads can be used to send a message to someone that you love. Blow the seeds off the head in their direction and visualize the message travelling to them. It is said that you can find out how long you will live by blowing on a seed head. Blow the seeds off and you will live for as many years as the number of seeds that remain on the head. It may be prudent not to blow too hard!

Suggestion for the home apothecary

Dandelion 'Sun' and 'Moon' tinctures

Make two tinctures, one of the fresh flowers in 50% ABV alcohol and the other of the seed heads, also in 50% ABV alcohol. Once the tinctures are ready, take 5 drops in a little water daily of either one or the other, according to how you are feeling. The flower (Sun) preparation is to lift the mood and energy; the seed head (Moon) preparation is to calm and cool down. If you feel totally in balance, you can take 2 drops of each.

Dock 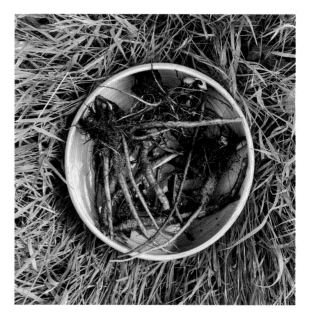 *Rumex crispus/R. obtusifolius*

'Dock is a gentle and consistent laxative and alterative. It is especially indicated for those with a rusty red hue in their cheeks.'

My Western herbal teacher, Ifanca, taught me to look for the sign of Yellow Dock (*Rumex crispus*) in a patient's complexion. The ripe seeds of this plant have a very particular rusty red hue. Sometimes we see a patient, often middle-aged or elderly, who is perhaps a bit out of shape, and we notice that exact same colour in their cheeks. This is always a good prompt to investigate to see whether Yellow Dock is indicated. It usually is.

Medicinal part
- Roots
- Leaves

Roots mostly, but sometimes leaves for topical application

Physiological actions

Summary
- Bitter
- Cholagogue
- Alterative
- Laxative
- Astringent
- Tonic

Physiological virtues

Dock is most often thought of as a liver herb and an alterative. It contains anthraquinones, which stimulate the bowel. However, in Dock root, the action of these plant chemicals is moderated somewhat by the presence of toning and anti-inflammatory tannins. This combination makes Yellow Dock root a gentle and consistent laxative. Yellow Dock would not be my first choice of herb for a patient with chronic constipation, though – a change of lifestyle and diet would be my priority.

Consider Yellow Dock for liver congestion and poor fat digestion, especially when there is a feeling of heaviness that comes on after eating.

I find Yellow Dock most useful where there is a build-up of waste products in the system, which leads to skin eruptions, itchiness, and joint inflammation. Combine it with Burdock in these cases. As a topical treatment, Dock leaves make a good soothing compress to ease itching.

Dock is also a totally fantastic herb to build up healthy iron levels in the blood where there is anaemia. Low iron levels are a very common presentation, menstruating women being especially vulnerable, along with anyone with compromised digestion and therefore poor absorption. Often those who have been taking proton pump inhibitors, such as Omeprazole and Lanzoprazole, over a long period of time, find that they are prone to low iron levels for this reason. Supplementing with additional iron, whether in an inorganic or natural form, will be of limited efficacy if better absorption is not encouraged.

Be cautious with Dock root in pregnancy, as a strongly laxative effect is to be avoided; likewise during lactation, as the effects can be transferred to the baby through the milk.

Energetics
Dock is bitter and astringent.

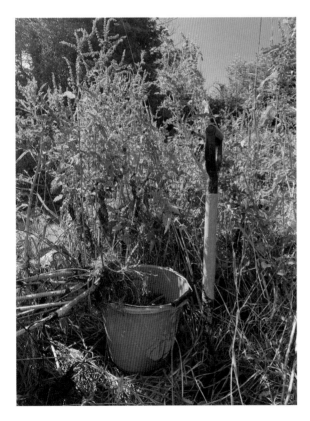

In Tibetan medicine
In Tibetan medicine the root of the species *Rumex nepalensis* is prescribed. Its Tibetan name is *Sho mang* [ཤོ་མང་]. Its taste is sweet and bitter, with a sweet post-digestive taste. Its potency is smooth, cool, and supple. It is considered to take the heat out of wounds, reduce inflammation, and treat hot disorders of the channels. It is antimicrobial.

In my dispensary
Dock root is a staple in my dispensary. I most often reach for it when supporting patients who have a tendency to be low in iron. I combine it with Spirulina, Nettle leaf, Dandelion leaf, and Ashwagandha root in a capsule formula to boost iron levels and build the blood. I usually prescribe the capsules alongside a tailor-made tincture or infusion designed to treat the root cause of the problem – for example, a weak digestive system or heavy periods. As ever, appropriate lifestyle and dietary changes are essential if a sustainable cure is to be achieved.

Historical applications
Gerard described one of the Docks as '*Bloudwort*', writing that it: '*is best knowne unto all of the stocke or kindred of Dockes: it hath long thin leaves sometimes red in every part therof, and often striped here and there with lines and strakes of dark red colour: among which rise upstiffe brittle stalkes of the same colour. . . . The root is likewise red or of a bloudy colour . . . it is an excellent wholesome potherb, for being out into the pottage in some reasonable quantitie, it helps the jaundice, and such like diseases proceeding of cold causes . . . it purifieth the bloud and makes young wenches look faire and cherry-like.*'

Magical
Dock is associated with attracting money and promoting fertility. It is said that if it is made into an infusion and sprinkled about a business

premises, it will attract customers. It is also said that if the seeds of a Dock are tied to a woman's left arm, they will help her to conceive.

Suggestion for the home apothecary

Dock root tincture

Take dried dock roots and fill one third of a jar with them. Pour over 45% ABV alcohol, and leave for at least 4 weeks before straining, pressing, and bottling. Take ¼ tsp in a little hot water daily for 6 weeks if you wish to build up your iron levels.

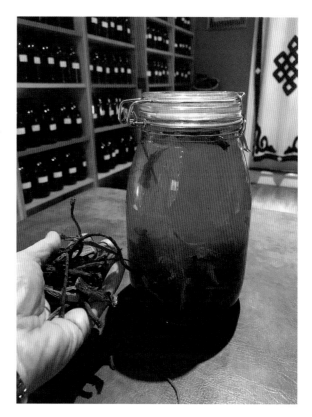

Echinacea   *Echinacea purpurea/E. angustifolia/E. pallida*

'Echinacea supports us while teaching us not to exploit our bodies.'

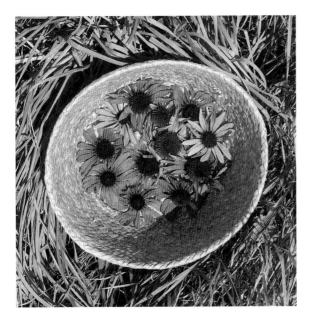

The name 'Echinacea' comes from the Greek *echinos,* which is a word used to describe a hedgehog or sea urchin. The plant that those of European descent call Echinacea is a medicine known for generations by indigenous Americans. It was prescribed mostly for cleaning the blood, for rheumatism, and for snake bites. Over time this traditional healing knowledge passed to settlers. In the late 1880s a German doctor from Nebraska, a Dr Meyer, developed a 'cure-all' formula based on Echinacea, which he sold from his travelling medicine wagon. Apparently, part of his sales pitch was to allow himself to be bitten by a rattlesnake and then to take the medicine immediately. It should be said here that history does not record how he eventually died. Despite – or maybe due to – his sales tech-

niques and his unshakeable faith in the power of Echinacea, Echinacea moved from being a curiosity – among Europeans, at least – to being a widely sought-after herbal remedy.

Echinacea is hugely popular and much overly self-prescribed these days. It is certainly very big business for supplement companies. I feel very lucky that we live in a world where we have access to this beautiful medicine; however, it is not a herb to take long-term as a preventive, and it is not always suitable in every situation. Please be mindful of the need to take it or to prescribe it wisely.

Good-quality liquid extractions of Echinacea produce a very pronounced tingling sensation in the mouth, which can be a bit disconcerting if you are not expecting it. But be happy if you do experience it, because it means that you have access to very good-quality medicine.

Medicinal parts
▷ Roots
▷ Flowers

Physiological actions

Summary
▷ Alterative
▷ Circulatory stimulant
▷ Immune tonic
▷ Antimicrobial

Physiological virtues

Echinacea is an alterative. It is in the group of blood-cleaning herbs known as snake-bite medicines. It is diffusive and stimulant, boosting not only the immune system in the form of increasing the number of white blood cells, but also invigorating the blood circulation to an affected area, so that the white blood cells can be efficiently transported to where they are needed.

Echinacea's virtues mean that it can support our immune system in the face of a tough challenge, helping to make the difference between experiencing a day or two of feeling 'off' and coming down with full-blown influenza. It can be helpful in cancer support as well as supporting the healing of deep infections caused by dog bites or puncture wounds. It is also worth considering for urinary-tract infections.

Echinacea is very good stuff and a very important herb in the dispensary; yet, I admit that the way that Echinacea is promoted and sold these days makes me quite uneasy. My Western herbal tutor, Ifanca, pointed out that over-use of Echinacea to boost a flagging immune system is counterproductive. It robs the chance for us to address the underlying lifestyle and dietary changes that need to be made, encouraging us to keep pushing ourselves to work longer hours in stressful situations, and it also results in over-harvesting. Ifanca always said to me 'Look at the red stem! It's a blood cleaner not a long-term immune tonic.'

I feel that taking Echinacea regularly as a preventive is exploitative. I use the word 'exploitative' in two ways. First, it exploits our own bodily resources by pushing our immune systems into a state of readiness over potentially quite long periods. The support that Echinacea generously offers us can also encourage us to exploit our bodies by continuing to work long hours in stressful situations, skipping meals, or eating out of packets. This beautiful medicinal being gives itself up to help us, and we 'use' it to support an unsustainable way of living.

Second, unnecessary prescribing of this plant is 'exploitative' of a precious medicine that, when taken appropriately, can save people's lives. If we take Echinacea as a crutch without being mindful of its true value, we are contributing to over-harvesting and could be diverting supplies away from those who are in real need of its life-saving properties.

As a topical treatment, Echinacea is excellent to resolve wounds, boils, and abscesses. It can be helpful to heal infections, psoriasis, and acne. I find the flowers excellent for topical preparations and more sustainable if you do not have an abundance of it in your herb garden. However, for these indications you may also wish to consider other more plentiful and sustainably sourced herbs, such as Calendula, or resins, such as propolis, instead.

Energetics

Echinacea is bitter and hot. It is associated with increasing our power, promoting our immune response, and increasing the quality of our blood through 'cleaning it'. It is a herb of strength and amplification. Taken within a spiritually mindful context, it is the most amazing healer for human beings – yet unfortunately Echinacea has become far removed from its context. It has probably been commercialized above any other herb, and, as human beings, our relationship with Echinacea has become largely exploitative rather than respectful. This, in turn, has led to the development of an exploitative attitude to our own bodies more usually associated with allopathic healthcare modalities.

In my dispensary

As I believe that this herb is generally over-exploited, I am especially mindful with how I prescribe it. I do reach for it when it is clear that a patient needs its blood-cleaning action, but I prefer to save its immune stimulating properties for short-term acute situations. Even then I tend to blend it with other suitable herbs – for example, Thyme and Honeysuckle for upper respiratory infections. I strongly believe that appropriate dietary and lifestyle changes make heroic doses of Echinacea unnecessary. The most common example is a persistent cold or cough with mucus, which patients say they cannot 'shake off'. It is very often the case that these patients are not changing their lifestyle and diet. They continue to exploit their bodies and expect the Echinacea to 'make them better'. They may be staying up late and indulging in a diet rich in mucus-forming foods such as dairy products, laying the ground for the infection to be perpetuated. A commitment to rest and a break from mucus-forming foods allows

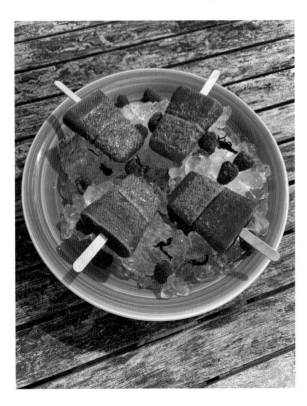

a short course of Echinacea to bring welcome results.

Echinacea should not be taken over a long period without a break, as it can cause the immune response to become depleted through over-stimulation. A couple of other cautions about Echinacea are worth noting. It may trigger flare-ups in some people with autoimmune conditions such as lupus or multiple sclerosis. Also, if you are taking Echinacea because you have a tooth abscess, be aware that taking large doses could increase the amount of pus that is formed as the immune system is boosted. This could potentially lead to greatly increased pain levels if the abscess is in a position where it cannot easily come to a head.

Historical applications

The plains Indians of North America used to smoke Echinacea, and they also took it to make themselves more able to endure high temperatures, such as those within a sweat lodge. There are tales of people being able to hold live coals in their mouths at medicine shows thanks to previously coating their mouths with macerated Echinacea roots.

The Eclectics prescribed it for syphilis, gonorrhoea, and typhoid.

Magical

Indigenous American peoples traditionally chose Echinacea as an offering to the spirits to strengthen spells. Nowadays it is considered protective and to have the ability to strengthen powers of clairvoyance.

Suggestion for the home apothecary

Echinacea, Hibiscus, and Raspberry iced lollies

You'll need:

» *1 tbsp, heaped, of chopped dried Echinacea root*
» *1 tbsp, heaped, of dried Hibiscus calyces*

» *2 cups water*
» *1 cup fresh or frozen Raspberries*
» *½ cup honey (or to taste)*
» *⅓ cup coconut milk*

Gently simmer the Echinacea and Hibiscus for 20 minutes in the water, then strain and reserve the decoction. Allow to cool. In a food processor, blend the fresh or frozen raspberries with the cooled decoction, then add coconut milk and honey to taste. Pour the mixture into ice lolly moulds and freeze.

These are ideal for children with sore throats, tonsillitis, or feverish colds. Give one, or even two, each day, as needed. Do not give daily over a long period: these are for acute illnesses not as a 'preventive'.

Elder 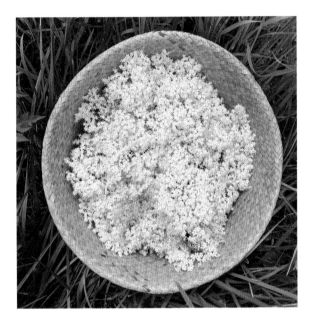 *Sambucus nigra*

'Elder disperses and brings movement, both physiologically and emotionally.'

The name 'Elder' derives from the Anglo-Saxon word *aeld*, which means to fan the flames of a fire by blowing on it. This is presumably a reference to the use of the hollow stems for this purpose. In Tibetan medicine, Elder 'opens the channels'; in Western herbal medicine it helps to support the peripheral circulation. The element of Fire is associated with growth and movement. Elder may not be a strongly warming remedy, but it definitely brings movement to sluggish areas, whether in the body or in the mind.

The hollow stems could be considered to represent the circulatory system as well as the respiratory system. When made into musical instruments, Elder stems help us to be heard. These same stems can be thought of as a portal to other worlds, especially when you think of their association with Pan's pipes. Whichever way we interact with Elder, it encourages us to move forward and look beyond our own narrow viewpoint of life.

Medicinal parts

- ▷ Flowers
- ▷ Fruits

The leaves are no longer taken internally. Bark was also considered medicinal in the past, but caution is advised.

Physiological actions

Summary

- ▷ Expectorant
- ▷ Anticatarrhal
- ▷ Peripheral circulatory stimulant
- ▷ Diaphoretic
- ▷ Sudorific
- ▷ Diuretic
- ▷ Laxative
- ▷ Antiviral
- ▷ Galactagogue (see caution)
- ▷ Astringent

Physiological virtues

Elderflowers open the airways, clear catarrh, and resolve sinus issues. The tea helps to promote expectoration in cases of pleurisy and other pulmonary or bronchial diseases. It is a very good first treatment for the onset of influenza, often combined with Peppermint and Yarrow. The flowers also reduce the symptoms of hay fever. For this, drink the tea mixed with Nettle and Plantain in the weeks leading up to the allergen season and throughout the period when the challenge is greatest.

Elderflowers are diaphoretic, supporting the peripheral circulation and encouraging healthy sweating. This is especially helpful in order to bring down a fever but can also assist elimination from the skin when that requires support, for example when people do not sweat normally. For this reason, Elderflowers were traditionally prescribed for eruptive diseases such as scarlet fever and measles.

They are also diuretic and gently laxative. By supporting elimination through skin, bowels, and kidneys, they are a wonderful tonic to the system when gentle extra support is needed. They can act as a galactagogue, although they should be taken with great caution while lactating.

Cooled Elderflower tea can be used topically as an eye wash.

Elderberries are significantly antiviral and are traditionally made into a Vitamin-C-rich winter tonic for this purpose. They are best heat-treated before ingestion in significant quantities, hence cooked preparations such as decoction or syrups are preferable. As well as their nutritional benefit, it seems that Elderberries may prevent viruses from attaching themselves to the mucus membranes of the nose and throat, therefore enabling us to resist infection in the first place. Beyond their immune-supporting action, the berries were traditionally prescribed to ease migraine, trigeminal neuralgia, and muscle and joint pain.

Bear in mind that high doses of the fruit are laxative. Very excessive doses of Elderflower could, in theory, cause vomiting due to low levels of hydrogen cyanide (sambunigrin), but I have never heard of anyone experiencing this, so the dosage required must be extremely large. It is an effect that is more pronounced when taking the leaves or bark, both of which are rarely prescribed these days.

Energetics

Elderflower is bitter, slightly sweet, and cooling. It is dispersing, not only physiologically but also emotionally, encouraging us to look beyond and to widen our existing viewpoint on life.

In Tibetan medicine

Elder is known in Tibetan medicine as *Yu Gu Shing Nakpo* [ཡུ་གུ་ཤིང་ནགཔོ།]. The species referred to in the pharmacopoeia as *nakpo,* which means black or dark, is usually considered to be *Sambucus adnata.* This has pinky flowers. There is also a white form referred to as *Yugu Shing Karpo* (*Sambucus wightiana*), which has white flowers.

Sambucus has a taste that is bitter and slightly sweet, with a post-digestive taste that is bitter. Its potency is neutral to cooling, slow-acting, light, and rough.

Its primary action is 'to clear the blockage of channels', a reference to its circulation-supporting effect. It is, however, mostly thought of as a topical treatment. It heals wounds, sets broken bones, and reduces swelling. The external application of concentrated extracts of a combination of leaf, flower, and fruits is effective for treating psoriasis and skin diseases, and it is traditionally applied as a cure for blisters that have become abscessed.

In my dispensary

In my clinic I generally work with the flowers. This is not to say that I do not respect the enormous value of the berries, but I prefer to encourage people to gather and make their own Elderberry medicine.

As a gentle circulatory support, Elder is specific for those people who develop purple 'leopard print' markings on their legs when they exert themselves in cold weather. Many of us will have noticed this either on ourselves or on the legs of fellow team members during outdoor sports. When several signs point towards Elderflower being needed within the prescription, I often ask the patient whether they notice a 'leopard print' tendency on their legs during exertion in cold weather. They may need to think back to their school days to give an answer, but it is uncanny how often it is the case that they say yes. With these patients, even if poor circulation is not reported to be 'an issue', we can be sure that the gentle improvements to the circulation brought by Elder are going to help resolve the underlying causes of the case.

Let us take the case of 'Lindsey' as an example. When she came for her first consultation, she was in her late 60s and ran a small business with her husband. As they were both at retirement-age, they were working towards selling the business as a going concern. This involved quite a bit of extra work in making preparations for a smooth sale and handover. The administration and accounts were the responsibility of Lindsey, and she was feeling the strain. Her energy levels had been very low for a few years, and she was not sleeping well. She had very frequent headaches, a tendency to post-nasal drip, and sinusitis. Underlying all of this, she had quite a bit of anxiety and often complained of cold hands and feet. I asked her about whether she had 'leopard print' legs when she exercised, and she said that she had not had the energy to exercise for many years and really could not be sure about whether this was the case, but she thought that she might have done when she was at school. What she could say with certainty is that when she exercised, she never sweated – in fact, she never really sweated at all. When she said that, I knew that her prescription was crying out for the inclusion of Elderflower.

Her digestion was sluggish, and she was not drinking enough water, so I encouraged her to make changes to her diet and lifestyle to rectify this. Her prescription contained gentle digestive support as well as some nourishing and calming herbs, such as Wild Oat and Ashwagandha. Elderflower was included too. She took on board the changes I recommended, and she took her herbal medicine religiously. Within 3 months, her energy levels had bounced back, her sleep was much better than it had been for many years, and her post-nasal drip was completely resolved. On top of this, she had not had any symptoms of sinusitis and was now completely free of headaches, previously having had a headache on waking every day for years. She reported that her anxiety was much more manageable and was reducing all of the time. Her cold hands and feet had completely gone, and she now had the energy to once again incorporate a healthy exercise regime into her life. All of this was truly excellent news, but you may ask how could I say that the Elderflower had played such an important role in all of this. My answer is that when I asked her if she now sweated, she looked at me and said: 'Oh. My goodness, I hadn't really noticed but yes, I'm now sweating normally now when I exercise.' That, in my opinion, had to be the Elderflower.

Historical applications

The bark is strongly purgative and was used in the past for that purpose, but it is quite a violent remedy and has fallen out of favour these days. The leaves used to be made into an ointment called 'green elder ointment', which was a domestic remedy for bruises, sprains, chilblains, haemorrhoids, and applying to wounds. It was considered best to harvest the leaves on the last day of April. Elder leaves are emetic and purgative and no longer prescribed internally. They were once thought to be very efficacious for dropsy.

Magical

Elder is traditionally known as 'Pipe Tree' and 'Ellhorn'. It has a wealth of magical associations. It is the tree of the Celtic religion, of witches, sprites, and faeries. It symbolizes the revival of the Faerie realm. It is often associated with death and rebirth. You can look at this positively or with dread, depending on your conditioning and culture. I see Elder as a tree of new beginnings and rebirth.

It is considered to be protective and so was often planted by the corner of a country dwelling to protect it from lightning strike and other misfortunes. If worn, Elder wood wards off psychic or physical attackers. It was hung over doorways and windows to keep evil from entering the house. It is said to also have the power to force the breaking of enchantments or spells that may have been cast against you. In England, in the days when all hearses were horse-drawn, the drivers carried whips with handles made of Elder wood in order to protect themselves from possible bad intentions of the spirits of the dead. It is also worth noting that Elder was found in long barrows, so must have a very long history of being used in burial rites.

Elder is so strongly associated with the faerie realm that it was considered ill-advised to make a baby's cradle out of Elder wood as the faeries would likely come and steal the baby away, perhaps replacing it with a changeling. If you stand under an Elder tree at midnight on midsummer's eve, it is said that you will see members of the faerie kingdom processing past you. This is not something I have yet tried myself, but it is on my bucket list.

Within the tree resides an aspect of the Elder Mother, a guardian spirit who haunts anyone cutting a tree without seeking proper permission. This tradition is especially strong in Denmark, where she is known as *Hylde-Moer*. It was wise to ask permission and placate the resident spirits before cutting the wood from an Elder tree. The traditional recitation was as follows:

> *'Lady Ellhorn, give me of thy wood,*
> *And I will give thee of mine,*
> *When I become a tree.'*
>
> [Geoffrey Grigson, *The Englishman's Flora*]

This is recited kneeling before the tree, prior to making the first cut, and allows the witch or spirit residing in the tree time to vacate.

Elders bleed red sap when cut, and this is thought to be the blood of the magical beings that inhabit the tree. The hollow stems lend themselves to the making of magical pipes, the reason why one of its country names is Pipe Tree. These flutes were used to summon spirits. It is a long-time favourite for the making of wands. I once crafted a bow made from an Elder stick, which I have to this day. It was quite an experience working slowly and gently with that magical wood. I am honoured that my project worked out well and the arrows fly so true from it.

There are some medical magical associations associated with Elder. For example, to lose a fever, poke an Elder twig into the ground while remaining completely silent. Toothaches, which were once believed to be caused by evil spirits, were treated by the patient chewing on an Elder twig, then placing it in a wall while saying 'Depart thou evil spirit!' Rheumatism was prevented by tying a twig of Elder into three or four knots and carrying it in one's pocket. Warts were cured by rubbing them with a green Elder twig and then burying it into the ground.

Suggestion for the home apothecary

Elderflower, Yarrow, and Peppermint tea for colds

Combine equal parts of Yarrow, Peppermint, and Elderflower to make a tea or inhalation blend that is very helpful for colds and 'flu. Keep some ready blended in your medicine cabinet so that you can take it straight away if you succumb to influenza.

Elecampane 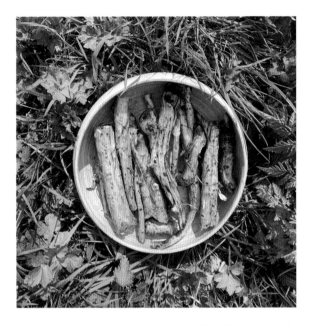 *Inula helenium*

'Elecampane supports the digestion, opens the lungs and sustains the spirits.'

I grow Tibetan Elecampane (*Inula racemosa*), which is very similar to European Elecampane (*Inula helenium*). Elecampane was known as 'Horse Heal' and was grown in every cottage and physic garden. People say that the name 'Horse Heal' comes from it being used to treat horses, but actually the word 'horse' in a herb's name implies that it is 'large' or 'rough': think of Horseradish and Horse Chestnut, for example.

In the West we consider Elecampane to be primarily a respiratory-system-supporting herb that also encourages improved digestion. It has a very strong bitter and aromatic taste, which I really love, but not everyone is a fan.

Medicinal parts
 ▷ Roots

These are harvested in the second or third year.

Physiological actions

Summary
 ▷ Expectorant
 ▷ Antitussive
 ▷ Bitter
 ▷ Tonic
 ▷ Diaphoretic
 ▷ Diuretic
 ▷ Alterative
 ▷ Antimicrobial

Physiological virtues

Elecampane is most often thought of as an expectorant and antitussive, although it has a myriad other medicinal virtues. As an expectorant, it loosens phlegm and helps to clear congested lungs. Its antitussive action calms coughs, being helpful in bronchitis, asthma, and whooping cough.

It is an excellent bitter digestive tonic, encouraging improved levels of stomach acid, which, in turn, reduce mucus production. With strong digestive systems we are in the best position to get well again and stay well. In fact, Elecampane is my first choice as a tonic for weakness following a bout of influenza or bronchitis. Traditionally this kind of post-viral malaise was thought of as being caused by malicious elves, and the affected person was said to have 'elf shot'. Elecampane is considered to be an effective cure for 'elf shot'.

It helps to ripen and resolve lingering fevers, being a stimulant and a diaphoretic. It is also alterative and diuretic. This means that it can support the body in detoxification and recovery after illness.

Elecampane is excellent to treat deep-seated

infections, especially when these are cold and damp, since it is warming in nature, and it is directly antimicrobial. As an astringent, it is anti-inflammatory and healing. This is a herb that truly supports patients on many levels.

Energetics

Elecampane has a sweet, bitter, and hot taste. It opens the lungs on more than just a purely physiological level. I find that it can be very helpful where long-held grief is causing tension in the lungs. It is also specific for when someone is struggling to settle in a new place after relocating.

In Tibetan medicine

The species included within the Tibetan *Materia medica* is *Inula racemosa*. In Tibetan, Elecampane is known as *Manu* [ཨ་རུ]. Its taste is sweet, bitter, and hot, while its post-digestive taste is sweet. Its potency is light, rough, and cooling, but it also has a warming and drying action.

It is considered to cure the onset of *rLung* disorders where there are undesirable interactions between *rLung* and blood. It is specific for tumours that arise below the xiphoid process and is described as the best remedy for 'pains in the ribcage'. *Manu* also helps to generate digestive heat and restores the appetite. A decoction cures diseases caused by an excess of the *Pekén* humour, especially when there is fever and inflammation within such a presentation.

It is the primary ingredient in the formula known as *Manu Zhi Thang* [ཨ་རུ་བཞི་ཐང]. This formula is considered very good when a fever has become mixed with another disease or is 'hidden'. In these circumstances a patient can have a very long-standing lingering cold or cough that never fully resolves. *Manu Zhi Thang* allows the fever to be separated from the underlying disease, so that it can be properly treated. This is described as 'ripening the fever'.

I make a decocted tincture, so the medicine is quickly available and has a good shelf life.

In my dispensary

I work with Elecampane as a tincture, decoction, and in respiratory-system-supporting capsule blends. It is such a helpful herb in many circumstances.

Here is an example: 'Sonia' was a very active lady in her early 70s when she first attended the clinic for treatment. She had suffered a close personal bereavement two years previously, and this seemed to have triggered the development of late-onset asthma. She was prescribed inhalers, which helped to manage her asthma, but she continued to suffer from tightness in the chest and a burning sensation when walking up hills. One year later, after suffering from a very bad cold, she suddenly lost all sense of taste and smell. She told me that she could not even taste Chilli. She also had digestive problems, with a tendency to acid reflux and some mild IBS symptoms.

It was clear that there was a link between Sonia's grief and the start of her respiratory issues, so Elecampane immediately stood out clearly as a herb that I should include in her prescription. Elecampane would help to open her lungs and release the tension that she was holding there, as well as resolving the build-up of catarrh in her upper respiratory system. It would also strengthen her digestive system, so that she did not produce so much mucus. Sonia embraced the dietary changes that I recommended, cutting out all dairy products from her diet, since these were too mucus-forming for her rather weak digestion. She also committed to drinking fewer caffeine-containing hot drinks and increasing her hydration. I gave her a herbal tincture prescription that included Elecampane, Thyme, Mullein, Usnea, and a little Chilli. She also had some of my sinus ointment to apply to the areas of her face that overlaid her sinuses.

Within four weeks of treatment the tightness and burning sensation in her lungs had completely disappeared, and on one occasion she thought that she could actually smell some freshly baked bread. She noticed that some mucus was being released and draining down her throat, which she saw as a positive sign. Four weeks later her digestion was much improved, and her sense of taste and smell was definitely returning. She continued to follow the herbal treatment for several more months, until her sense of taste and smell had fully recovered.

Historical applications

Pliny described how Elecampane would help the digestion and cause mirth.

There is an old Latin rhyming couplet that says, '*Enula campana reddit praecordia sana*', which means 'Elecampane will the spirits sustain'.

Galen recommended it for '*passions of the hucklebone called sciatica*'.

Culpeper wrote: '*The fresh roots of Elecampane, preserved with sugar, or made into a syrup or conserve, is very good to warm a cold and windy stomach, or the prickling therein, and stitches in the sides, caused by the spleen; also to help a cough, shortness of breath, and wheezing in the lungs . . . the dried root is profitable for those who have their urine stopped; likewise to prevent stoppages of the menstrua, the pains of the mother, and of the stone in the reins, kidneys or bladder.*' He went on to describe its beneficial action against venom and '*worms in the belly*', its ability to fasten loose teeth, its ability to strengthen eyesight and to guard against the plague, and its pain-relieving properties in cases of gout, sciatica, and joint injuries. He even adds that it has anticonvulsant properties. Finally, he describes how, as a topical wash, it will heal skin conditions such as the scab or itch.

Magical

Elecampane is known as 'Elf Wort' or 'Elf Dock'. Its Anglo-Saxon names are 'Eolone' and 'Sperewort'. This is a herb that has a long-standing association with protection and was traditionally chosen to treat 'elf shot' – a condition associated with unexplained failure to thrive. Elecampane is still an excellent choice within a herbal prescription for a patient who is failing to thrive.

The leaves or flowers are sewn into a pink cloth that is made into a sachet and carried to attract love or for protection. The herb, smouldered on charcoal, is said to aid in sharpening psychic powers, particularly when scrying.

Elecampane tea will soothe sorrow at having to leave one's home and be far away in a strange place. Legend has it that it originally sprang from Helen of Troy's tears when she was abducted.

Suggestion for the home apothecary

Elecampane honey

Chunks of Elecampane root preserved in honey are a delicious cough-calming and lung-clearing treat to nibble on. First, you need access to fresh Elecampane root. If it is a plant not yet in your herb collection, now is the time to add it. Be generous with the number of plants you make space for, so that in the autumn you can harvest one or two and leave the others to grow to maturity.

Thoroughly wash your roots, scrubbing them but do not peel away the skin. Leave them on a tray covered with kitchen paper for 24 hours to air dry. Once the surface washing water has evaporated, cut the roots into even-sized slices or chunks. Take great care to remove any woody bits present in older roots. These bits are still medicinal and would be used if you are making a tincture or decoction, but as you will be eating the chunks preserved in the honey, it is nicer if they are tender. While you cut the roots up,

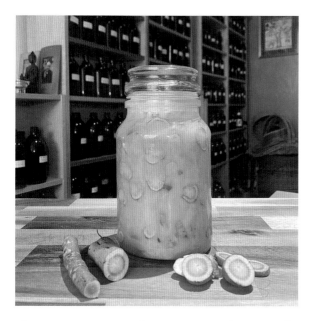

also remove any surface crevasses that contain remnants of soil or roots that are damaged and discoloured. Put the root pieces into a clean Kilner jar and cover them with honey. Leave them for at least a month. Top up the level of honey as needed to make sure that they are thoroughly covered. Roots not covered will be prone to moulding. Store in a refrigerator and stir regularly.

Manu Zhi Thang [ཨ་ནུ་བཞི་ཐང་] *decocted tincture*

This is a decocted tincture. It means you have the benefit of a slow aqueous extraction combined with the keeping qualities of a tincture. It does require high-strength alcohol to make successfully.

You will need:
» *4 parts dried Tibetan Elecampane root (Inula racemosa) (Manu)* [ཨ་ནུ།]
» *1 part dried Raspberry cane inner bark (Rubus idaeus) (Kandakari)* [གཎྜ་ཀ་རི]
» *1 part Clove buds (Syzygium aromaticum) (Lishi)* [ལི་ཤི]
» *1 part dried Ginger root (Zingiber officinalis) (Gaja)* [ས་ག]

To make it, combine the herbs and add to cold water. Bring slowly to the boil and simmer until the volume is reduced by a half. The quantities of herb you choose will depend on the volume of water you choose. For 500 ml (which will end up as 250 ml) you could add around 28 g of dried herb: 16 g *Manu* and 4 g each of the other three. Once the decoction is cooled, strain into a measuring jug, reserving the herbs, as these are needed for the tincture phase. Make a note of the final volume of the decoction and place it into a large tincturing jar with the herbs. Add the same volume again of high-percentage alcohol (at least 60% ABV), so that the final tincture will be at least 30% ABV and will have a good shelf life as well as efficient extraction of oil-soluble constituents. Leave for at least four weeks in a cool, dark place, then strain, press, and bottle.

Take 5 ml in hot water to ripen a cold or lingering low-grade unresolved fever. Rest and allow your body to do its work.

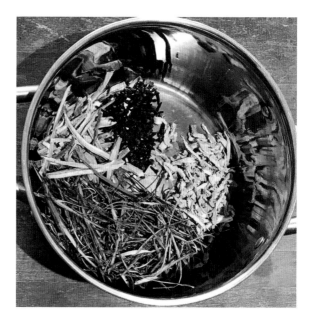

Eyebright 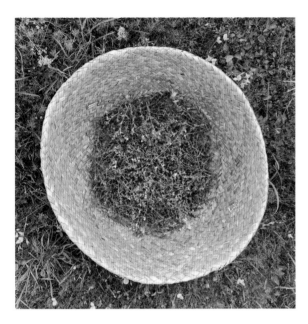 *Euphrasia officinalis*

'Eyebright has a special affinity for irritated eyes.'

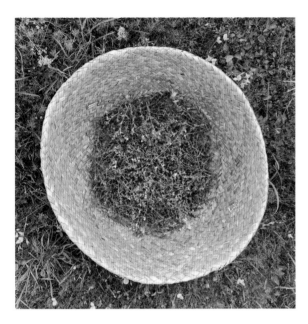

The name *Euphrasia* derives from the Greek *Euphrosyne*, which means gladness. Euphrosyne was one of the three graces who was especially associated with joy and mirth. *Euphrasia* is a very variable genus containing around 20 different species of Eyebright, which are all interchangeable in terms of medicinal properties.

Eyebright is a herb that is prescribed for eye inflammation in many different parts of the temperate world. I still marvel at how plant knowledge often spans cultures and continents. I do wonder whether some of this is because physicians travelled the world in ancient times and shared plant knowledge with each other. Mostly, though, I feel that being around the plants and working with them allows them to transmit the information to us directly. This is all the more reason for us to strive to maintain a hands-on relationship with herbs and to look carefully after their wild populations.

Medicinal parts
▷ Aerial parts
These are harvested when the plant is in flower.

Physiological actions
Summary
▷ Astringent
▷ Anti-inflammatory

Physiological virtues
Eyebright is astringent and has a particular affinity for the eyes in Western herbal medicine. A cooled infusion applied topically will bring immediate relief for tired, itchy, or irritated eyes. It is also absolutely excellent as an anti-inflammatory treatment for hay fever, allergies, sinusitis, and bronchial conditions. It can be helpful in some cases of vertigo and labyrinthitis, especially where these are associated with a build-up of mucus.

Energetics
Eyebright is astringent and bitter.

In Tibetan medicine
Eyebright's Tibetan name is *Zhim thik sangyae chu jib* [ཞིམ་ཐིག་སངས་རྒྱས་ཆུ་འཇིབ]. It has a bitter and astringent taste with a post-digestive taste that is bitter. Its potency is cool, slow-acting, and light. This makes it well suited to treatment of

reactive conditions associated with heat. It is good in cases of bronchitis, chronic lung disorders, constipation, diabetes, and lymphatic congestion. It is a tonic, rejuvenative and aphrodisiac. Eyebright is also favoured for the eyes, but the *Gyudzhi* lists another action of this plant as being to treat difficulty in passing urine and urinary retention.

I vividly remember the moment when my dear Tibetan medicine teacher, Khenpo Troru Tsenam, reached down into the grass in a meadow near the Samye Ling Tibetan Centre in Scotland and carefully picked a stem of Eyebright. He grinned broadly and said, 'We have a very similar plant in Tibet, and it treats eye diseases.'

In my dispensary

Eyebright is a very important herb in my dispensary. I most often prescribe it as part of an eye-drop tincture blend. I also include it in prescriptions for patients suffering with hay fever, allergies, and streaming eyes, either as a tincture or within a capsule blend.

'Ginnie' was 17 years old. Each spring and summer she suffered with very severe hay fever and had to take antihistamines daily during the summer. Her main reason for attending my clinic was because she suffered with very painful periods, and we were working on this with dietary changes and herbs. Although I believed that the dietary changes would in time reduce the hay fever, we decided that Ginnie would take two capsules daily containing a blend of Eyebright, Elderflower, and Nettle leaf, starting two months before the hay fever usually started and continuing throughout the season. That year her hay fever symptoms were minimal, and alongside that, the herbal treatment for her painful periods had also been very effective. She was delighted.

Historical applications

Gerard wrote that '*It is very much commended for the eis. Being taken it selfe alone, or any way else, it preserves the sight, and being feeble & lost it restores the same: it is given most fitly being beaten into pouder; oftentimes a like quantitie of Fennell seed is added thereto, and a little mace, to which is put so much sugar as the weight of them all cometh to. . . . Eyebright stamped and laid upon the eyes, or the juice thereof mixed with white Wine, and dropped into the eyes, or the distilled water, taketh away the darknesse and dimnesse of the eyes, and cleareth the sight.*'

Culpeper said that Eyebright fortifies the brain. He said it improves memory and treats dizziness.

Magical

Eyebright is associated with promoting mental acuity as well as visual clarity. You could also extend this to promoting foresight and intuition. It is said that the infusion applied to the eyelids on cotton pads over an extended period of time induces magical clairvoyance. Drinking Eyebright tea clears the mind and aids the memory.

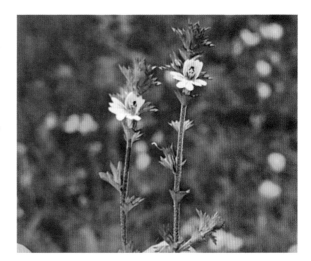

Suggestion for the home apothecary

Eyebright eye wash for inflamed and sore eyes

First make a tincture. Note that you only need a very small amount for the home apothecary.

Take a small jar and loosely fill it with fresh Eyebright. Cover with 50% ABV alcohol, and leave in the dark for 4 weeks, making sure that the plant material is completely covered. Strain and bottle. Add 3 drops of the tincture to an eyebath of cooled boiled water and bathe the eye twice a day. If both eyes are affected, use a separate eye bath for each eye. You can also mix equal parts Eyebright and Calendula tinctures for this eye lotion, still adding 3 drops of the blend to an eye bath of cooled, boiled water. Do not put undiluted tinctures into your eyes.

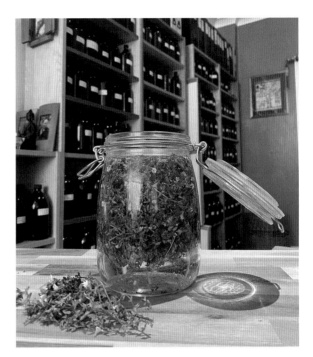

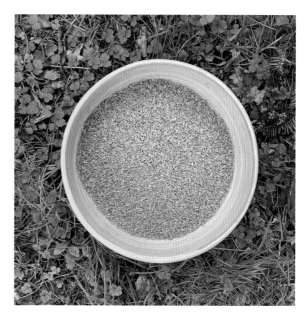
'Fennel is specific for painful spasms which are made worse by worry.'

Fennel is most often thought of as a digestive aid, relieving colic and gripes, but it has many other excellent virtues. The seed has a warming, oily, and nutritious nature, so it tends to counteract excess *rLung* in the body, which, in turn, calms the mind. That is why I consider Fennel a specific for painful spasms made worse by worrying about them.

Medicinal parts
▷ Seeds

Physiological actions

Summary
▷ Carminative
▷ Galactagogue
▷ Antiemetic
▷ Expectorant
▷ Anti-inflammatory
▷ Oestrogenic

Physiological virtues

Fennel is an aromatic and a carminative, being perhaps best known as the main ingredient of Gripe Water, a traditional compound that helps to relieve colic in babies. It is also popular with breastfeeding mothers, as it is a galactagogue and helps to maintain an abundant supply of good-quality milk. A side benefit is that the Fennel comes through in the milk and helps to reduce painful colic in the infant. If stronger help is called for, you can add some cooled Fennel tea to the baby's bath water, allowing its carminative virtues to be delivered transdermally. This is an especially effective method for babies because of their delicate skins.

For adult patients, Fennel is commonly prescribed alongside purgatives in order to alleviate the potential griping they may cause. It can also be a good herb to consider where there is nausea, but please be cautious when taking it during pregnancy.

Fennel is a stimulating expectorant, helpful in bronchial asthma, wheezing, and hoarseness. As a mild remedy it is well indicated for children's bronchial complaints. It has also long been associated as a herb to support the eye. A compress of cooled Fennel tea is a good home remedy for blepharitis and conjunctivitis.

You will often see mention of Fennel tea to assist with weight loss. It is true that Fennel can reduce hunger cravings and is a diuretic, so it can be helpful as part of a weight-loss regime if it suits the individual patient.

Fennel contains phytoestrogens and has a significant influence on the female reproductive system. It can help to stimulate menstruation when this is absent or scanty and can also be a great support during menopause to alleviate symptoms that arise as the body is adjusting to lower oestrogen levels. Made into a pessary or ointment and applied daily, Fennel seed can be extremely effective at restoring vaginal tissue tone in patients suffering from dryness and vaginal atrophy.

Energetics

Fennel is hot, sweet, and bitter. It has an oily quality and is both stimulating and relaxing.

In Tibetan medicine

Fennel is called *Seera karpo* [ཟི་ར་དཀར་པོ]. It is bitter, pungent, and warming, with an oily nature, and this, combined with its warming qualities, makes it excellent to counteract raised *rLung*. It is a wonderful digestive support, increasing stomach and spleen heat without aggravating *Tripa*. It calms stomach pains and relaxes cramps. Due to its *rLung*-reducing nature, it is a very good first aid treatment for someone whose anxiety about their stomach pains is making them much worse. In Tibetan medicine, Fennel is also considered helpful for fevers associated with the respiratory system.

In my dispensary

I prescribe Fennel in tincture, tea, and ointment form. Years ago, after reading about research that showed that Fennel seed extract could bring lasting relief from perimenopausal vaginal atrophy, I started making Fennel seed ointment for my patients. The feedback has been absolutely amazing, and it remains a very popular off-the-shelf product at my drop-in clinics.

This is a typical example where Fennel has helped a woman who was experiencing vaginal atrophy: 'Jade' was 62, happily married, and in pretty good health; however, she was intensely disappointed and upset about the increasing discomfort she was experiencing during intercourse. I advised her to increase her hydration levels, and I prescribed her a digestive and mucous-membrane-supporting tincture blend. I also sent her home with a pot of my Fennel seed ointment with the instruction to apply approximately half a teaspoon's worth to the inside of the vagina daily. She was also to apply an extra 'dollop' prior to intercourse. Within four weeks things were beginning to feel a lot more comfortable, and she made sure she got another pot of 'the miracle ointment' at her next appointment. She continued to improve and was delighted to be feeling much more like her old self after a couple more months.

Historical applications

Hildegard of Bingen wrote of Fennel's ability to positively influence a person's state of mind, saying that it brings a person back into a state of joyfulness. This, in my view, is in complete accordance with its abilities to ground and balance an excess of the *rLung* in Tibetan medicine. On a purely physiological level, Hildegard recommended Fennel seeds for the digestion: '*Eaten daily on an empty stomach, they reduce mucus and all rottenness, take away halitosis and clear the eyes.*' She also said: '*Whoever eats fried meat, fried fish, or anything else fried, and suffers pain from it should eat Fennel or Fennel seeds and will have less pain.*'

Many of the old herbalists talk about Fennel's ability to clear the sight. Pliny wrote that '*serpents eat it when they cast their old skins, and they sharpen their sight with the juice by rubbing against the plant*'.

Parkinson wrote of Fennel's abilities to support digestion: '*The leaves, seede and rootes are both for meate and medicine; . . . which being sweet and somewhat hot helpeth to digest the crude qualitie of fish and other viscous meats.*'

William Coles, in his *Nature's Paradise* of 1650, wrote of its abilities to help reduce excess body weight: '*both the seeds, leaves and root of our Garden Fennel are much used in drinks and broths for those that have grown fat, to abate their unwieldiness and cause them to grow more gaunt and lank*'.

Culpeper wrote that '*Fennel expels wind, provokes urine, and eases the pains of the stone, and helps to break it. . . . the seed and roots . . help to open obstructions of the liver, spleen, and the yellow jaundice, as also the gout and cramp.*' He also alluded to Fennel's relaxing expectorant qualities: '*The seed is of good use in medicines for shortness of breath and wheezing, by stoppings of the lungs.*'

Lyte, in his *New Herball,* has a lot to say about Fennel. He describes it as '*hot in the third degree and dry in the first*', and, when moving on to its '*vertues*', he starts with its galactagogue properties. He writes: '*The seed therof drunken . . . filleth womens breasts . . . with milke*' and that '*the decoction . . . drunken, easeth the payne of the kidneys, causeth one to make water, and to avoid the stone and bringeth down the floures. The root is good . . . against the dropsy to be boiled in wine and drunken.*' Note: I think that the word '*floures*' here may refer to urinary gravel.

Lyte goes on to describe Fennel's ability to reduce stomach pain and nausea as well as its usefulness in '*opening obstructions*' in the lungs, liver, and kidneys. When mixed with honey, Fennel was considered a useful topical treatment for bites by mad dogs.

Magical

In Greek mythology, Prometheus stole fire from the gods, carrying it in a hollow Fennel stem in order to present it to mankind. In mediaeval times Fennel was considered to protect against witchcraft. At Midsummer it was hung, with St John's Wort, over doors in order to ward off evil spirits. It seemed to have repellent properties in the earthly realm too: wearing a sprig of Fennel inside your left shoe was believed to repel ticks and prevent their bites.

Fennel is one of the nine herbs that make up the Anglo-Saxon 'Nine Herbs Charm', sharing a verse with Chervil, as follows:

'*Chervil and Fennel, most mighty two,*
those worts were shaped by the witty Drighten,
holy in the heavens, where he hung;
set and sent into seven worlds
for the wretched and the wealthy for all a cure.
Stands she against pain, stuneth she against
  venom,
that prevails against three and against thirty,
against the fiend's hand and against far-braiding
against maskering by evil wights.'

Suggestion for the home apothecary

Fennel ointment for vaginal atrophy and dryness

Take a cup of Fennel seeds and put them into either a double boiler or a slow cooker with a warm setting with one litre of mild and light olive oil. The important thing is not to directly heat the oil, so you want to warm the oil for an hour or so in the double boiler or turn the slow cooker onto 'warm' and warm the oil in there for just an hour or two. A slow cooker with only 'high or low' is not suitable, as 'low' is much too hot. If you do not have a double boiler, you can balance a Pyrex bowl on top of a pan of simmering water.

Once the oil is infused, strain it through a funnel lined with a coffee filter paper. It will take a while to go through so come back to it and keep tipping a little more in whenever you go past it. This may take a few hours. There is no rush.

Once the oil is filtered, measure the final volume by pouring it into a measuring jug. Get some clean dry glass jars ready, enough to take

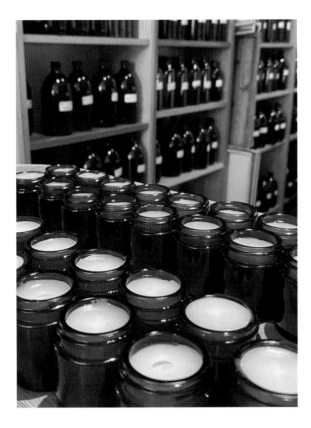

the volume that you are left with plus a little more. Pour the filtered Fennel-infused oil into your clean double boiler and warm it through again. Add 1 g beeswax for each 7 ml of oil. Stir until it is melted, then pour it into the jars. It is easiest to do this by transferring the oil and melted wax mixture into a jug, so that it pours more readily. Leave the filled jars undisturbed until the contents are fully set. Put on the lids, label, and store in a dark cupboard.

Apply approximately half a teaspoon's worth into the vagina each night, and extra prior to intercourse.

You can buy beeswax granules from herbal suppliers. The granules melt more quickly than a big lump of wax. If you want to make a vegan version, infuse the Fennel seeds into Coconut oil instead, since this is usually solid at room temperature, or can be stored in the refrigerator.

Feverfew ❦ *Tanacetum parthenium*

'Traditionally a migraine herb, but it also has other virtues to offer us.'

In the 1970s and 1980s Feverfew rose to prominence as a herb to prevent migraines. It was then that a lady called Ann Jenkins discovered how valuable Feverfew was as a migraine preventer after suffering from regular episodes of migraine for fifty years. She tried eating a few leaves of Feverfew every day, and it completely prevented them. As a result of this, Dr Stewart Johnson carried out research to investigate Feverfew further. He found that it was indeed of value for migraine prevention.

Medicinal parts

▷ Aerial parts

Leaves harvested before flowering are preferable.

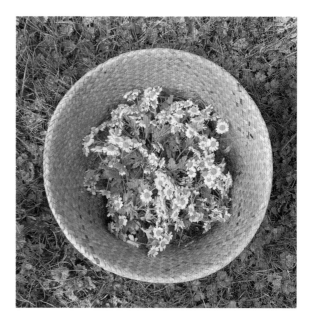

Physiological actions

Summary

▷ Bitter
▷ Aromatic
▷ Peripheral circulatory stimulant
▷ Diaphoretic
▷ Anti-inflammatory
▷ Analgesic
▷ Emmenagogue
▷ Vermifuge

Physiological virtues

Feverfew is an aromatic bitter that relaxes the blood vessels. This may influence the circulation to the head, playing a part in its well-publicized action against migraine. In old times Feverfew was considered a specific for giddiness and vertigo, which makes sense, given its influence on the circulation to the head. Perhaps this is something that we should consider again.

Feverfew influences the body's ability to disperse heat and is a good febrifuge, as its name suggests. It is anti-inflammatory, which makes it good to consider in cases of rheumatoid arthritis as well as asthma. It has pain-relieving properties and is an effective emmenagogue, being helpful not only to stimulate menstruation, but also to relieve period pain. One way of benefitting from its emmenagogue virtues is to prepare it as a vaginal steam. Simply fill a bowl with a steaming decoction of the fresh leaves and squat over it.

As a strongly bitter herb, Feverfew stimulates the liver and digestion and is a vermifuge. Many report that it helps to lift their mood and therefore reduces depression.

Avoid in pregnancy or if on blood thinners.

Energetics

Feverfew is bitter, warming, and drying.

In my dispensary

I find Feverfew absolutely invaluable for those patients who have a combination of migraines that are relieved by warm packs, along with a tendency to joint inflammation. It is prescribed either as a small part of a daily personalized prescription, or the patient is given a dropper bottle of pure Feverfew tincture and instructed to take 10 drops prior to the onset of an attack, repeating the dose every 2 hours, as needed.

The following case, where there were frequent migraines and poor circulation, is a typical example of when Feverfew can make a big difference. 'Angie' was 40 years old and suffered with frequent (twice-weekly) migraines. She had a healthy diet, made sure she had a good work–life balance, and always tried to minimize the allopathic medications that she took. The migraines had started when she was a child. Her tongue was quite coated, and she had signs of a sluggish digestive system, she was not hungry in the morning, she often suffered with bloating, and her bowels were not regular. She tended to have cold hands and feet but described a tendency for her head to overheat. She had a history of vertigo.

She had a tailor-made blend that supported her digestion and liver, alongside gentle circulatory support from Yarrow, Elderflower, and Lime flower. I included Feverfew at a rate of one-tenth of the blend. Four weeks later, although the migraines had not yet reduced, her tongue was much less coated, her appetite was better in the morning, and her bowels were more regular. Another two months later her circulation was getting better and, although the migraines were still occurring at the same

frequency, each one was lasting only half a day instead of two days. Two months after that the migraines were much less frequent and often did not develop into a full attack. She continues to improve steadily.

Historical applications

Feverfew was a fragrant strewing herb with helpful insect-repellent properties. Since Roman times, it has been considered to be an effective emmenagogue, inducing menstruation and assisting with the expulsion of the placenta.

Gerard wrote of Feverfew as a remedy for vertigo: '*Feverfew dried and made into pouder, and two drams of it taken with hony or sweet wine, purgeth by siege melancholy and flegme; wherefore it is very good for them that are giddie in the head, or which have turning called Vertigo, that is a swimming and turning in the head. Also it is good for such as be melancholik, sad, pensive and without speech.*'

Culpeper described Feverfew's powers against the ague: '*the herb bruised and applied to the wrists before the coming of the ague fits, does take them away*'. He also wrote about Feverfew being an antidepressant, saying that Feverfew in wine might help those who were '*troubled with melancholy and heaviness or sadness of spirits*'. He also described it as being '*effective for all pains in the head*'.

In *A Welsh Botanology*, published in 1813, there is a description of a woman who cured her tendency to migraine by drinking regular infusions of Feverfew. Perhaps this is what inspired Anne Jenkins to try Feverfew for her own migraines over 150 years later.

Magical

Feverfew is associated with protection against colds and fevers, as well as accidents. Carry it with you in an amulet.

Suggestion for the home apothecary

Feverfew sandwiches

Take 2–3 medium-sized fresh leaves daily in a sandwich. Taking the leaves in a sandwich can help to protect the mucous membranes of the mouth, as eating the leaves on their own can cause mouth ulcers in sensitive people. Some people find that this is reduced by lightly frying the leaves before ingestion.

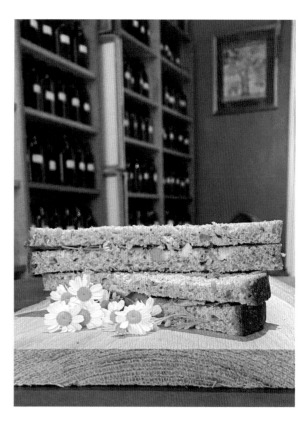

Garlic 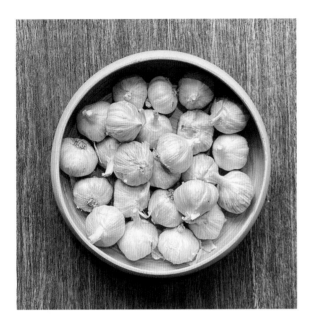 *Allium sativum*

'Garlic protects us against invasion and counteracts the rLung *humour.'*

Garlic has been a mainstay of our human herbal medicine chest for thousands of years. It was famously found in the tomb of Tutankhamun, but it was never just a medicine for kings. Those tough souls that built the pyramids were fed Garlic daily to keep them strong and healthy. Later on, Galen referred to Garlic as the '*peasants' theriac*' – that is, a medicine that cures everything. In Chaucer's time Garlic was known as '*poor man's treacle*'.

Garlic protects us against invasion from various microorganisms and parasites. It is a great antiviral, antibacterial, antifungal, and vermifuge. It enlivens blood flow, which, in turn, helps its protective influence to get to harder-to-reach areas of the body, such as the extremities, the lower respiratory tract, and around slow-healing wounds in elderly patients. It is an effective and easily accessible expectorant, so this, combined with its antiviral action, makes it a perfect first aid herb for colds and influenza. Garlic also protects us from our own patterns of instability – the distressing highs and lows of blood sugar swings and unstable mood associated with an excess of *rLung* in Tibetan medicine. It is a popular over-the-counter supplement due to its ability to reduce harmful blood cholesterol levels.

Medicinal parts
- Cloves within bulb

Physiological actions

Summary
- Antimicrobial
- Antifungal
- Antiviral
- Vermifuge
- Expectorant
- Diaphoretic

Physiological virtues

Garlic is absolutely packed with beneficial medicinal constituents. It contains vitamins, minerals, and sulphur compounds, which are responsible for the characteristic taste and odour. When fresh Garlic is chewed or crushed, a compound called alliin is converted to allicin, and this, in turn, is converted to diallyl disulphide. This diallyl disulphide, produced by our chewing, chopping, or crushing of fresh Garlic, has antibacterial properties against both gram-negative and gram-positive bacteria. This is well worth remembering in a world where antibiotic resistance is becoming increasingly frequent. In both World Wars, Garlic was included in wound dressings to prevent gangrene.

It is significantly antiviral, helping to protect people from influenza and making their recovery from it much quicker. It is also expectorant and acts directly to reduce bronchial and nasal congestion and is one of the key ingredients in Fire Cider. It has been prescribed successfully in the treatment of pulmonary tuberculosis, whooping cough, and asthma. Antiviral and antimicrobial properties of Garlic are much more pronounced when raw Garlic is consumed. To make the most of this, add freshly chopped Garlic to your food after cooking, or make Garlic Honey. If you are laid low with a viral infection and cannot manage to consume sufficient Garlic, place a sliced clove in your socks and go to bed with them on. The Garlic will enter your system through your skin and work its medicinal magic. You can also make a chest rub with fresh Garlic to help relieve severe coughs. Traditionally this was made by bruising cloves and mixing them with lard, but infusing in a suitable oil, such as olive oil, or mixing with coconut oil would be just as good. Apply to the chest and between the shoulder blades.

Topically, Garlic can be a helpful foot treatment. Its antiviral properties treat warts and verrucae, and its antifungal virtues make it suitable for fungal infections such as athlete's foot. Mash fresh cloves and apply to the affected areas regularly, while also increasing consumption of Garlic within the diet. A clove of fresh Garlic can also be a good topical application for skin infections and acne.

Garlic is a vermifuge: in the case of worm infestations one should aim to eat 3–6 raw cloves daily. If there is a particular problem with recurrent infestations of threadworms (where the eggs survive in the rectum), a peeled uncut clove of Garlic inserted into the rectum overnight can help to break the cycle of infestation. If trying this, make absolutely sure that the clove is whole, as any cut surface will be too irritant and cause discomfort.

Garlic stimulates the circulation, acting as a diaphoretic and thinning the blood. It can be helpful for people with concerns about excessive blood clotting; however, too much Garlic is not a good idea if you are taking prescribed blood thinners. It is, on the other hand, an excellent dietary addition for people with insulin resistance and Type II diabetes, as it helps to balance blood sugar levels.

Garlic is very heating and can irritate the stomach of sensitive people. Be cautious if trying large increases of Garlic within the diet.

Energetics

Garlic tastes hot and sweet, with a bitter and hot post-digestive taste and a hot, drying, stimulating, fast-acting, oily, and heavy potency. It protects us from invasion. It is familiar and accessible. It is a herb that can make us feel grounded, safe, and secure.

In Tibetan medicine

Garlic is known as *Gokcha* [སྒོག་སྐྱ]. Since *Gokcha* is hot as well as being oily, it is excellent to counteract an excess of *rLung*; in fact Garlic is suggested as one of the best medicines for an excess of *rLung* in the *Gyudzhi*. Interestingly, Garlic's effectiveness at calming and grounding us makes it contraindicated as a food or medicine during certain spiritual practices within the Vajrayana Buddhist tradition, because it may make the practitioner feel heavier and duller of mind during the long periods of intense meditation and visualization required.

Gokcha counteracts sleep deprivation, loss of appetite, loss of digestive heat, leprosy, disorders of serous fluid, vitiligo, hair loss, haemorrhoids, and upper respiratory tract infections. It is often described as counteracting animalcules (infectious microorganisms) associated with *rLung* disorders, as well as poisoning and diseases caused by evil spirits.

For some medicinal compounds intended for curing *rLung*, dried *Gokcha* is placed in a lidded clay pot, then sealed with a type of mud, then placed in a pit, and covered with wet sand; a fire is lit above. When it is cooked and cooled, it is black and sparkles. This *Gokcha* is added to certain formulae.

In my dispensary

Since Garlic is so specific to counteract *rLung*, I add it to my special *rLung* calming tincture blend, along with a lot of warming and oily

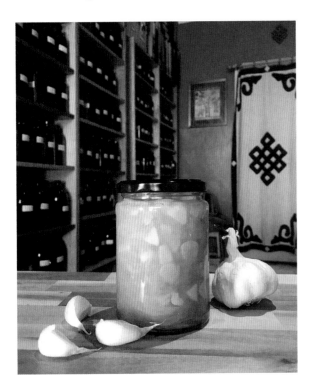

spices, such as Cloves, Caraway, Nutmeg, and Cardamom. In most cases, lifestyle changes are the most effective and sustainable approach, but sometimes patients are unable to incorporate richer, oilier, and more nutritious foods into their diets, and they have unstable lifestyles that take time to be changed. In these cases, stronger herbal support is needed in order to start the rebalancing process. The Garlic contained in my *rLung* mix tincture is a valuable and effective part of this strategy.

When I first created my *rLung* mix, I wondered whether Westerners would object to the garlicky taste, but I need not have worried. It is pretty much universally loved, with people telling me that they genuinely look forward to their next dose. In fact, the spicy taste and the quick results that it brings can sometimes make it quite difficult to persuade people that they no longer need it. Please note that warming, oily, nutritious blends aimed at counteracting *rLung* are not appropriate for patients with *Tripa* or *Pekén* disorders.

Historical applications

Garlic has a very long medicinal history. Galen referred to it as the '*peasants' theriac*' – that is, a medicine that cures everything. In Chaucer's time, Garlic was known as '*poor man's treacle*'.

Culpeper considered it to be a herb that should be taken with caution by those people with a melancholic constitution: '*in men oppressed by melancholy it will . . . send up . . . many strange visions to the head: therefore, inwardly, let it be taken with great moderation.*'

Maud Grieve reports that Garlic is an old cure for dropsy, removing the oedema and guarding against its recurrence. She also writes that sniffed into the nostrils, it will revive someone who is hysterical. From my Tibetan medicine perspective, I cannot help but associate this with its *rLung* calming virtues.

Magical

Garlic is protective, on an etheric level as well as a physiological one. It was worn to guard against the plague, and it was considered to be able to absorb diseases. It was rubbed onto the affected part, then thrown into running water.

Garlic was traditionally placed in the home to protect against the intrusion of evil and to keep out thieves and envious people. Rubbed into pots and pans before cooking, it is considered to remove negative influences that might otherwise contaminate the food. Roman soldiers ate it to give them courage, and sailors carried it to protect against shipwrecks.

The ancient Greeks left cloves of Garlic at crossroads as food for the goddess Hecate.

Suggestion for the home apothecary

Garlic honey

Take vibrant, fresh, unblemished Garlic cloves, and peel and chop roughly. Place in a clean jar or ramekin, and cover completely with honey. Leave overnight, and in the morning the honey will have become much more liquid and infused with medicinal Garlic juice. Take teaspoons of the juice as an immune-boosting and expectorant support. You can also eat chunks of the Garlic.

If you are making more than will be used in one day, then you will need to store this in the refrigerator. It will remain in good condition for many months, even over a year.

Ginger 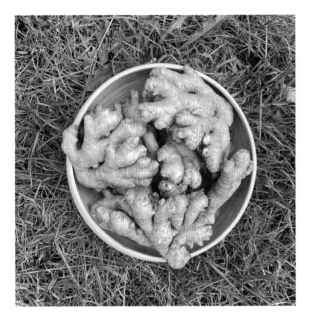 *Zingiber officinalis*

'Ginger is warming and invigorating.'

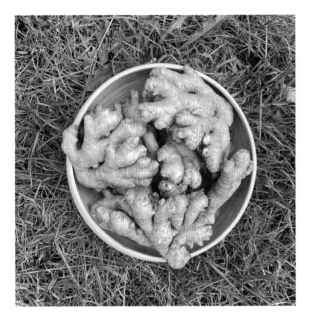

In Ayurveda, Ginger is known as *vishwaghesaj*, which means 'universal medicine'. It is aptly named, since it has virtues that help all systems of the body. It brings the element of Fire to our bodies, warming us and invigorating us while relaxing smooth muscle with its aromatic compounds.

Medicinal part
- Rhizome

Physiological actions

Summary
- Circulatory stimulant
- Diaphoretic
- Expectorant
- Antitussive
- Digestive
- Carminative
- Antiemetic
- Anti-inflammatory
- Antimicrobial

Physiological virtues

In the digestive tract, Ginger increases stomach secretions and is a carminative. This makes it a good first aid choice for digestive colic, heartburn, and flatulence. It is considered especially valuable in cases of alcoholic gastritis. When there is diarrhoea due to the bowel being too relaxed, it can be helpful, but only if there is no inflammation. It has significant antimicrobial properties, so consider it in cases of gastrointestinal infections such as bacillary dysentery.

It is a circulatory stimulant, warming the body and increasing the blood flow to the periphery. Consider Ginger for patients who feel the cold and suffer with cold hands and feet or chilblains. It opens up the circulation and can improve a number of conditions, including hypertension and haemorrhoids. It acts as a diaphoretic: it stimulates sweating and helps to reduce fever. It is also antitussive, so can help the patient feel more comfortable if they are affected by a cough. Large doses can bring on menstruation, so pregnant women should be careful to keep consumption low, especially if there is a history of miscarriage. Ginger is famous for relieving nausea associated with travel or pregnancy sickness, so pregnant women should be especially aware of keeping their intake moderate. It can be very helpful for dysmenorrhea associated with uterine congestion and poor circulation. Drink the tea or apply a compress made with grated root to the abdomen. Do not leave the root in direct contact with the skin for long periods.

Ginger is significantly anti-inflammatory and is a good choice to include in prescriptions for chronic joint inflammation associated with poor circulation. It should not be prescribed for acute hot phases of inflammation. There is emerging evidence that Ginger may help to reduce cholesterol levels. This is perhaps linked to its anti-inflammatory action on the blood vessels, as well as its ability to invigorate the circulatory system.

Medicinal doses of Ginger can be taken as a decoction (1–2 slices added to a mug of water and simmered for 10 minutes), in capsule blends, as a passive infusion (it is best grated for this), as a tincture, an oxymel, or glycerite. The tincture is commonly added in small proportions to certain prescription tincture blends in order to encourage the herbs to be better absorbed and circulated in the body. It is better tolerated than Cayenne for this purpose. It should be prescribed with caution for people with a dry constitution or a sensitive stomach prone to ulcers. If you are not sure whether Ginger will be tolerated in medicinal doses, start slowly (gingerly!) and advise that it is taken with food rather than on an empty stomach.

Ginger can be applied topically as a foot or wrist bath, fomentation, compress, or infused oil. A Ginger hand-and-wrist-bath is a really good option for carpal tunnel syndrome or repetitive strain injuries in the hands or wrists. It can also be invaluable for martial artists who have to practice painful wrist locks. It is a rubefacient when applied to the skin. Avoid applying Ginger to areas that are already hot or inflamed. Although it is anti-inflammatory, it will be too heating in those circumstances.

In Tibetan and Chinese medicine, fresh and dried Ginger are considered different in action.

Fresh Ginger is preferred for colds, diarrhoea, and vomiting, while dried Ginger is prescribed for chronic bronchitis and coldness associated with shock. In Western herbal medicine Ginger is primarily considered to be a warming circulatory stimulant and a good anti-inflammatory.

Energetics

Ginger is hot and sweet, stimulating and dispersing. If your life feels stagnant, you may wish to connect with the warmth and fieriness of Ginger. If you are not able to consume much of it, just carry a piece around with you in your pocket and hold it in your hand regularly.

In Tibetan medicine

Ginger is known by various names within Tibetan medicine, according to how it is prepared. Dried Ginger is called *Menga* [སྨན་སྒ]. It has a hot and astringent taste with a bitter post-digestive taste. Its potency is hot, warm and fast-acting. It increases digestive heat and allows patients to ingest food when otherwise they would have felt nauseous. It treats *Pekén* and *rLung* disorders.

Medicinal Ginger, prepared by steaming, is called *Gajja* [སྒ་བྱ]. It is similar to *Menga,* as its taste is hot and astringent, and it has a bitter post-digestive taste. Its potency is also described as hot, warm, and fast-acting. It treats *Pekén* and *rLung* combinational disorders. It is said to thin the blood in diseases of cold blood, and it increases digestive heat. Semi-dried but still moist Ginger is called *Gasher.*

Fresh Ginger is considered to be sweet and sharp, with a potency that is hot and oily. It increases heat in the body and stimulates the digestion. It will increase the *Tripa* humour and counteract an excess of *Pékén.* It thins the blood, reduces pain and gas, as well as clearing the sinuses.

In my dispensary

I prescribe Ginger in individual tincture blends, tea blends, and capsule blends, as well as in topical applications. When patients need a bit of warmth and movement in their blends, I often choose Ginger at a rate of no more than 10% of the mix. I also include it in a circulation-supporting capsule blend alongside other stimulants, such as Prickly Ash, and antispasmodics, such as Cramp Bark. Ginger really is a very important and versatile herb in my dispensary.

This case illustrates Ginger's effectiveness as part of a capsule blend: 'Julia' was 69 years old and had been suffering with intermittent claudication for the past couple of years. On exertion she experienced intense pain in her lower legs, and it was preventing her from doing the things she loved. Her circulation had always been 'terrible', and she constantly had cold hands and feet. I prescribed two of my circulation-supporting herbs each day alongside a tincture blend containing Hawthorn and Ginger, among others. Within four weeks she noticed that she was able to walk further before the pain started; another couple of months later she was pain-free and feeling much lighter in herself. Her cold hands and feet were much better too.

'Susan' was 70 and recovering after chemotherapy treatment for endometrial cancer. She was doing well but was suffering with very uncomfortable peripheral neuropathy in the form of pain and numbness in her feet – so much so that she was feeling quite unsteady. I suggested that she had Ginger footbaths for 20 minutes daily. She reported a month later that her pain and numbness were already starting to feel much better.

Historical applications

The word for Ginger is similar in a great many different languages. This is because it would seem to have its roots in an ancestral language spoken by 'Austronesians'. The Austronesian people lived 6,000 years ago and migrated south from southern China across the Pacific to New Zealand, and west to Madagascar. They must have valued their Ginger greatly, taken it with them to new lands, and included its name in new languages as they developed.

The Romans considered Ginger to be a very precious commodity and taxed it. They brought it to Northern Europe: it is mentioned in Anglo-Saxon herbals from the ninth century. It was revered as a medicine and was thought to have come from the Garden of Eden. The Greeks used to wrap a piece of Ginger root in bread and eat it as a cure for indigestion. This is the origin of gingerbread.

Gerard wrote: '*Ginger, as Dioscorides reporteth, is right good with meat in sauces, or otherwise in conditures; for it is of an heating and digesting qualitie, and is profitable for the stomache, and effectually opposeth it selfe against all darknesse of the sight; answering the qualities and effects of Pepper.*'

Magical

Ginger is associated with fieriness, success, and power. Eating Ginger before performing spells is considered to increase their power. If you carry some Ginger in your pocket with intention, it will attract wealth. Alternatively, you can grow it, but do look after your plant if you are growing it as a symbol of attracting wealth.

Suggestions for the home apothecary

Ginger tincture

Thinly slice fresh Ginger root, and loosely fill a jar halfway. Cover with the highest percentage strength alcohol you can obtain, preferably at least 80% ABV. If you make your tincture with dried Ginger, you can get away with a lower-percentage alcohol, but, the main medicinal constituents being oil soluble, a higher percentage will result in a much better extraction. Leave to macerate in a cool, dark place for at least four weeks before draining, pressing and bottling.

Take 2.5 ml in hot water when you are in need of Ginger's warming and digestion-supporting virtues.

Ginger wrist soak or foot bath

Slice 5 cm of fresh Ginger and add to 1 litre of cold water. Slowly bring to the boil. Reduce the heat, and simmer gently for 20 minutes, with a lid on. Cool until comfortable and use as a wrist soak or foot bath, leaving the affected part in the decoction for 15–20 minutes. This preparation is excellent for relieving the discomfort of carpal tunnel syndrome or peripheral neuropathy.

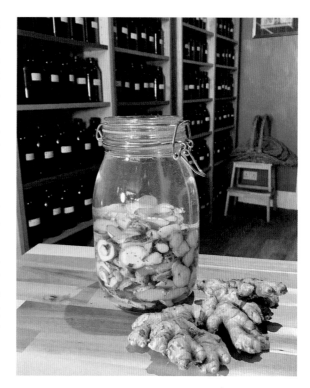

Ginkgo/Maidenhair Tree   🦋   *Ginkgo biloba*

'Ginkgo supports passage of the blood within the small vessels.'

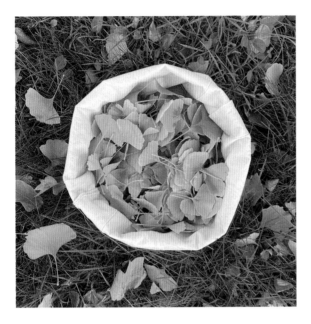

Ginkgo is our most ancient tree species, having existed in its current form for at least the last 270 million years. It is also the only seed-bearing plant to have fan shaped leaves with veins that radiate out to the edges. It is often considered to be a deciduous conifer, but it is actually in its own genus, called the *Ginkgoopsida*. Here in Europe, Ginkgo is often planted as an ornamental, so we are lucky to be able to connect with some lovely large specimens in parks and gardens. It even thrives as street trees in many of our cities.

Medicinal parts
▷ Leaves
▷ Seeds

Leaves are gathered when golden in the Autumn, and seeds are gathered for Chinese medicine.

Physiological actions

Summary
▷ Anti-inflammatory
▷ Antispasmodic
▷ Anticoagulant
▷ Peripheral circulatory stimulant

Physiological virtues

Ginkgo leaves are anti-inflammatory, relaxing the blood vessels, stimulating the circulation, and thinning the blood. They contain flavone glycosides (including ginkgolides), bioflavones, sitosterol, lactones, and anthocyanin. They are especially helpful where increased blood flow to the small vessels within the brain, eyes, and ears is an aim of herbal treatment. In general, Ginkgo has a reputation of helping to safeguard against memory loss as well as helping with deafness, tinnitus, vertigo, and failing eyesight. It can be a good choice to support patients with Raynaud's disease, as it stimulates the peripheral circulation. It is also worth considering for varicose veins, haemorrhoids, and where there are slow-healing leg ulcers. It can be prescribed topically as well as internally for these cases.

Herbalists generally work with whole herbs rather than isolated compounds, but it is interesting to note that ginkgolides have been shown to have a positive effect on treating severely irregular heartbeat as well as inhibiting the body's allergic response. These compounds may also protect against damage to nerve cells.

In traditional Chinese medicine the seeds are prescribed to support the lungs and kidneys, but I do not have experience of working with the seeds myself.

I was taught that Ginkgo should always be prescribed with great care, as it has a significant blood-thinning action. If a patient has fragile blood vessels or is on blood-thinning medication, long-term intake of Ginkgo is probably not a good idea. My clinical herbal tutor used to say that long-term intake of Ginkgo could put elderly patients at risk of a haemorrhagic stroke. The tone of my tutor's words when she said this has always stuck with me, and as a result, I am always quite cautious when considering Ginkgo for patients.

These days Ginkgo is widely promoted as a preventive against Alzheimer's disease and as a treatment for dementia, and I would urge that its suitability should be assessed in each case rather than being considered a blanket suggestion. Ironically, Ginkgo is also popular as a herb to aid recovery after a stroke, but this is usually over a time-limited period such as just three months. I would say that this strategy is best for cases of ischaemic rather than haemorrhagic stroke.

As always, it is important to consider the individual circumstances of each patient and to weigh up whether a herb is appropriate to that patient at that time. Simply viewing herbs as being good for particular named conditions may suit those selling health supplements, but it is not a good way of working with herbs for long-term chronic conditions. Acute conditions are a different matter.

Energetics
Ginkgo is sweet, bitter, astringent, neutral, dry.

In my dispensary
Ginkgo is not for everyone and certainly not something to take for many years without being sure it is suitable. Ideally any herb should only be taken for a short time, to support a patient while they adjust lifestyle and diet and while their body moves back into healthful balance. I admit that I find it disconcerting when new patients report that they have been self-prescribing Ginkgo for many years without any professional assessment as to its suitability for them. When I ask them why, they tell me 'I thought it would help safeguard my memory' or 'I wanted to improve my eyesight'. They say that the shop assistant in the health-food shop or the online vendor's website did not mention any reasons for caution. After such long-term intake, I often encourage these patients to switch to a handful of red and purple berries each day in their diet instead.

Ginkgo should be treated with respect. If you have been taking it for a long time, perhaps now is a good moment to take a good hard look at your lifestyle and make positive changes there instead. Definitely do not take Ginkgo if you are on blood-thinning or antiplatelet medication or if you are pregnant.

Here is a case where Ginkgo played a very positive role in supporting blood circulation to the brain: 'Michael' was 12 years old. When he was 5 years old, he had been in an accident in which he had received a severe blow to his head. This had unfortunately resulted in him sustaining an acquired brain injury. His motor skills were adversely affected, and he had a lot of difficulty remembering things and maintaining his focus. Michael's mum was very organized and showed me the notes and the brain scans from the time of his injury. The neurological consultants had explained that he was left with scarring and reduced blood flow to certain areas of his brain. While he would always be affected by his injury, his mum wanted to see if herbal medicine could help improve his short-term memory and his attention span. We decided to work with capsules, as he was used to taking pills and did not mind doing so. I prescribed a capsule blend containing Ginkgo along with St John's Wort, Wild Oats, and Yarrow. Michael was to take two size '0' capsules in the morning and another two at night.

He kept going with the regime, and his mum kept me posted: seven months after starting the herbal capsules, he had his annual review at the special school that he attended. Apparently, the teaching and support staff were very impressed with how, for the past three months, there had been a positive change in his behaviour. He seemed to be much more adult and sensible in his behaviour, and his attention span and recall were improving significantly. His mum said that she had also noticed quite a change in him at home. She knew that she was never going 'to get him back to how he had been before the accident', but she was very pleased at how the herbs were supporting him and making his life easier.

Historical applications

Ginkgos are treated with reverence in China and Japan, where they are often planted at sacred sites such as in the grounds of temples. In China the fruit symbolizes longevity and is eaten at weddings. In general, the East has a much longer lineage of understanding the medicinal virtues of Ginkgo, whereas Western herbal medicine's understanding of Ginkgo seems to be largely based on reductionist research that has been carried out since the 1960s. I would love to spend more time considering Eastern ways of working with Ginkgo to improve my under-

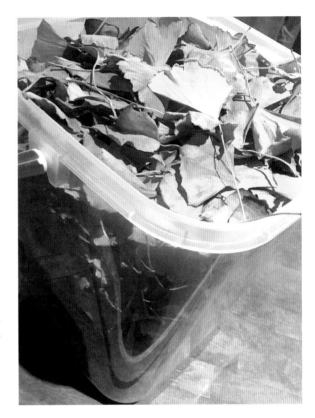

standing of this beautiful medicine. Learning about herbs is never-ending.

Suggestion for the home apothecary

Ginkgo tea

Add 2 tsp dried Ginkgo or 5 fresh leaves per cup, pour on boiling water, steep for 10 minutes. Drink occasionally if suffering from failing memory, poor eyesight, or tinnitus. Alternatively add a leaf to your daily tea blend every so often.

'Goat's Rue teaches us about moderation and excess.'

Goat's Rue is a beautiful and valuable plant in my herb garden. It grows well in deep moisture-retentive soil, and, being a legume, it brings extra fertility to the soil through its ability to fix nitrogen from the atmosphere. The beautiful lilac-coloured flowers have only a slight fragrance when still on the plant; however, once bruised, the leaves and stems emit a distinctive musky odour. Perhaps because of this odour, it is known as *Herba Rutae Caprariae* in the old herbals. Alternatively, this may be because it was fed to goats in order to encourage their milk production. It is an exuberant plant, self-seeding very readily; it has a tendency to take over the herb garden if not kept in check.

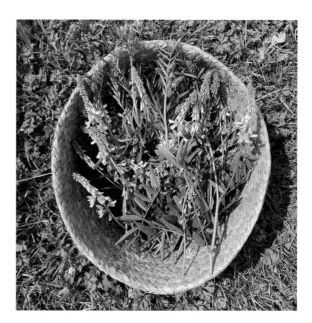

Medicinal parts
▷ Aerial parts

These are gathered while the plant is in flower.

Physiological actions

Summary
▷ Galactagogue
▷ Hypoglycaemic/blood sugar balancer
▷ Bitter
▷ Diaphoretic
▷ Vermifuge

Physiological virtues

King's American Dispensatory, 1905, stated that it has: '*a disagreeably bitter taste, and upon being chewed it imparts a dark yellowish colour to the saliva*'. They describe it as a diaphoretic that was prescribed to treat the plague and pestilential fevers, such as typhoid. They also mention its vermifuge properties and the fact that it was considered to be a stimulant to the nervous system. I find it a bit surprising that they add that '*it is seldom, if ever, prescribed in practice*'.

These days most people think of it as a galactagogue, helping to improve the quality and quantity of breast milk, but I was taught that it is primarily a herb to consider where there is a need to address high blood sugar states. Goat's Rue is rich in guanidine, which in 1918 was found to effectively lower blood glucose levels. The Type II diabetes drug, dimethylbiguanide – that is, Metformin – is a derivative of guanidine. Goat's Rue was instrumental in the development of various guanidine-derivative diabetes drugs, some of which were later discontinued due to toxicity and the potential side effects associated with the increased availability of insulin.

To me, Goat's Rue teaches us about excess and being happy when we have enough. This is especially appropriate when we think of its ability to stabilize blood sugar in those who have become insulin-resistant. It helps the cells of the body become more sensitive to insulin again and to recognize when the blood sugar is moving beyond a healthy level. In order to heal ourselves from a tendency to insulin resistance, we also have to change our diet and our attitude to food. We need to choose lower-glycaemic-index foods and look at our portion sizes. Goat's Rue helps to reverse our tendency to want more and more.

As a galactagogue, it helps our body in its drive to look after our baby and give it maximum nourishment through an increase in breast milk production. It takes a lot of energy to create breast milk, and Goat's Rue can help us to do this while still leaving a little energy for ourselves. Caution is required, as this is a herb that will lower blood sugar. I do not recommend taking it as a simple. Try it mixed in with other galactagogue herbs, so that the amount you are prescribing, or taking, is not too great.

People sometimes ask me whether it is safe to work with Goat's Rue due to the presence of biguanides. My answer to this is that it is very different to work with a whole plant rather than isolated, concentrated extracts. In addition, Goat's Rue is prescribed carefully with other herbs in a personalized prescription, so the dose of each herb is not as large as when prescribed as a simple.

Goat's Rue, as a whole-herb preparation, can even play a supportive role for Type I diabetics who have been injecting insulin for many years. Over time, in these cases, insulin resistance tends to creep in, and the patient begins to respond less effectively to their dose of insulin, leading to higher and higher blood sugar levels. Goats Rue, prescribed cautiously with appropri-

ate patient monitoring, can be a game changer. I must emphasize here that it is not intended to replace insulin therapy, but it will help patients to respond better to it.

Goat's Rue can also play a supportive role in the treatment of patients suffering with polycystic ovary syndrome. We know that Metformin is prescribed allopathically to reduce insulin secretion and blood sugar levels in such patients, so it is worth considering Goat's Rue in a multiple herb prescription as a temporary support while addressing the underlying root causes of the problem.

Energetics
Goat's Rue is bitter and astringent, and cooling. It helps us to helps us to recognize that moderation is a healthy trait and to appreciate and value what we already have. If you have a tendency to strong cravings, whether for sugar or for other non-food objects, you may want to consider introducing a little Goat's Rue into your life for a short time.

In Tibetan medicine
As a cooling bitter, this is a herb that is especially indicated in conditions of excess *Tripa*, where digestive support is needed. It should be prescribed in moderation in all cases, especially where there is a tendency to an excess of *rLung*.

In my dispensary
I most often prescribe Goat's Rue to help patients lower their blood sugar when there is insulin resistance or Type II diabetes. I have had very good results by working with it in this way. I also tend to prescribe it, in personalized blends, to patients suffering with polycystic ovary syndrome. Here it plays its part with other herbs as well as lifestyle and dietary changes, so it can be harder to single out the action of Goat's Rue

for particular praise. However, I believe that its influence is very important to the success of the treatment as a whole, and I would not want to be without it in my dispensary.

This case illustrates very well the influence that Goat's Rue's can have. 'Julia' was 70 years old and was a Type II diabetic. She was not doing well on her regime of Metformin, saying that it did not seem to be working and that she felt sick much of the time. She was too exhausted to exercise, and her mood was low. She was trying to eat a low-glycaemic-index diet with plenty of protein, but she admitted that she had a sweet tooth and often turned to biscuits and pastries as a 'pick me up' when she felt tired. She often liked to make herself cheese on toast as an easy meal, because she was so tired. Matters were made worse by the fact that she was not drinking enough water. I explained about the importance of sticking to a low glycaemic index diet and drinking plenty of water, and she agreed that she would do her best to change her ways. She had a prescription herbal tea blend rather than a tincture blend, as she wished to avoid alcohol. Goat's Rue formed 10% of the blend alongside other digestive and circulation-supporting herbs. She was to drink two cups each day. Four weeks later she was feeling much less exhausted, and the sickness had completely gone. She had found it much easier than expected to quit the sweet biscuits and pastries, and she was drinking more water. She realized that her well-being was worth making an effort for, and she was rewarded with better

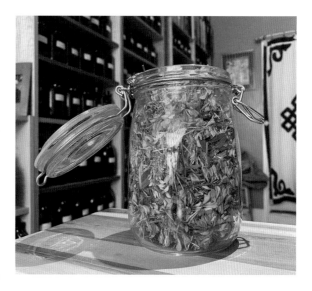

mental clarity, more energy, and an increasingly positive outlook on life.

Historical applications

In old times Goat's Rue was much prescribed for '*malignant fevers*' and the '*plague*', since it encourages sweating. This is why one of its old names is '*Pestilenzkraut*'. It was also a favourite for getting rid of parasitic worms and as a cure for the bites of serpents.

Culpeper wrote: '*A bath made of it is very refreshing to wash the feet of persons tired with over-walking. In the northern countries they use this herb for making their cheeses instead of Rennet.*'

Magical

It is said that placing Goat's Rue into a shoe cures and prevents rheumatism.

Goji 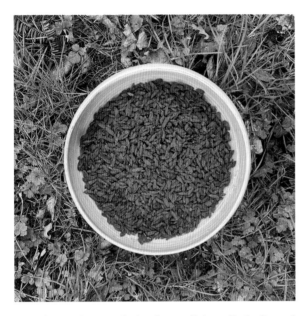 *Lycium barbarum*

'Goji berry restores and protects the liver.'

Goji berry is a tonic herb, traditionally believed to promote long life. Its name is linked to the Chinese character *Gou*, which means 'wolf': hence its other name, 'Wolfberry'. Therapeutically, it is primarily a tonic liver-protective herb. Through its positive action on the liver, it improves many areas of our health, including our eyesight. It is especially valuable to protect the liver when taken during harsh allopathic treatment regimes, such as chemotherapy.

Medicinal parts
▷ Berries

Physiological actions

Summary
▷ Hepatic/hepato-protective
▷ Tonic
▷ Adaptogen
▷ Blood sugar balancing

Physiological virtues

Goji berries are a blood and liver tonic, improving the circulation and encouraging better uptake of nutrients into cells. They are a good choice for those suffering with symptoms of weakness and debility, such as vertigo, tinnitus, or recurrent headaches. Goji berries are helpful in cases of low libido and sexual dysfunction. They are also well indicated as a general support during convalescence or in later life. They bring colour to the cheeks and restore strength.

They are rich in xanthophyll carotenoids, which support liver function. They help to balance blood sugar and bring the liver back towards health if it is diseased. While cases of chronic hepatitis B, liver cirrhosis, and hepatocellular carcinoma may not be curable, Goji berries can play a very helpful role in managing these conditions and supporting patients who suffer with them. They are also hepato-protective for patients undergoing potentially harsh treatments, such as chemotherapy. The carotenoids protect the liver cells from damage caused by exposure to toxic compounds. As well as being a liver tonic, they are also considered a kidney tonic. I think that this can sometimes be due to encouraging better liver function, which, in turn, supports the kidneys when they have been having to compensate.

Consider Goji berries for those with failing eyesight. They contain taurine, an amino acid with antioxidant, anti-inflammatory and immune-modulating properties that also supports retinal health. In Tibetan medicine there is a traditional understanding of the link between liver health and eye health, so it is not surprising that Goji berries are an excellent eye tonic as well as a liver support.

In Tibetan and Chinese medicine Goji berries have long been prescribed to reduce and resolve tumours.

Goji berries can be taken as a food, being added to smoothies or included in soups, muesli, or porridge. They can easily be prepared as a tea, by simply infusing 1 tsp, heaped, in a cup of boiling water. It is probably better to take them as a decoction, though, especially when they are being taken for medicinal purposes. They form part of my Fu Zheng decoction, a slow extraction of various adaptogens and tonic herbs with traditional liver-protective and tumour-reducing actions. I also make Goji berry tincture and prescribe it in personalized blends, as needed.

Energetics
Goji berry is sweet, sour, neutral, and moist.

In Tibetan medicine
Goji berry is known as *De tserma* [འདྲེ་ཙེར་མ།] in Tibetan. It has a sweet-to-sour taste and a post-digestive taste that is sweet. Its potency is neutral. *De tserma* is described as treating anaemia, loss of kidney and liver strength, dizziness, and blurred vision in Tibetan medicine. As a medicine with a sweet and sour taste, it is well suited to patients who are deficient in the grounding energies of Earth and Water – that is, those patients who have an excess of *rLung*. Since *rLung* conditions also tend to be dry, the moistening aspect of Goji berry is also very helpful.

In my dispensary
I usually prescribe Goji berry as a tincture or as part of a Fu Zheng decoction designed to support patients going through cancer treatments. I also often reach for Goji when people need building up after a long period of stress. Goji seems to help people feel more grounded and less 'hollow'. (For more information on the Fu Zheng decoction, see Ashwagandha.)

Historical applications
Goji berries have long been part of Chinese culture. There are many folk tales circulating about the power of Goji berries to enormously lengthen people's lifespan. Whether or not these can be taken literally does not matter to me, since Goji berries are a very positive and supportive adaptogen for most people. I think it is fair to say that they will prolong life and quality of life if taken in the context of a healthy lifestyle.

Suggestion for the home apothecary
Goji berry tincture
Fill a jar one third full with Goji berries and fill to the top with 25% ABV alcohol. Leave in a dark place for at least four weeks, then drain, press, and bottle. Take 5 ml in a little hot water daily, or make a blend with other suitable adaptogens and take 5 ml of the blend.

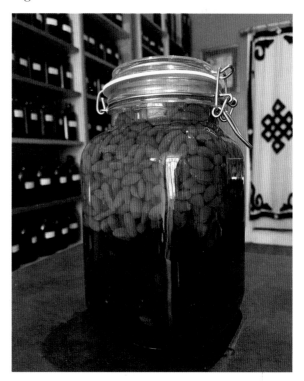

Goldenrod 🍃 *Solidago canadensis/S. virgaurea*

'Solidago makes us whole again.'

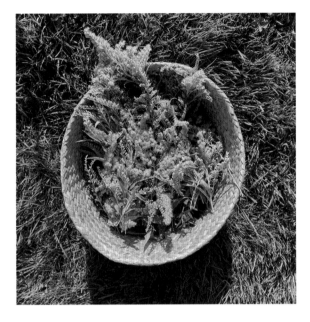

The specific name of Goldenrod, '*Solidago*', comes from the Latin *solidare* – to make whole, and one of its country names is 'Woundwort'. It is a medicine chest in itself. When you look at all its very many medicinal virtues, you can see that it is very aptly named. If you only have a handful of herbs in your home dispensary, this should be one of them.

Medicinal parts
- Leaves
- Flowers

Physiological actions

Summary
- Diuretic
- Astringent
- Anticatarrhal
- Antiseptic
- Diaphoretic
- Carminative
- Stimulant

Physiological virtues

This gorgeous aromatic herb has a very wide range of virtues. It is astringent and diuretic and is a good choice to help the passing of bladder stones. Its astringency reduces inflammation, and it has antiseptic properties, making it excellent for urinary-tract infections such as cystitis, urethritis, and nephritis. As well as improving kidney function, it contains flavonoids (rutin, quercetin, and quercitrin), which protect the capillaries within the kidneys and decrease the secretion of proteins in the urine. Weiss, in his book, *Herbal Medicine*, considers it specific for when anuria or oliguria develop in acute nephritis, but a different strategy is required for chronic or sub-acute conditions, when increasing kidney output is not always desirable.

Its virtue of encouraging more efficient elimination of toxins via the kidneys makes it helpful to consider for arthritis. It is also helpful for skin disorders such as eczema, a strong infusion being applied topically along with a weaker one (made with approximately 1 gram of the fresh herb per cup), being taken internally. As a gargle it soothes inflammations of the mouth, and it makes a good douche for flare-ups of thrush, the saponins present being specific against Candida infection. In the past it was a herb of choice to treat diphtheria, being prescribed as a spray, as well as internally.

Goldenrod is anticatarrhal and is therefore a good choice for upper respiratory infections or for allergic rhinitis accompanied by a build-up of catarrh. It is stimulant, boosting the metabolism, and, when taken as a warm infusion, it acts as a diaphoretic. It is also carminative, easing spasms of the smooth muscle in the digestive tract while enlivening the digestion and increasing the production of bile. Its astringency makes it a good first aid treatment for diarrhoea. On top of all of that, it helps to relieve period pain and treats amenorrhoea.

Energetics

Goldenrod is bitter and astringent.

In Tibetan medicine

As a herb with a bitter and astringent taste, Goldenrod is well suited to treating imbalances of *Tripa*. *Tripa* is counteracted by blends of herbs that are bitter, astringent, and sweet: its qualities of being diaphoretic, anti-inflammatory, and antimicrobial bear this out.

In my dispensary

The two *Solidagos* mentioned can be prescribed interchangeably. I tend to work with *S. canadensis*, because that is what I have growing in my herb garden. I was given the original plant by my herbal tutor, Barbara, and it reminds me of her to have it there.

Goldenrod is a key ingredient in my kidney-supporting tea blend and capsule blend. I frequently prescribe it to patients in their individual prescription when their presentation calls for it. I really would not want to be without it.

Historical applications

Gerard said that '*Goldenrod has in times past been had in greater estimation and regard than in these days, I have known the dried herb that came from beyond the seas sold. . . for half a crown an ounce. But since it was found in Hampstead Wood. . . no man will give half a crown for a hundredweight of it: which plainly setteth forth our inconsistency and sudden mutability, esteeming no longer of any thing*

(how precious soever it may be) than while it is strange and rare.'

Magical

Goldenrod is associated with divination and money. It is said that if you wish to see your future love you should wear a piece of Goldenrod: he or she will appear the next day. A flowering stem of Goldenrod can be used for divination. If you hold it in your hand, the flower nods in the direction of hidden or lost objects, or where buried treasure lies. Also, if a Goldenrod plant springs up by the door of the house, the family living there will soon have unexpected good fortune. Perhaps not surprisingly, Goldenrod is chosen for money spells.

Suggestion for the home apothecary

Goldenrod tea

Dry Goldenrod for medicinal teas and external washes throughout the year.

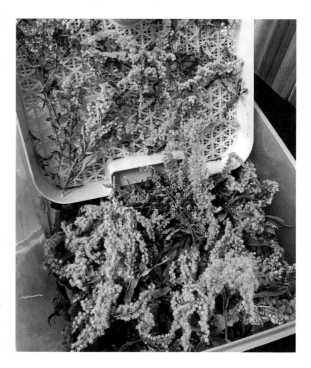

Goldenseal 🌿 *Hydrastis canadensis*

'Goldenseal is an excellent mucous membrane tonic which must be sourced sustainably and prescribed sparingly.'

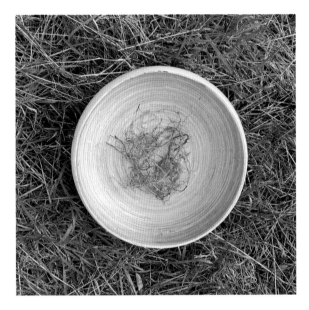

Goldenseal is a species native to North America, and the indigenous peoples there are the knowledge holders for this wonderful and precious herb. I am sure that my understanding of its actions is woefully inadequate compared to that of the original knowledge-holders, so please do not take my words to be comprehensive as regards what this plant can offer as a herbal medicine.

The name 'Hydrastis' comes from two Greek words, referring to water and 'to accomplish', and perhaps this signifies its primary action as a mucous membrane tonic. Its common name, 'Goldenseal', refers to the markings that form on its dormant rhizomes after the stems have died down. Where each stem had grown, a small depression is formed. With the rhizome being such a bright golden colour, the depression has the appearance of sealing wax that has been stamped with a round seal.

Goldenseal is a valuable medicine that has become much too scarce to be sourced from wild harvesting. If we want to take it or prescribe it, we should find a sustainably cultivated source or aim to grow our own supplies. We should also think very hard about whether it is appropriate in our circumstances and whether we are planning to work with it holistically or allopathically.

Medicinal parts
▹ Rhizomes
▹ Roots

Physiological actions

Summary
▹ Bitter
▹ Mucous membrane tonic
▹ Antimicrobial
▹ Anti-inflammatory
▹ Astringent
▹ Styptic
▹ Uterine stimulant

Physiological virtues

Goldenseal is an outstanding mucous membrane tonic. It has a healing affinity with the eyes, nose, throat, and ears. It is also a very effective support for the mucous membranes of the stomach, intestines, and vagina. When prepared as a dilute infusion or decoction, it is an excellent eye wash or mouthwash. Dilute preparations can also be applied as a douche to treat vaginal infections, or as a topical skin treatment for psoriasis. They can also be helpful for haemorrhoids.

The colour of the bright yellow roots is indicative of high levels of berberine. Berberine is an isoquinoline alkaloid that is antibacterial. These antibacterial properties make Goldenseal a highly sought-after herb. Sadly, I have seen an increasing tendency for people to self-prescribe Goldenseal as a natural 'antibiotic' and antifungal over long periods of time. They tell me that they are taking it daily for gut flora imbalances such as Candida overgrowth, or as a preventive, but at the same time they do not support this with appropriate dietary and lifestyle changes. This is an exploitative way to work with such a precious plant. Taking it in this way will not produce the desired results and will lead to the same problems as taking allopathic antibiotics inappropriately.

Goldenseal is bitter and stimulates the digestive system. Its bitterness means that it can act as a mild laxative (but there are plenty of other more abundant herbs to choose for this). It is an excellent anti-inflammatory and styptic for the digestive mucous membranes. This means that it can be a very good short-term support for gastritis, ulcers, or IBS. As with its exploitation for its antibiotic actions, there is also a widespread tendency for people to take it over long periods to 'manage' digestive tract inflammation and lesions. This is not holistic; it should not be necessary if appropriate dietary and lifestyle changes are made. If long-term herbal support is absolutely unavoidable, more abundant herbs, such as Oregon Grape, Meadowsweet, and Calendula, should be considered.

Goldenseal contains the alkaloid canadine, which stimulates the uterus. This is the reason why Goldenseal should be avoided in pregnancy. It also contains hydrastine, which constricts the blood vessels and stimulates the autonomic nervous system. It can raise the blood pressure, so should be avoided by people with hypertension.

Energetics
Goldenseal is bitter and astringent.

In my dispensary
I do work with Goldenseal in my clinic but reserve it for short-term support of patients who need it. I love its mucous-membrane-toning actions and choose it as an ingredient in mouth and eye washes for acute presentations. I also add it, in a small proportion, to acute mixes for viral and bacterial infections.

Historical applications
The Cherokee mixed it with bear fat and prescribed it topically as a treatment for wounds, ulcers, and inflamed eyes; the Iroquois prescribed it internally, for whooping cough, fevers, and heart problems.

Magical
Goldenseal is precious and is therefore a potent symbol of wealth, health, and abundance.

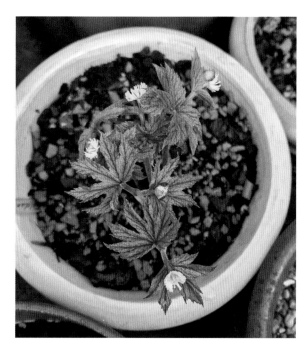

Greater Celandine 🌿 *Chelidonium majus*

'Greater Celandine helps us to clear away obstructions and to escape entrapment.'

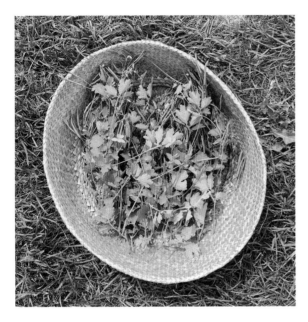

Greater Celandine is an unassuming member of the Poppy family, but it demands to be noticed, because the slightest brush against it will leave a bright yellow stain of sap on our skin or clothes. It is this sap that is the acrid, bitter, active part of the herb.

Medicinal parts

▷ Aerial parts

These should be fresh, with sap.

Physiological actions

Summary

▷ Bitter
▷ Cholagogue
▷ Purgative
▷ Diuretic
▷ Alterative

Physiological virtues

Greater Celandine is most often thought of as a very intense bitter, helpful to stimulate bile production and therefore helping to remove obstructions in the gallbladder and to resolve jaundice. It is also purgative, diuretic, and alterative, cleansing toxins from the body through enhancing the production of bile as well as stimulating sweating and diuresis. It can be prescribed as a tincture in drop doses or as a small proportion in a blend, or it can be taken by the wineglassful when prepared as an infusion. This is made by steeping one ounce (28 g) of dried herb in 570 ml/1 pint of boiling water. This is taken in wineglassful doses to treat jaundice, eczema, and scrofulous diseases. It is extremely bitter but should not be sweetened.

The bright orange/yellow sap is a traditional and effective topical remedy for warts and verrucas. The sap added to milk is said to be an effective treatment to remove white opaque spots from the cornea but I do not have experience of this myself.

In the United Kingdom, Greater Celandine is on the Schedule 20 list of potentially toxic herbs, the prescribing of which is strictly controlled. Practicing medical herbalists have to keep within particular low-dosage limits.

Energetics

Greater Celandine is bitter and cooling.

In my dispensary

Greater Celandine is a herb that needs to be prescribed with some caution as an internal medicine. I do call on it where gallbladder support is needed, but I make sure it is in small amounts within a personalized prescription blend. The bitterness of Greater Celandine helps to stimulate bile production and relax spasms of the bile duct, assisting with flushing out small stones or obstructions.

I make a wart and verruca ointment with fresh Greater Celandine tops infused into olive oil with Lavender and Tree of Life foliage. It is a popular off-the-shelf product in my clinic and very often effective when other wart treatments have failed. Persistent application over a couple of weeks is required for best results. I see it as helping our immune systems to recognize that a wart or verruca is present and that action is needed. Perhaps this is a physical manifestation of its connection with releasing us from entrapment.

Historical applications

Pliny named it 'Chelidonium' from the Greek word *Chelidon*, which means swallow, because it comes into flower when the swallows arrive, and it fades when they leave. It is also associated with swallows because the acrid juice can be applied to the cornea of the eye in order to remove any film that has developed there. Pliny writes that this property was discovered by the swallows. On this Gerard wrote: '*The juice of the herbe is good to sharpen the sight, for it clenseth and consumeth away slimie things that cleave about the ball of the eye, and hinder the sight, and especially being boiled in hony in a brasen vessel, as Dioscorides teacheth.*'

He also wrote that '*The root being chewed is reported to be good against the tooth-ache. . . . The juice must be drawn forth in the beginning of Summer, and dried in the sunne, saith Dioscorides recommended it for Hawks, saying: "The root cut into small pieces is good to be given unto Hauks against sundry diseases, whereunto they are subject."*'

Maud Grieve's entry for Celandine mentions that in the fourteenth century a drink made from it was considered '*good for the blood*'.

Parkinson described it as: '*hot and dry in the third degree, and of a clensing facultie*'. . . . '*It openeth the obstructions of the Liver and Gall, and thereby helpeth the yellow Iaundies, the herbe or the rootes being boyled in white wine with a few Anniseedes and drunke: Mattiolus saith that if the greene herbe be worne in their shoes that have the yellow Iaundies, so as their bare feet may tread thereon, it will helpe them of it. . . . The juice thereof taken fasting, is held to bee of singular good use against the Plague or Pestilence.*' He also recommended it for fungal infections, warts and growths: '*The juice often applied to tetters, ringworms or other such like spreading Cancers, will quickly kill their sharpnesse and heale them also: the same rubbed often upon warts will take them away.*'

Magical

Celandine is said to help us escape entrapment or imprisonment, whether that is physical, emotional, or psychic. It is worn next to the skin and should be replaced every three days for this purpose. Its reputation for helping people to avoid

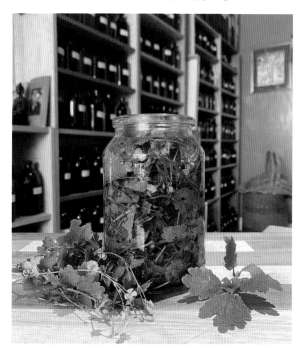

imprisonment meant that defendants used to wear it in court in order to win the favour of the judge or jury.

Suggestion for the home apothecary

Infused oil for warts and verrucae

Take fresh Greater Celandine, cut it up, and put it into a jar. Cover with mild olive oil and leave for four weeks before straining and bottling. When straining, be careful to decant the oil fraction only, leaving any watery layer in the bottom of the jar. Apply to warts and verrucae twice a day. The oil can be set into an ointment for convenience. Only make enough for one year, as Greater Celandine preparations (including tinctures) deteriorate 12 months after extraction.

Hawthorn 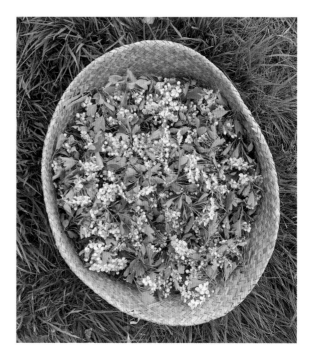 *Crataegus monogyna*

'Hawthorn supports the circulatory system and helps us to maintain boundaries.'

Imagine the triumphalism that would accompany the discovery of a drug that treats congestive heart failure, coronary artery disease, and associated conditions such as hypertension and angina completely safely and without side effects. Imagine the television advertising, the press launches, and the awards. The company responsible for the development of this wonder drug would be proud to point out that it was able to dilate the coronary arteries, improving cardiac circulation, and was even able to offer a protective effect against the build-up of atheroma in the entire cardiovascular system. It is ironic that all of these properties and more exist in the humble Hawthorn, yet in many countries it continues to be overlooked as an option for patients who would benefit from it. Luckily its true value is recognized in Brazil, China, the Czech Republic, Slovakia, France, Germany, Hungary, Russia, and Switzerland, where it is included in their official pharmacopoeias and is prescribed often.

Medicinal parts

  ▷ Blossom
  ▷ Leaves
  ▷ Berries

Physiological actions

Summary

  ▷ Cardiotonic
  ▷ Cardiovascular tonic
  ▷ Astringent
  ▷ Nervine

Physiological virtues

Hawthorn is an excellent herb for toning the cardiovascular system and therefore supporting the circulation. It increases coronary blood flow, helping the heart to beat more strongly in the presence of less oxygen, and it decreases blood pressure through reducing peripheral vascular resistance. It can also gently raise low blood pressure through its toning action on peripheral vessels: a wonderful example of amphoteric action, the herb helping our system to move to a healthier norm rather than forcing a change on the body.

It can reduce or resolve arrhythmia, and it can treat congestive heart failure, coronary artery disease, and associated conditions, such as hypertension and angina.

It seems that taking Hawthorn regularly actually enables the body to reduce a build-up of atheroma in the vessels, as well as enabling the heart to function more efficiently in the presence of less oxygen through improving myocardial tolerance of oxygen deficiency. This is a particularly useful property in a patient who is suffering from atherosclerosis, where the supply of oxygenated blood to the heart could be significantly reduced. Hawthorn also acts to lower blood pressure, and it is a good remedy to consider where there is any form of arrhythmia or possibility of heart weakness.

Hawthorn supports us slowly and steadily, low doses usually being prescribed over a long period of time. Care should be taken when considering Hawthorn for patients who are already taking allopathic heart medication, especially Digitalis drugs.

As well as supporting the heart and central cardiovascular system, Hawthorn is also especially helpful for peripheral circulatory disorders. I often think of Hawthorn for intermittent claudication, venous stasis, and hypertension. Through its effects on promoting a more vibrant circulatory system it is also worth considering in cases of senile dementia and Raynaud's syndrome.

The astringency of Hawthorn needs to be considered carefully in cases where there is excessive tension and dryness in the digestive tract, leading to habitually sluggish bowel. Too much Hawthorn could worsen the problem. In these circumstances prescribe in low doses or choose a blend, rather than prescribing it as a simple, for example. I generally prescribe herbs in blends in any case.

Energetics

Hawthorn berries are sour, astringent, and sweet; Hawthorn blossom is astringent and cooling. As well as its well-researched physiological cardiovascular benefits, Hawthorn brings a powerful emotional and energetic message of healing to the body. It has a soft, loving, heart-healing aspect, helping people to release long-held hurt and trauma. Over the years I have seen many patients who report improvements in their ability to 'digest and accept' bereavement, trauma, and other distressing 'heartbreaks' after taking Hawthorn.

Hawthorn may be gentle and healing, but it is also strong and thorny. It can help us to enforce firm and confident boundaries in our lives. As the inner boundaries of our circulatory system become less inflamed and more toned, so we feel more able to enforce our own external boundaries. People who need Hawthorn usually do not realise that they need to create firmer boundaries. Hawthorn helps us to see the need for boundaries more clearly. Sometimes those boundaries are with ourselves in moderating excessive demands that we place upon ourselves. Contrast this with the energetic property of Shepherd's Purse, where the person realizes that they are giving too much away but are too drained and exhausted to do anything about it.

Again and again, I hear from patients who are feeling able to say 'no' for the first time after a course of Hawthorn. How can we heal ourselves and fulfil our true life's purpose if we feel unable to stay on track and say 'no' to things that will scatter our energy and distract us from our path?

In Tibetan medicine

Astringency is helpful in *Tripa* and *Pekén* disorders but should be prescribed in moderation for those with an excess of *rLung*. The astringent taste brings Air and Earth elements into the body. Better, in cases of excess *rLung*, to choose the berries, with their predominantly sour taste, bringing Fire and Earth into the body. *rLung* is best counteracted by sweet, sour, and salty-tasting herbs.

In my dispensary

I tend to make Hawthorn tincture from the berries alone and reserve the blossom for teas and capsules. Mostly, patients needing Hawthorn will receive it as a berry tincture in a blend designed for their unique circumstances. I do prescribe Hawthorn blossom capsules for patients with excess *rLung*, provided that their diet and lifestyle have been addressed and they are taking significant steps to balance their previously 'light and rough' behaviours and diet.

I feel that the case of 58-year-old 'Colin' is a good illustration of the power of Hawthorn. He had been diagnosed with congestive heart failure and atrial fibrillation about eighteen months prior to our first meeting. At the time of his diagnosis, his cardiac consultant had told him that he should not expect to live much beyond a further two years. As his predicted end of life approached, Colin had got in touch with me. He explained that he was seeking herbal support, with the hope of 'staying alive for longer'.

When he first became a patient, he was on a multitude of cardiovascular-system-supporting drugs, including Warfarin (a blood thinner) and digoxin. As I took his case history, there were two major points that struck me. First, he complained that the drugs were making him feel unwell, and he wanted to see if he could cope without them. He had, in my view, the rather dangerous expectation that he would be able to quit his medication as soon as he started taking herbal medicine. Given his medical circumstances, his attitude made me a quite nervous. The second thing that struck me about Colin's case was that he seemed quite angry about various things that had happened during his life. He told me that he did not want to die before he had been able to resolve his issues.

I really wanted to do what I could to help him. I emphasized the importance of him sticking to his allopathic drug regime alongside the herbal medicines that I would be prescribing. I explained that we would have to take a slow and steady approach in order to avoid any adverse herb drug interactions. He agreed this strategy, and we started with drop doses of Hawthorn, Motherwort, and Rose, with a view to increasing this gradually, under close monitoring from both his allopathic team and me. After a year of treatment, he was not only still living, but he was feeling very much better. He had noticed that his energy levels were improving, and he was able to walk further and do more than he had been able to before he started herbal treatment. He had (with the full blessing of his GP), been able to cease some of the original drugs that he had been prescribed and reduce others. Over time, the herbs in his prescription stayed the same, but the dosage gradually increased, from just a few drops at first to 5 ml a day two years after commencing treatment. It was clear that the herbs had supported him physiologically in improving his circulation, helping to reduce his atrial fibrillation and strengthening his heart. As well as physical improvements, he also experienced a softening of his attitude. You could say that there had been a 'heart-opening' effect. He was able to continue with his efforts to reconcile and forgive the wrongs he had experienced in his life.

The following is another case that illustrates Hawthorn's ability to heal the physical and the

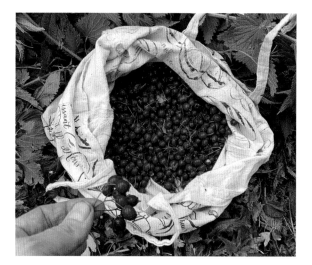

emotional heart. 'Victoria' was 67 years old. She was exhausted all the time, and suffering with angina and hypertension. On top of that, she had severe anxiety and regular panic attacks. The anxiety had started when, a few months previously, she had lost a younger sibling to a massive heart attack. She was grieving and very frightened that she, too, was at risk of a similar outcome. Victoria was taking various hypotensive drugs, but her blood pressure remained too high, and she was under pressure from her GP to increase her medication. She wanted to try herbs alongside instead.

We had a long chat about the likely role that grief and fear were playing in perpetuating her symptoms, and we agreed that I would give her Hawthorn berry tincture as a simple and a blend of calming nervine herbs to support her. Four weeks later she was feeling much less anxious, and her chest pains had lessened. After another four weeks, her blood pressure had come down to 140/88, and she was no longer experiencing any chest pains. Her energy levels were better; she was feeling much more positive and was more trusting in her body. Over the next few months she continued to do well, and we gradually reduced her herbal regime down to two Hawthorn blossom and Rose petal capsules each day. One month after starting the Hawthorn and Rose capsules, she told me that she had quite suddenly been able to face clearing her late sibling's flat, a task that she had been delaying for over a year. The Hawthorn and Rose blend had produced a significant emotional shift now that her cardiovascular symptoms had eased.

Historical applications

Lyte, in his *New Herball*, referred to it as White Thorne, saying: '*The fruit of White Thorne is drie and astringent . . . as some of the latter writers affirme, it is good against the gravell and the stone.*'

Later it became known as a heart medicine. Lloyd and Felter, in their *King's American Dispensatory* of 1905, wrote of *Crataegus oxycantha*: '*The fruit and bark of this shrub, or small tree, have been introduced into medicine as a heart remedy. . . . Claims are made for this drug as a curative remedy for organic and functional heart disorders, including cardiac hypertrophy, with mitral regurgitation from valvular insufficiency, and angina pectoris. Sometimes spinal hyperemia is associated with the latter, when both are said to be relieved by drug.*' The drug should be studied with a view to its adaptability to cases '*characterized by pain, precordial oppression, dyspnoea, rapid and feeble heart action, evidence of cardiac hypertrophy, valvular insufficiency, and marked anaemia. Prof J A Jeancon MD, employs it for venous stasis.*'

Magical

One of its names is Hagthorn, because each plant was believed to be a witch who had transformed themselves into a tree. It is also known as 'Huath', 'Bread and Cheese', 'May Blossom', and 'Mayflower', and it is traditionally chosen to decorate Maypoles. The blossom is believed to enhance fertility, while the leaves are believed to maintain chastity or celibacy.

If worn as an amulet, it promotes happiness and alleviates depression and sadness. It protects against lightning, and, if kept in a house, no evil ghosts may enter. Placed in a crib, it will guard the child from evil spells.

Suggestion for the home apothecary

Hawthorn blossom capsules

You will need thoroughly dried Hawthorn blossom and empty vegetarian capsules, which can be sourced from various herbal retailers. I choose size '0'. Take dried Hawthorn blossom and powder it in a food processor or a coffee grinder that you keep just for herbal medicine.

Pass the powder through a fine sieve, saving the coarser pieces for tea or for later regrinding. Put the fine powder into a small bowl deep enough to contain about 2.5 cm of powder. Separate the two halves of each capsule, and dab the large section into the powder until it is full. It is easiest to keep the open end of the capsule below the surface of the powder between each dab to start with, otherwise the powder can fall out as you go. Once the capsule is properly full, the powder is more amenable to staying in place. Place the capsule 'lid' on securely, and pop the capsule into your storage jar. Repeat until all the powder has been encapsulated, or you have made as many capsules as you need. Store any spare powder separately in a labelled, airtight jar. Take 1–2 capsules each day, if suitable for your circumstances.

If there is an element of unresolved grief or trauma held in the heart area, mix powders of Hawthorn blossom with Rose petals in equal parts. Take 2 a day when you are feeling ready to start to release and process it.

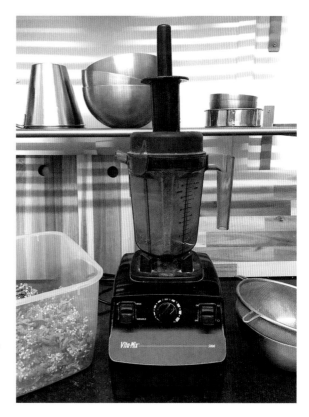

Honeysuckle 🍃 *Lonicera periclymenum*

'Honeysuckle is cooling and antiviral, being especially supportive to the respiratory system.'

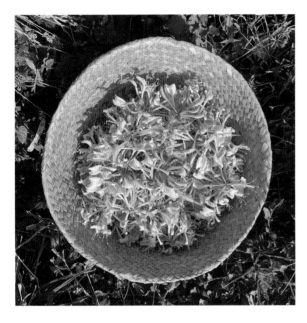

Honeysuckle is a beautiful wild climbing plant which flowers in June. If you are out walking, you will smell it before you see it. The flowers have a fabulous and slightly intoxicating fragrance. Gathering Honeysuckle is one of the highlights of my foraging year. It is known as Honeysuckle because it is rich in very sweet nectar, something that country children know. Other county names are Woodbine and Goat's Leaf.

Medicinal parts
- Flowers

There are many different species of Honeysuckle, so plant parts can vary between different species. In the United Kingdom, only the flowers of *Lonicera periclymenum* are harvested, being careful to avoid including leaves, seeds, or berries because of their significant emetic and cathartic properties.

Physiological actions

Summary
- Anti-inflammatory
- Antiviral
- Antibacterial
- Sudorific
- Antispasmodic
- Expectorant
- Nervine

Physiological virtues

The flowers are antiviral, antibacterial, and anti-inflammatory. They are sudorific (induce sweating), which means that their action can cool the body and can be helpful as part of a strategy for easing fever, menopausal hot flushes, or other over-heated conditions.

They are very supportive of the respiratory system, both in easing the symptoms of colds and flu, but also in relaxing the bronchi and bronchioles, so helping with asthma, croup, or bronchitis. Honeysuckle's significant antispasmodic properties mean that it has traditionally played a part in reducing convulsions and tremors. Emily Elizabeth Waller reported that *'a decoction of the flowers has been celebrated as an excellent antispasmodic and recommended in asthma of the nervous kind. An elegant water may be distilled from these flowers which has been recommended for a nervous headache.'*

Energetics

Traditional Chinese medicine considers Honeysuckle to be a cooling herb that can help to clear excess heat from the body. Here in the West, the old herbalists, Gerard, Parkinson, and Culpeper, considered Honeysuckle to be heating, and therefore contraindicated for inflammation and fevers. I wonder whether these energetic differences arise due to differences between *Lonicera japonica* (a herb in traditional Chinese medicine) and *L. periclymenum*, which is in the European pharmacopoeia.

In Bach's flower essences, Honeysuckle is considered to help people to resolve feelings of homesickness and nostalgia when these are dominating a person's thoughts. My own feeling is that Honeysuckle encourages us to be in the present moment. Anyone who has ever caught the fragrance of Honeysuckle in a June hedgerow will instinctively understand this. There is no need to yearn for the past when we understand that our past experiences have shaped us and will always remain in the fabric of our being. We can let go of that yearning and see that there is so much to appreciate and experience in the here and now.

In Tibetan medicine

In the Tibetan pharmacopoeia, the fruits of the beautiful Lilac-Flowered Honeysuckle *Lonicera syringantha* is the species most often prescribed. It is known as *Pang mé drebu* [པང་མའི་འབྲས་བུ།]. It has a sweet taste and a cool, rough, light potency. It is considered to cure heart fevers and some gynaecological disorders.

In my dispensary

In my clinic I work with Honeysuckle in tincture, tea, and capsule form. I most often call on it to help patients who need respiratory support. This can be both in acute situations such as in colds or influenza, or in longstanding chronic conditions such as asthma, where its antispasmodic influence is very helpful.

Historical applications

Dioscorides recommended that '*the ripe seed gathered and dried in the shadow and drunk for four days together, doth waste and consume away the hardness of the spleen and removeth wearisomeness, helpeth the shortness and difficulty of breathing, cureth the hicket (hiccough) etc. A syrup made of the flowers is good to be drunk against diseases of the lungs and spleen.*'

Gerard considered the flowers to be: '*neither cold nor binding, but hot and attenuating or making thin*' and that '*The floures steeped in oile, and set in the Sun, are good to anoint the body that is benumbed, and growne very cold.*'

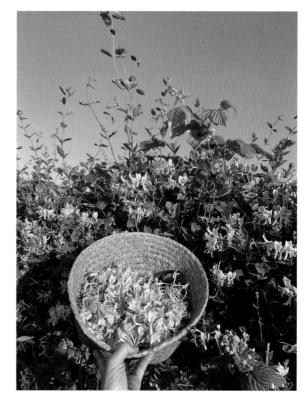

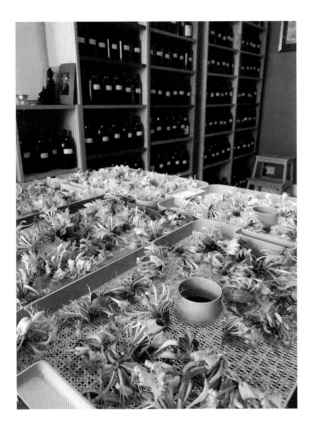

Culpeper said: '*I know of no better cure for the asthma than this.*' He also recommended it to procure '*speedy delivery of women in travail*'. He was vehemently against prescribing Honeysuckle for inflammatory states, since he considered it to be heating.

Honeysuckle has a long history of being utilized in topical beauty products to clear away freckles or other 'skin discolourations'. As interesting as that is, I very much hope that these days people have learnt to love their freckles.

Magical

Honeysuckle is associated with psychic powers, protection, and attracting wealth. A Honeysuckle vine growing near to one's house is considered to bring good luck.

Suggestion for the home apothecary

Honeysuckle flower tea

Dry Honeysuckle flowers so that you can add them to your winter herbal tea blends when you feel in need of extra antiviral or respiratory support. Make sure they are thoroughly dry, and store them in an airtight jar in the dark.

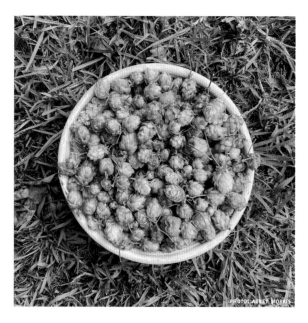
'Hops help us to unwind. They are sedative, bitter and oestrogenic.'

Hops grow on a vine that reaches up to 12 metres in height, spiralling around from left to right in order to support itself on other vegetation or the supports it has been provided with. Pliny named it the 'Willow Wolf', and this gave rise to its specific name, 'lupulus'. The vine is dioicous, male and female flowers being produced on different plants.

Medicinal parts
▷ Flowers

Female flowers, the strobiles, are ideally harvested in late August or early September, before they have been pollinated, as this is when the medicinally active constituents are at their height.

Physiological actions

Summary

▷ Nervine
▷ Bitter
▷ Sedative
▷ Antispasmodic
▷ Diuretic
▷ Antibacterial
▷ Oestrogenic

Physiological virtues

Hops are best known as being a bitter nervine and a sedative. They help to encourage restful sleep and are generally calming, as they are significantly antispasmodic. Hops are therefore worth considering as part of a prescription for patients whose symptoms are worsened by tension – for example, period pain, asthma, or tension headaches. They are also well indicated for digestive gripes associated with IBS.

Hops act as a mild depressant on the higher nerve centres, and this means that they are contraindicated in states of depression. As they age, the constituents of Hops change and oxidize, becoming more rancid-smelling and changing in action from sedating to stimulating. For this reason, in the dispensary Hops are best replaced each year.

They have antibacterial properties and can therefore be a good choice when there is ulceration in the upper digestive tract, especially when this is associated with digestive insufficiency and tension. They are diuretic and are a traditional remedy for kidney gravel.

Hops are oestrogenic in nature. This was first discovered when female Hop pickers reported disruption to their menstrual cycle, the medicinal constituents being readily absorbed through the skin. This oestrogenic action can also cause unwanted side effects in males. Think of the symptoms commonly associated with heavy beer drinkers: erectile dysfunction, also known as 'brewer's droop', loss of libido, and gynecomastia (the development of breasts).

Hops are bitter, and this bitterness makes them a good general support to the liver and digestive system. Since menopausal symptoms are worsened by poor liver clearance, Hops are an excellent herb to consider for menopausal women who are not sleeping well. You can say that they work on three main levels: liver support, relaxing sedation, and the delivery of helpful phytoestrogens.

Energetics
Hops are bitter and cooling.

In my dispensary
I prescribe Hops in the form of tincture and teas. The following case shows how I typically work with Hops.

'Marianne' was 58 years old and had been prone to insomnia since she was a child. Her sleep had deteriorated further since she had been through the menopause. She would wake up at 3:00 am every morning and lie awake with churning thoughts. Usually she was unable to get back to sleep at all and felt exhausted most of the time. As well as lack of sleep, she suffered with weak digestion, being sensitive to many foods and often experiencing gripes and bloating. I asked her to eat more regularly, to reduce sugary snacks, and to introduce daily bone broth. Her individual herbal prescription contained Hops for their sedative, digestive stimulating and antispasmodic properties, as well as some gentle oestrogenic support. She also had Passionflower, Lemon Balm, and Lime blossom. After four weeks she reported that, although

she was still waking at 3.00 am, she was now able to go back to sleep again. Her digestion was also much more comfortable, with hardly any bloating and griping. After several more months of a concerted effort with the dietary changes and consistent herbal support, she was getting better sleep and was even beginning to sleep right through the night.

Historical applications
Hops have been used in brewing since the eleventh century but were never included in traditional English ale. Gerard wrote: '*The floures are used to season Beere . . . and too many do cause bitternesse thereof, and are ill for the head. . . The manifold vertues of Hops do manifest argue the wholesomeness of beere above ale, for the hops rather make it a physical drinke to keep*

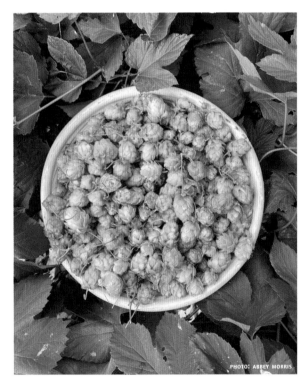

PHOTO: ABBEY MORRIS

the body in health, than an ordinary drinke for the quenching of our thirst.'

Culpeper wrote: '*This physician operates in opening obstructions of the liver and spleen, cleansing the blood, loosening the belly, expelling the gravel, and provoking he urine; the decoction of the tops of the hops, whether tame or wild, worketh these effects.*'

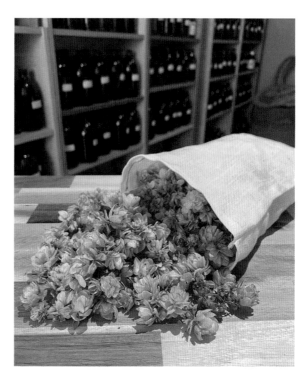

Suggestion for the home apothecary

Hop pillow

Take dried Hops that are not more than one year old. Stuff them into a cotton pocket, and sew up the open end to form a little pillow. Place it by your pillow to aid restful sleep.

Old, dried Hops do not have the same sedative properties as recently dried ones, so you need to make a new pillow at least each year. However, if you have tackled the root cause of your poor sleep, you probably will not need it.

Horse Chestnut   *Aesculus hippocastanum*

'Horse Chestnut heals weak boundaries.'

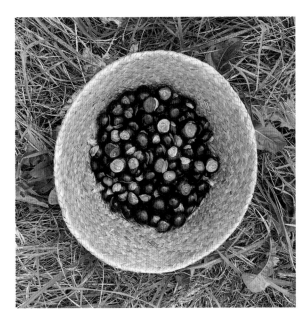

When I was a kid, I used to love gathering conkers. There is so much magic in filling a basket with bright, shiny nuts and taking them home as treasure. My own children used to gather them to play the game called 'conkers', where you thread them on a string and swing them against your opponent's chestnut. These days I gather these nuts for medicine.

Medicinal parts
▷ Seeds/nuts
▷ Bark

The seeds or nuts are known as 'conkers' or 'buckeyes'. Some herbal practitioners work with the bark of young twigs and the flowers, but I have not tried this myself.

Physiological actions

Summary
▷ Astringent
▷ Anti-inflammatory

Physiological virtues

Horse Chestnuts are astringent and help to strengthen the walls of the venous circulatory system. This makes them excellent for chronic venous insufficiency, slow-healing ulcers, varicose veins, haemorrhoids, and broken veins.

They contain a significant amount of aescin saponins, which make them a reasonable alternative to chemical laundry liquids. The nuts also contain flavonoids, coumarins, and condensed tannins. The saponins are anti-inflammatory, and, together with the flavonoids, reduce the tendency to spasm in the vessels and help to dilate them. Coumarins improve the resistance of the vascular walls, toning them, encouraging better blood flow, and reducing the risk of deep vein thrombosis. Toning the venous system reduces 'leakiness', reducing, in turn, varicose eczema and ulcers. Weiss, in his book *Herbal Medicine*, reports that Horse Chestnut can reduce potential secondary brain injuries by helping to disperse suffusions of blood.

When taken internally in more than a very small dose, Horse Chestnut can be toxic. For this reason, the usual method of working with Horse Chestnut is to make it into topical treatments, such as ointments, creams, suppositories, and fomentations. These are often prescribed for varicose veins, haemorrhoids, phlebitis, and even to reduce swelling in the feet and ankles during long-distance air travel. Herbalist and author, Christina Stapley, describes infusing the fresh flowers into olive oil as a pain-relieving massage treatment specifically for dull, throbbing pain.

As well as prescribing topical treatments made with the nuts, I often prescribe Horse Chestnut internally at very low doses in the form of a tincture. Added to a patient's prescription as a very small proportion, it can work absolute wonders to tone the venous system. It is not suitable for everyone and particular care is needed for those who are prone to constipation. Horse Chestnut should not be ingested during pregnancy.

Energetics

Horse Chestnut is primarily astringent. Since the internal state of our bodies reflects our experience of the outside world, weak veins can be associated with difficulty in establishing and maintaining healthy personal boundaries. I have lost count of the number of times that I have treated a patient for chronic venous insufficiency and they have come for a follow-up appointment revelling in an unexpected ability to enforce better boundaries in their life. I believe that Horse Chestnut is almost always the main instigator of this change when the change is relatively fast and pronounced. Compare this to the boundary-enforcing action of the Rose family – such as Hawthorn – which is slower and more gradual.

Within the Bach flower essences system, Horse Chestnut essence is associated with failure to learn from past mistakes – a negative pattern often strongly linked to poor boundary setting.

In my dispensary

When the pulse of a patient seems to have no pause between beats – that is, it is 'running into itself' – this is usually a sign that they would benefit from inclusion of a little Horse Chestnut in their prescription. Often, they will have physiological signs such as varicose veins or haemorrhoids, but this is not always the case. If I feel this type of pulse, I tend to ask the patient how their personal boundaries are. More often than not the patient's answer confirms the need for Horse Chestnut.

The following case is typical of how Horse Chestnut's virtues can help those who need it. 'Esther' was 65 years old and suffered with swollen and painful varicose veins. Her pulse was running into itself, and so I was not surprised when she told me that she found it very hard to say 'no' to the demands of others, especially family members. She wanted to spend time developing her own creative projects, but she felt unable to as she had taken on a lot of extra commitments. I prescribed Horse Chestnut in her personalized tincture blend of circulatory and digestion-supporting herbs, and she also had an ointment to apply topically. Within four weeks her varicose veins were feeling more comfortable, and within twelve weeks they were much less visible. She had also been able to tactfully reduce her commitments and was happily developing her new projects.

'Jilly' was 56 years old and, despite being healthy and active, had swollen and painful varicose veins on her lower legs. The pain and throbbing was beginning to keep her awake at night, and she was at her wits' end. She hoped that herbal medicine could reverse the venous deterioration she was experiencing. I included Horse Chestnut in her personalized blend at a very low level (about 3%), alongside the herbal digestive and nervine support that she needed. She also had a Horse Chestnut and Witch Hazel ointment to apply daily. Within four weeks the appearance of the veins had dramatically reduced, and the painful throbbing had ceased.

Historical applications

Maud Grieve, in her *Modern Herbal*, writes that Horse Chestnut bark has tonic, narcotic, and febrifuge properties, and that it was prescribed for intermittent fevers. It was prepared as an infusion, made with 30 g of bark to 570 ml of water, and given in tablespoon doses three or four times daily.

Magical

Conkers are associated with success and wealth, and people would carry one in their pocket to attract these. Some said it was more effective if you wrapped some paper money around the conker. Country folk also used to carry them to ward off rheumatism, backaches, arthritis, and chills. If you carried three it was said to guard against giddiness.

Suggestion for the home apothecary

Varicose vein oil

Roughly crush dried Horse Chestnuts with a pestle and mortar or a mallet, with the nuts in a pillowcase. Place into a slow cooker pot with an equal volume of dried Witch Hazel bark and dried Pilewort (also known as Lesser Celandine). If you do not have Pilewort, just add the other two. Cover with mild olive oil. Set it to warm very gently on the 'warm' setting only. If you choose the 'low' setting, this would be too hot. Leave it for one hour on 'warm' and then let it cool down again before giving it the next exposure to gentle heat. In practice I find

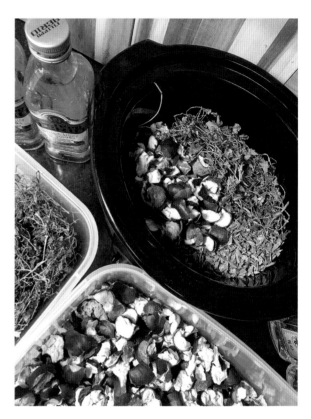

it most convenient to do this over a few days, giving it just one hour a day on the 'warm' setting. Once it is ready to bottle, strain the oil through a jelly bag or a coffee filter and store in clean, dry bottles. The oil can be set into an ointment in jars if that is more convenient. Massage into the affected area morning and night. It will also be helpful for varicose veins if the patient sleeps with the foot end of the bed elevated slightly.

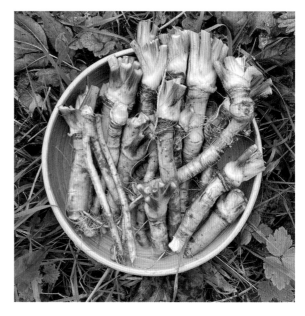
'Horseradish brings fire and movement to the system.'

Horseradish is not native to Britain but has been here for a long time. Gerard wrote about it, being the first to coin the name 'Horse Radish'. Lyte, in his *New Herball*, referred to it as 'Mountain Radish' or 'Rayfort' (from the French for 'strong root: *raifort*'). It is perhaps best known medicinally these days as an important ingredient in the oxymel known as 'Fire Cider'. It is a freely available and easily grown hot herb for our dispensaries for those of us who live in temperate climates.

Medicinal parts

▷ Roots

Physiological actions

Summary

▷ Circulatory stimulant
▷ Expectorant
▷ Antimicrobial
▷ Diuretic
▷ Aperient

Physiological virtues

Horseradish is antimicrobial and particularly helpful in supporting patients with either upper respiratory or urinary-tract infections. It is stimulant, encouraging a more vibrant blood circulation, whether taken internally or applied topically as a rubefacient. It supports healthy digestion, stimulating the digestive process and acting as a mild aperient. It is also a very strong diuretic and is a good choice to clear urinary calculus and bladder stones. It resolves oedema and was prescribed for dropsy in days gone by.

Horseradish is an expectorant, opening up the airways and allowing us to breathe more freely. This is helpful if we have chronic respiratory challenges such as asthma or acute issues such as bronchitis or pneumonia. It is a specific to clear congested sinuses too. As a topical application, it can help to relieve the pain of arthritis, rheumatism, and sciatica. All in all, Horseradish's many wide-ranging medicinal virtues make it a great warming winter tonic remedy.

Horseradish contains pungent glucosinolates, which are broken down in the body to powerful derivatives called isothiocyanates and indoles. These are believed to have a significant cancer-preventive action. It also contains a relatively high level of Vitamin C, and in old times was employed in the treatment of scurvy.

Horseradish is a Brassica and, like other members of this plant family, may inhibit the function of the thyroid gland. For this reason, it is not recommended at high doses or for long periods for patients with hypothyroidism. Prolonged topical application may cause skin irritation. Be cautious until you discover your own level of tolerance.

Energetics

Horseradish is hot and sweet. If you feel that you are slipping into apathy and stagnancy in your life, try introducing some Horseradish into your dietary or herbal routine.

In Tibetan medicine

As a very hot herb, Horseradish is helpful to treat cold conditions, but it is contraindicated for patients with hot conditions, such as inflammatory conditions of the digestive tract.

In my dispensary

I often include Horseradish, as a fresh tincture, in prescriptions for patients with long-standing sinus issues. The Horseradish helps to resolve stagnancy in the circulation to the sinus area and shifts stubborn long-standing infections. I also encourage my patients to make Fire Cider, and I make some each year for those who are unable to make their own.

I remember when I first learnt about the properties of Horseradish. I was a herbal student and attending a seminar at my tutor, Barbara Howe's, garden and clinic. Barbara had finely chopped a Horseradish root in a food processor, and she passed it around the group, so that we could get a sense of just how pungent it is when freshly chopped. She warned us not to stick our faces into the food processor container or to inhale too deeply. My dear friend and a truly excellent herbalist, Jeremy Griffiths, wanted to get the full Horseradish experience and decided to do just that. He moved closer to the container and inhaled deeply. Immediately he turned bright red, his eyes streamed copi-

ously, and he started coughing and spluttering for a minute or two before, quite impressively, recovering himself. I will admit that the rest of us found it highly amusing, but we were very much in awe of Jeremy's willingness to engage properly with this formidable medicine.

Historical applications

According to Greek mythology, the Oracle at Delphi told Apollo that Horseradish is worth its weight in gold. It has been used medicinally for more than 3,000 years. The Greeks and Romans prescribed it topically as a poultice to ease pain, such as in backaches and menstrual cramps. Internally, it was used to relieve coughs and as an aphrodisiac. Starting in the Middle Ages (ca. 1000–1300 AD), Horseradish was incorporated

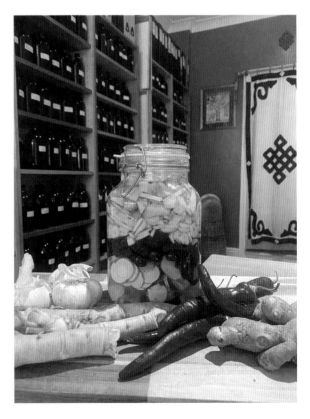

into the Jewish Passover Seder as one of the '*maror*', or bitter herbs (along with Coriander, Horehound, Lettuce, and Nettle).

Magical

Horseradish has magical associations with cleansing and driving out evil influences. There is an old tradition of sprinkling dried root around the house to clear out unwanted energies and to remove negative spells.

Suggestion for the home apothecary

Fire cider

Chop fresh Garlic, fresh Ginger, fresh Chillies and fresh Horseradish. Choose the proportions to suit your preference, and add other respiratory herbs if you like – there is no exact recipe. Fill a Kilner jar or other large jar with the herbs. If you are using a jar with a metal lid, you will need to protect it with waxed paper. Pour organic Apple Cider Vinegar into the jar so that the herbs are completely covered. Label and place in a dark cupboard for at least two weeks, preferably four. After it has steeped, drain and press out the liquid, putting the spent herbs on the compost heap with gratitude and respect. Add honey to the vinegary liquid to taste. I tend to add honey at a rate equivalent to approximately one third the volume of the vinegar – so for 1 litre of vinegar I would add around 300 ml to 400 ml runny honey. Stir thoroughly, put into clean bottles, and label. This will keep well on the shelf for more than a year.

Take 1 tbsp daily to ward off colds. Use 1 tsp three times a day if you have a cold. Fire Cider can also be used as delicious salad dressing or drizzled over stir fries.

Horsetail 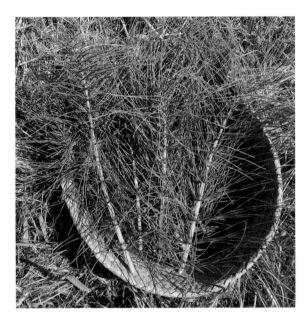 *Equisetum arvense*

'Horsetail supports strength and structure in weak tissues.'

Horsetail is an ancient plant: it has been living on our planet since the Palaeozoic era. It is tough, with coarse, brittle, leafless, jointed stems. Its country names include 'Shave Grass', 'Pewterwort', or 'Bottlebrush', since the stems have the appearance of a bottlebrush and, in the past, some types of Horsetail were sold for polishing metal. In the spring it produces fertile stems, which bear cone-like catkins at their tips. Later in the season these are replaced by the main medicinal stems. It is a very invasive plant and is not generally welcomed into cultivated areas. There are various species of Horsetail, but it is the Field Horsetail that is most often gathered for medicinal purposes.

Medicinal parts
  ▷ Stems
The barren stems are harvested after the fruiting stems have died down.

Physiological actions

Summary
  ▷ Diuretic
  ▷ Astringent
  ▷ Styptic

Physiological virtues

Horsetail has a high proportion of silica in its tissues. It is therefore a plant to consider where there is a lack of structure or strength in the body. It can be helpful to support patients with osteoporosis or who are recovering from broken bones, as well as those with weak or brittle nails and hair.

Horsetail is diuretic and astringent. It is beneficial in all sorts of urinary system disorders, in particular assisting with the passing of gravel, reducing oedema, or helping to resolve infections such as cystitis. It is styptic and anti-inflammatory, which makes it well indicated when there is ulceration in the urinary passages or blood in the urine. In general, it helps to tone and strengthen the bladder and the urethra. A strong decoction acts as an emmenagogue.

Horsetail is also well suited to being added to bath water as a topical treatment for skin lesions or inflammation. The cooled decoction is also excellent to reduce swelling of the eyelids.

As an internal medicine, it can be irritant in large or prolonged doses, so it is a good idea to prescribe it in short courses and to combine it with demulcent herbs, such as Marshmallow. It also contains thiaminase, which breaks down Vitamin B1, so prolonged large doses could potentially deplete this vitamin in the body.

Energetics

Horsetail is sweet, bitter, astringent, cooling.

In Tibetan medicine

Equisetum arvense is known as *Khujug tsa jang menpa* [ཁུ་བྱུག་རྩ་བྱང་དམན་པ།]. It has a sweet taste and a sweet post-digestive taste, with a cool and rough potency. It is considered to stop bleeding and cure oedema.

In my dispensary

I prescribe Horsetail in short courses for patients as needed, usually in a tea or a capsule blend. It is especially helpful for people who need help with improving the strength of the structures in their body.

Historical applications

Horsetail is strongly astringent and was a battlefield herb, helping to staunch the bleeding from deep wounds. Parkinson wrote: '*It is very powerfull to staunch bleedings . . . eyther inward or outward, the juice or decoction thereof being drunk, or . . . applied outwardly.*'

Culpeper quotes Galen, who said: '*it will heal sinews though they be cut in sunder*'.

Culpeper also wrote that '*It is very powerful to stop bleeding, either inward or outward, the juice or the decoction being drunk, or the juice, decoction or distilled water applied outwardly. . . . It also heals inward ulcers…it solders together the tops of green wounds and cures all ruptures in children. The decoction taken in wine helps stone and strangury.*'

In Gerard's time Horsetail was used to scour pewter and other kitchen utensils; and fletchers used it to polish their arrows.

Magical

Horsetail is associated with snake charming. It is said that whistles made of Horsetail stems, when played, will attract snakes. It is also considered to promote fertility when added to magical formulations.

Hyssop 🌿 *Hyssopus officinalis*

'Purge me with Hyssop, and I shall be clean.'

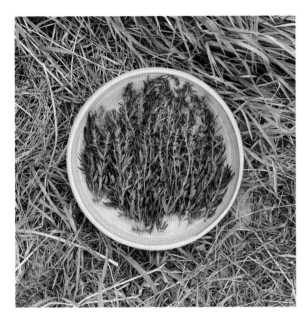

Hyssop was named originally from *azob* (holy herb), as it was used for cleaning sacred spaces; hence the quote: *'Purge me with Hyssop, and I shall be clean.'* Our body is a sacred space too. Hyssop has an extraordinary ability to cut through phlegm and support expectoration. Its bitterness stimulates the liver and aids in the process of systemic detoxification. I feel that there is much more to it than that, though. Hyssop seems to be a herb that acts on a higher level. Perhaps by moving stagnation in the body, it encourages new beginnings, a renewed breath of life, and a willingness to commit to a more spiritually nourishing path when we have been consumed by worldly and materialistic concerns.

Medicinal parts
- Aerial parts

These are harvested when in flower.

Physiological actions

Summary
- Bitter
- Expectorant
- Anticatarrhal
- Diaphoretic
- Anti-inflammatory
- Vulnerary

Physiological virtues

Hyssop is mostly considered a respiratory-system-supporting herb, it being a very effective expectorant and anticatarrhal. It is helpful to treat influenza, bronchitis, coughs, colds, and catarrh, as well as being excellent for chronic conditions, such as asthma. It has diaphoretic properties, so it can help reduce a fever, making it especially good for feverish colds.

As a topical treatment, it is helpful for bruises and burns. Traditionally, a topical treatment was prescribed to ease rheumatism.

It is antiviral with a particular activity against the cold-sore-causing *Herpes simplex* virus.

Hyssop contains pino-camphone, which can, in very high doses, cause convulsions. Avoid it in large doses for patients who are epileptic or suffer from other types of convulsions.

Energetics
Hyssop is bitter, slightly warming, and dry.

In my dispensary
I prescribe Hyssop as a tincture, in teas and capsules, and it is an important ingredient in my rum cough elixir. When I first moved my clinic to Somerset, I was asked to give a talk to a gathering in the Market House, the beautiful

historic community building in the centre of Castle Cary. On the day of the talk I had come down with a very persistent, irritating cough, which was made worse by speaking. I did not want to cancel the talk, as I felt that it would not give the best impression for the business that I was launching in town, so I took along a little bottle and explained to my audience that I needed to sip this herbal cough medicine during my talk, as I had a rather tickly cough. With help from a few strategic sips of the rum cough elixir, I got through an hour's talk and answered plenty of interesting questions. It really is very effective stuff, and many people tell me that it is now a staple in their home apothecary.

Historical applications

Hippocrates prescribed Hyssop for pleurisy, and Dioscorides recommended it for asthma and catarrh.

Hildegard of Bingen saw Hyssop as primarily a herb to support the digestion and treat melancholy. She wrote: '*If one eats hyssop often, one cleans the sick makers and stinkiness out of the foamy juices. . . . Hyssop is good in all foods. It is more useful powdered and cooked than raw. It makes the liver active and cleanses the lung somewhat. But if the liver is sick because of the person's sadness, the person should cook young chicken with hyssop before the sickness increases. The person should often eat this hyssop and chicken, and should also eat fresh hyssop laid in wine, and then drink the wine.*'

Parkinson places Hyssop first out of all the herbs that he writes about in *Theatrum Botanicum*: '*Dioscorides saith, that Hysope boiled with Rue and Hony, and drunke doth help those that are troubled with Coughes, shortnesse of breath, wheezing, and rheumaticke distillations upon the lungs: taken also with Oxymel, it purgeth grosse humours by the stoole, and with hony killeth the worms in the belly.*' He wrote: '*Matthiolus saith that our Hysope is of thinne*

parts, and that it cutteth and breaketh tough flegme, it rarifieth or maketh thinne that which is thich or grosse, it openeth that which is stopped, and cleanseth that which is corrupt, the oyle therof being annoynted killeth lice, and taketh away the itching of the head.' Here, Parkinson was referring to physician Pier Andrea Mattioli.

Gerard recommended that '*A decoction of Hyssope made with figges, water, honey and rue, and drunketh, helpeth the old cough.*'

Magical

Hyssop is widely chosen as a purification herb in magic. The dried herb can be added to sachets, and the infusion can be sprinkled on people and objects to cleanse them. Bunches of Hyssop can be hung up in the home to purge it of evil.

Suggestion for the home apothecary

Rum cough elixir

This is my recipe for this gorgeous and effective rum cough elixir. It is something that everyone needs to have in their home medicine chest. I choose rum as the base of this formula because it has antimicrobial properties as well as tasting pretty good. If you are someone who needs to avoid alcohol, you can use vinegar instead and add honey after draining it to make it into an oxymel – in the same way as when making Fire Cider. (See Horseradish for recipe.)

Respiratory, antitussive, and anticatarrhal herbs are steeped in rum for a period of 2–4 weeks, then drained and bottled. Your actual choice of herbs will depend on what you have available and what you prefer in terms of level of bitterness, but bitter is good when it comes to cough herbs, so do not be too sparing with those if you want a really effective mix. I also add some demulcent, soothing herbs such as Marshmallow leaves. There is so much choice and so much scope to vary the recipe according to your own circumstances. I like to choose dried herbs, but if you prefer working with fresh herbs, you can do that too: just make absolutely sure that they are totally surface-dry and make a much smaller batch, until you have learnt how well it will keep.

The herb measurements are in loose handfuls. If you prefer cups, then assume that a large handful is one cup, a handful is half a cup, and a small handful is one third of a cup.

» *1.5 litres of good-quality rum*
» *handful dried Hyssop*
» *small handful dried Liquorice*
» *small handful dried Elecampane root*
» *small handful dried Wild Cherry bark*
» *small handful dried White Horehound*
» *2 tsp, heaped, of Caraway seed*
» *large handful dried Marshmallow leaf*
» *large handful, dried Elderflowers*
» *handful dried Cowslip flowers*
» *handful dried Thyme*
» *large handful dried Mullein leaves*
» *handful dried Sage leaves*

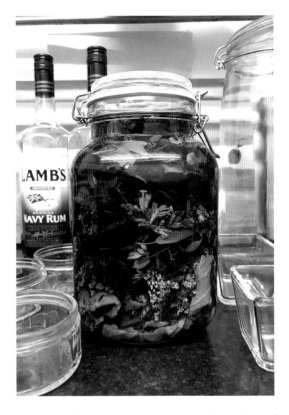

Chop the herbs and place into a jar large enough so that they loosely fill it but are not packed in tightly. Cover completely with rum; if necessary, add more than the amount suggested. It is important that the herbs are thoroughly covered. Leave in a cool, dark place for at least 14 days – preferably, for 1 month. Strain, press, bottle, and label. Take 1 tsp as needed when you have a troubling cough. You can put it in hot water and add honey if neat is too strong for you.

'Irish Moss is nutritious and soothing.'

I gather Irish Moss from my favourite beach on the Jurassic Coast. Although it is a very common seaweed of rock pools on Atlantic shores, it took me many years to find it. It turns out that it was there all along, but I had not figured out where to look. One of its special features is that it forms iridescent blue bubbles at the tips of its fronds in bright sunshine when growing in shallow water.

Medicinal parts
▷ Thallus

The thallus is snipped from its holdfast in situ.

Physiological actions

Summary
▷ Demulcent
▷ Anti-inflammatory
▷ Expectorant
▷ Laxative
▷ Tonic
▷ Nutritive

Physiological virtues

Irish Moss is filled with demulcent jelly-like compounds and is particularly helpful to soothe inflamed and irritated parts of the body. It is a good choice to soothe a sore and inflamed respiratory tract. Its high salt content also helps to loosen phlegm and assists with expectoration. Prompt treatment with Irish Moss can prevent colds from turning into pneumonia; in the past, it was widely prescribed in cases of tuberculosis. It is significantly antiviral and is a good way of helping to prevent influenza, sore throats, and chesty coughs.

Its soothing demulcent properties also play a helpful role in easing inflammation in the

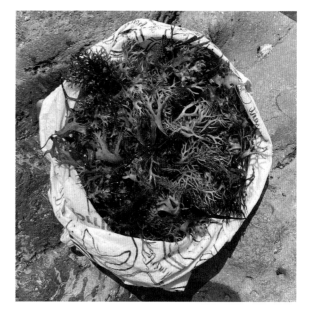

digestive tract. It has a high fibre content, and this, combined with its demulcency, makes it act as a gentle laxative. It reduces inflammation throughout the digestive tract, helping to soothe gastritis, dyspepsia, nausea (including pregnancy nausea), indigestion, and heartburn, as well as reducing the reactivity of the bowel in cases of irritable bowel syndrome. It is also a prebiotic. Irish Moss is an excellent herb to consider for an inflamed urinary tract too. A decoction should be drunk to soothe the discomfort of cystitis.

Irish Moss contains a compound called fucoxanthin, which gives it its beautiful bronze colour. Fucoxanthin is an antioxidant that also helps to counteract insulin resistance. This means that regular consumption of moderate amounts (2–4 tbsp/day) of Irish Moss can help to stabilize blood sugar. Irish Moss is widely considered a superfood. It can be used to thicken mousses and puddings, but do not confuse it with the laboratory-produced food additive called Carrageenan.

It is rich in minerals, especially iodine, and contains significant amounts of the compound Di-Iodothyronine (DIT), which is a precursor to the thyroid hormones thyroxin (T4) and tri-iodothyronine (T3). It can therefore be helpful in some thyroid imbalances, but care is needed here. It is best to seek professional advice to see whether it is appropriate in individual cases.

It is one of the best plant sources of Omega-3 fatty acids, so regular consumption can be very helpful for those recovering from cardiovascular disease or hypercholesterolaemia. It is a natural blood thinner, so avoid taking it if you are taking allopathic blood-thinning medication.

Irish Moss is an excellent convalescence food. It is nutritive and balancing, ideal to support recovery after major illness.

Topically, it is popular as a hair tonic and to help in dry skin conditions such as eczema and psoriasis.

Energetics
Irish Moss is salty and nourishing.

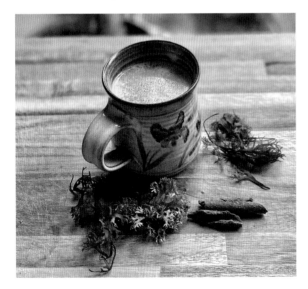

In my dispensary
My primary way of working with Irish Moss in a clinical setting is within capsule formulae for the respiratory and urinary systems.

Historical applications
Humans have been harvesting seaweed, like *Chondrus crispus*, for nearly 14,000 years. In China, evidence of the medicinal benefits of red seaweed can be traced back to 600 BC. In the British Isles, it was originally used as a food source around 400 BC. During the Irish potato famine in the nineteenth century, starving people survived by gathering and eating this seaweed. It became known as Irish Moss as a result. In America, the coastal town of Scituate in Massachusetts became the centre of the Irish Moss industry after an Irish immigrant, called Daniel Ward, noticed abundant Irish Moss growing in the waters off Boston in 1847. He started a thriving industry offering a living to a community of 'mossers', who gathered their haul and dried it on the beach. It was then sold to food manufacturers. Many Irish settlers came to Scituate in order to benefit from this successful entrepreneurial venture.

Magical
Irish Moss is associated with abundance and luck. Carry Irish Moss on your person to increase luck or to ensure a steady flow of money into the household or, to have the same effect, place it beneath rugs in the home.

Suggestion for the home apothecary
Irish Moss healing decoction

Soak 15 g of Irish Moss in cold water for 15 minutes, then simmer it in 1.5 litres of milk or water for 10–15 minutes. Strain and season with Liquorice, Lemon, or Cinnamon. Sweeten to taste. Can be taken freely.

Jerusalem Artichoke 🍂 *Helianthus tuberosum*

'Jerusalem Artichoke pushes out salivary and tonsil stones as well as supporting the digestion.'

Jerusalem Artichoke is a type of Sunflower, native to North America. It gets its common name from the Italian name for Sunflower, *girasole*. Apparently, Italian settlers in the United States named them *girasole*; when adopted by non-Italian speakers, this eventually morphed into the word 'Jerusalem'. The Artichoke part of the name is because its taste is reminiscent of a blend of Potato and Artichoke. The tuber is called *Topinambur* in French, German, Italian, Spanish, Polish, and Russian. It is said that this name arose in 1615, after a representative from a Brazilian coastal tribe, called the Topinambur, visited the Vatican while a sample of a tuber from Canada was on display. I guess that Brazil must have seemed very close to Canada in those days.

Jerusalem Artichoke is an important herbal medicine not often spoken about to herbal students these days. It is generally thought of as a helpful food stuff rich in prebiotic fibre, but it also has other very valuable medicinal attributes.

Medicinal parts
 ▷ Tubers

Physiological actions
Summary
 ▷ Bitter
 ▷ Sialagogue
 ▷ Cholagogue
 ▷ Alterative
 ▷ Prebiotic
 ▷ Antilithic

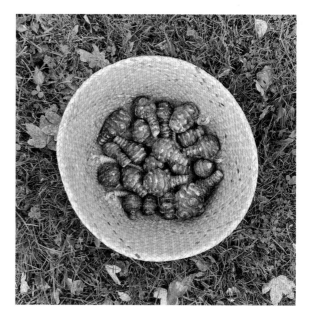

Physiological virtues

Jerusalem Artichoke is an alterative and digestive stimulant that is specific for the removal of stones in the digestive tract, particularly those that develop in the mouth. I mostly think of it when I see patients with salivary gland stones (sialoliths) and tonsil stones (tonsilloliths). It contains sesquiterpene lactone bitters that directly stimulate the digestive process through increasing saliva, bile, and other digestive secretions, such as stomach acid. The usual initial treatment for salivary gland stones is to stimulate the production of saliva, so it makes sense that Jerusalem Artichoke would be helpful.

Jerusalem Artichoke is rich in inulin, a fibre that is not digestible and acts as a beneficial prebiotic for bifidobacteria in the gut. Inulin also helps to reduce blood sugar spikes after eating and, through reducing fat absorption, can lower cholesterol levels in the body and help with weight reduction. A side effect of this is that, when eaten as food, Jerusalem Artichokes can cause gas and bloating, especially in those with a sensitive digestive system. A small quantity prescribed as medicine does not seem to have the same effect. Healthy gut bacteria help to improve calcium absorption, so eating Jerusalem Artichokes can help with maintaining healthy bones and speeding the healing of fractures.

Energetics
Jerusalem Artichoke is sweet and bitter.

In my dispensary
In my clinic, the presence of salivary or tonsil stones tends to crop up as a chronic presentation rather than an acute one. They are often mentioned as an aside during the consultation.

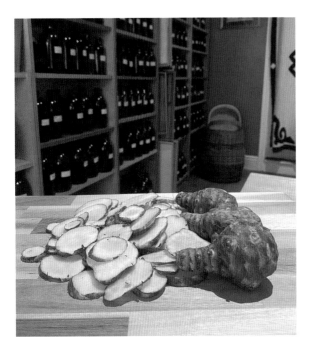

In these circumstances I usually add Jerusalem Artichoke to the patient's prescription. This may be in the form of tincture or capsules. I combine it with other herbs that are indicated for the case.

My tutor, Barbara Howe, used to tell a story about the action of Jerusalem Artichoke in getting rid of salivary stones. She had a patient who was looking forward to her daughter's wedding, but just a fortnight before the big day, she had developed a very painful salivary stone that had completely blocked her salivary duct. As well as being extremely uncomfortable, she was especially anxious about the prospect of having a very swollen face in the wedding photos. Barbara provided her with 40 capsules, advising her to take two each morning and two each night for the following ten days. The patient was impatient for a result and decided to go home and take all 40 capsules in one go, because they were 'just a food anyway'. The next morning, she noticed a little white nodule poking out of the swollen area below her tongue. She prodded about a bit and was able to pull out a 5-cm-long stone from her salivary gland. The swelling went down very quickly, and the patient was absolutely fine in time for the wedding.

A few years later I was in practice myself, and a patient mentioned that they had had a salivary stone for many years. It would flare up and cause swelling at odd times. She mentioned it as an aside to her main problem, which, I think, was tiredness and a tendency to colds. I included Jerusalem Artichoke in her mix and asked her to come back after a fortnight. When she returned for her follow-up, she reported that the stone had come out on its own within a week. She said that it felt as though it had been 'pushed out'. This description of the stone being 'pushed out' is one that I hear frequently from patients who take Jerusalem Artichoke.

Historical applications

John Parkinson, writing in 1629, said that when Jerusalem Artichokes had first arrived in England, the tubers were '*dainties for the Queen*', but that now they were so prolific in growth that they had become common and cheap and '*even the most vulgar begin to despise them*'.

Gerard did not rate the Jerusalem Artichoke as either medicine or food, quoting John Goodyer as saying: '*in my judgement which way soever they be drest and eaten, they stir and cause a filthy loathsome stinking wind within the body, thereby causing the belly to be pained and tormented, and are a meat more fit for swine than men*'.

Suggestion for the home apothecary

Raw Jerusalem Artichoke crisps

Slice fresh tubers into thin slices and lay out on dehydrator trays one layer thick. Dehydrate at 42°C/108°F for about 18 hours, or until they are very thoroughly dry and crisp. Sprinkle with herbal salt if desired before eating. Eat a couple a day to get the prebiotic benefits without upsetting the digestive system.

Karela 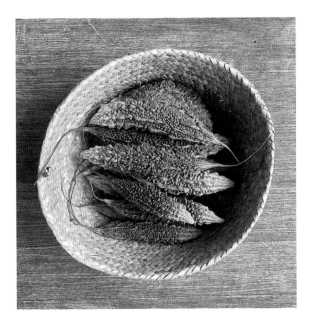 *Momordica charantia*

'Karela tones the digestion and supports blood sugar balance.'

Karela is also known as Bitter Melon or Bitter Gourd. As its common name suggests, it is very bitter – in fact, its generic name is derived from the word *mordio*, which means 'I bite'. Karela is a very important herb throughout the world for healing, ritual, and cleansing. I freely admit that my own experience of its wider properties is rather limited, but when I posted about Karela on Instagram, some of my Instagram family kindly shared their own experiences of how it is prescribed within their own cultures.

My tutor, Barbara Howe, taught me about Karela's affinity with balancing blood sugar and supporting the pancreas. She used to cut open a fruit and say how similar it looked to the images of pancreas cross-sections in medical textbooks. She had many tales of how Karela had made a huge difference to patients, and it had left a deep impression on me. Her teaching encouraged me to get to know Karela for myself.

Medicinal parts
> Fruit

Physiological actions

Summary
> Blood sugar balancer (hypoglycaemic)
> Bitter
> Topical vulnerary and astringent

Physiological virtues

Karela is a truly fabulous medicine for stabilising blood sugar. It supports pancreatic function and also seems to improve the sensitivity of the cells to insulin. It is very helpful in all sorts of blood sugar disorders, especially Type II diabetes and insulin resistance. Long-term use of insulin in Type I diabetes tends to be accompanied by the development of insulin resistance, so Karela can be a very good herbal support in these circumstances. Obviously, great care should be taken to avoid increasing the risk of hypoglycaemic episodes by upsetting the balance of a carefully calculated allopathic prescription dosage. Slow introduction and careful monitoring is essential.

Karela is great for patients who, despite conventional treatment and stringent dietary changes, seem to persistently have high blood sugar readings. It can kick start the process of rebalancing blood sugar, even when given alongside allopathic treatment.

Karela is far more than 'just' a blood sugar stabiliser. The following are some of the snippets of information that were kindly shared by people when I posted about Karela on my Instagram. I am very grateful to all of those who took the time to comment with their own stories. I hope that they will accept my apologies for not listing everyone individually.

In Guyana it is called *Kah-rye-la* or *Cerasee*. In Jamaica it is also called *Cerasee,* and it is prepared as a bitter tea, to be drunk a couple of times a week. In Trinidad and Tobago it is called *Carili.* One person shared how, while she was growing up, her grandmother encouraged the whole family to eat it regularly. She said it was especially important because they had Type II diabetes in the family. In Pakistan one way of benefiting from Karela's influence was to tread on the raw fruits with bare feet until a bitter taste was perceived in the mouth. In the Philippines it is prescribed as a soup for menstrual support. In the GaDangme tradition of Ghana it is known as *Nyanyara* and is an important plant for exorcism and cleansing. In Turkey the soft ripe fruits are put into a jar with olive oil and, after a few days, shaken until they dissolve. One or two teaspoons are consumed daily by those with stomach ulcers or diseases of the digestive tract. In central Asia it is prescribed as a tonic for sickly children who are not gaining weight. In Uganda it is juiced with spinach and cucumber as a calming blend for the digestive tract.

Maud Grieve describes a liniment being made by adding the deseeded, pulped fruit to almond oil. This preparation was helpful for haemorrhoids, burns, chapped hands, and other sores. The pulp could be applied as a poultice.

I know this is by no means an exhaustive list of Karela's virtues, but I hope that it helps to emphasize how wonderful and special it is.

Energetics
Karela is bitter and cooling.

In Tibetan medicine
Karela has a taste that is bitter and a post-digestive taste that is bitter. Its potency is cooling, slow-acting, rough, and mobile.

It is called *Sairji Metok* in Tibetan, which means 'Golden Flower' [གསེར་གྱི་མེ་ཏོག]. It is considered to treat fever of the hollow organs or fevers in the liver. It brings up and evacuates bile.

In my dispensary
I tend to prescribe Karela when there is insulin resistance.

'Charles' was a Type I diabetic in his 70s who had lost one of his legs to the disease ten years before I met him. He originally came to me for help in managing his blood sugar, as he was developing insulin resistance after many years of injecting insulin. He was on many allopathic medications as well as the insulin, and I was conscious of not wanting to upset things. I kept it simple, prescribing him one capsule of Karela per day to start with. At his next check-up, his diabetic nurse said that his blood sugar was much better than usual, and 'whatever he was doing he should keep doing it'.

At this point we increased his dose to two capsules of Karela per day, and at his next check-up his blood sugar was finally responding as it should to his insulin. His diabetic team were surprised and impressed, although they never knew the real reason for his improvement. Charles had many complex medical needs, including significant coronary disease, and, understandably at his age, he did not want to rock the boat with his medical team. He apologized to me, saying he preferred to give them the impression that he had achieved the improvement through dietary changes and more regular exercise. I did not mind at all, since for me herbal medicine is about getting my patients well again, not trying to score points with other health modalities.

If people feel more comfortable keeping quiet about their herbal medicine journey, it is entirely their choice.

Historical applications

Lyte talks of Karela, calling it '*Momordica*', and describes it as a '*marvellous apple*' the fruit being '*sharp pointed and rough without, like the fruit of the wilde Cowcumber . . . the leaves taken in wine are a present remedie for all paines, as well as within the bodie as without, and doth comfort the strength of such as take it in such sort, that no griefe may happen to them.*' I was quite surprised to find that it was known in the sixteenth century, when his *A New Herball* was written. Lyte said that it could be '*found in this countrie, in the gardens of certain Herboristes*'.

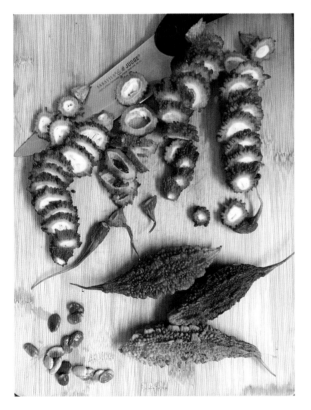

Magical

In the tropical lands where this plant is most at home, it has many magical and ceremonial associations. It seems that Karela is often chosen for cleansing rituals and protection, the vines being worn as ceremonial adornments as well as the medicine being consumed by the participants. There is so much richness to appreciate with Karela: I look forward to deepening my understanding of it as I continue to work with it and meet more people who have direct experience of its traditional roles in healing.

Suggestions for the home apothecary

Dried slices for capsules

Fresh Karela goes mouldy very quickly, so if you do not have access to regular fresh supplies that you can cook with, you may find it helpful to buy it in bulk and dry slices in a dehydrator. Once thoroughly dried, these slices can then be stored in an airtight container and powdered as needed for capsules. Although people usually say that bitter herbs work best when you taste them, we do also have many bitter receptors in our gut. I always prescribe this herb in capsule form and find this strategy very effective.

As soon as you have bought them, take your Karela fruits and cut them into slices about 4 mm thick. Place the slices on a dehydrator tray and dry them at 42°C for as long as needed, until thoroughly brittle. The time required varies according to ambient temperature, humidity, and the make of your dehydrator, but it is usually 12–36 hours. After the first 12 hours, check regularly to avoid over-drying. Store in an airtight container in the dark.

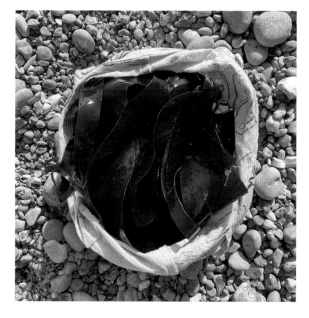
'Kelp counteracts depletion and restores us.'

There are various brown algae that are known as Kelp. The one that I gather is *Laminaria digitata*. 'Kombu' which is widely sold as an ingredient in miso soup and other Japanese dishes, is actually Kelp.

Kelp can be especially helpful for those people who are depleted. As well as being nourishing, it has a moistening, demulcent quality. In general, adding Kelp to the diet or taking it as medicine can help to boost the metabolism.

Medicinal parts
▷ Fronds (thalli)

Physiological actions

Summary
▷ Nutritive
▷ Tonic
▷ Demulcent
▷ Anti-inflammatory
▷ Prebiotic

Physiological virtues
Kelp is rich in minerals, especially iodine, so can be helpful for some people with hypothyroidism. In general, adding Kelp to the diet or taking it as medicine can help with boosting metabolism and support healthy weight loss – provided the diet is also healthy. However, taking a lot of Kelp over a long period could deliver too much iodine. Do not fall into the trap of thinking that the more you take, the better the result. Think of Kelp as a slow and steady support in moderate doses.

It also contains glutamic acid and plenty of helpful dietary fibre. It is traditionally chosen to help with joint inflammation, and its demulcent properties can be really fabulous in external treatments.

Energetics
Kelp is bitter, salty, sweet, cold, moist.

In my dispensary
A decoction or tincture of Kelp is not particularly palatable, so when Kelp is required, I often encourage my patients to add it to their own slow-cooked stews. For some patients, depending on their circumstances, I prescribe capsules, either of pure Kelp, or a formula based on Kelp, mixed with Nettle leaf and Wormwood. I tend to consider this blend for patients who are experiencing a sluggish metabolism while also having a tendency for their *rLung* to be raised. The salty and nourishing nature of the Kelp helps to counterbalance the *rLung*, and the formula as a

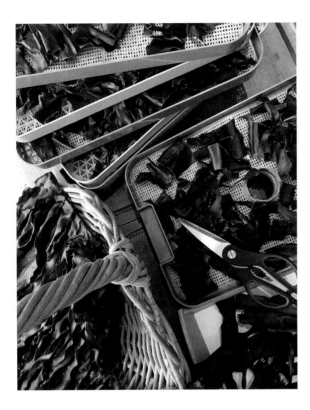

whole is nourishing, supporting the digestion and the thyroid. The advantage of powdering dried raw Kelp and prescribing it in capsules is that the constituents are delivered in a whole, unaltered state to the body.

Historical applications

According to Parkinson: '*All the kindes of Wrake, saith Dioscorides and Galen, doe coole and dry, and it is good to ease the Gout, and inflammations, being used fresh*', but Nicander of Colophon, a Greek physician and poet who lived in the second century BC, pronounced it to be more drying than cooling due to its high salt content.

Magical

Kelp is considered to be a protective talisman for long sea voyages.

Suggestion for the home apothecary

Dried Kelp for stews or capsules

Gather Kelp from under the water at low tide in an area with beautiful, clear, unpolluted seas. If you have any doubts, do not gather. Hang it to drip dry on a washing line for a day, then cut into pieces and lay out on trays in an airy place away from direct sunlight. You may need to finish the drying process in a dehydrator if the ambient humidity is high where you live. Store in an airtight jar in a cool, dark place. Add a couple of 7.5–10 cm pieces to slow-cooked stews.

Lady's Mantle   🍂   *Alchemilla vulgaris / A. mollis*

'Lady's Mantle tones and tightens the tissues as well as the spirit.'

Lady's Mantle was originally known as 'Greater Sanicle', Sanicle being the name for a wound-healing herb. When the Doctrine of Signatures (which states that herbs' appearance in terms of qualities, resemblance to parts of the body or other objects signals for which ailments they are effective) became influential in Western herbal medicine, the likeness of the leaves to a lady's waterproof cloak or mantle gave it a new name and a new emphasis. In the sixteenth century it became known as 'Alchemilla', which means 'little magical one' – a name that refers to the droplets of water that form on the leaves due to the process of 'guttation'. In the Scottish Highlands its name in Gaelic is *copan an druichd*, which means 'dew cup'.

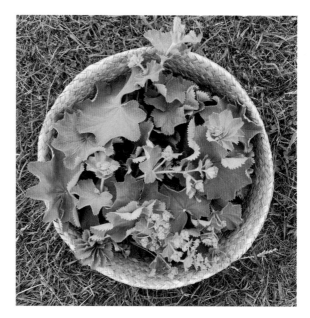

Medicinal parts
▷ Aerial parts

Physiological actions

Summary
▷ Astringent
▷ Anti-inflammatory
▷ Vulnerary

Physiological virtues

The main constituents of Lady's Mantle are tannins that help to tone and bind damaged, weak, or inflamed tissues. This herb has an affinity for the healing of torn membranes, and there are many cases describing its successful use in the healing of abdominal hernias and some of perforated eardrums. I have even read that in the sixteenth century it was used by young women to 'restore virginity'.

The toning and healing action of the leaves makes Lady's Mantle an ideal fomentation or sitz bath for post-partum healing, especially when there are tears to the perineum. It is also very helpful in treating incipient prolapse and improving the outcome of surgical prolapse treatments. A strong infusion is added to a sitz bath or bidet and the area is bathed daily. I grow a great deal of Lady's Mantle, so I can harvest enough to prescribe in sitz baths.

It is excellent taken internally as an infusion or tincture to tone and remove inflammation from the female reproductive tract, therefore helping to reduce period pain and excessive bleeding. Be careful if prescribing to a patient who has a sluggish bowel. This is something often accompanying a tendency to prolapse. In these cases, only include a small amount in a wider herbal prescription and work on regularizing the bowel as a matter of priority. If you feel that taking Lady's Mantle internally could introduce too much astringency to the gut, its virtues may be better accessed in the form of regular sitz baths or fomentations.

Energetics

Lady's Mantle is astringent and bitter. It works not only physically but also on the emotional and spiritual aspects of our being. For those patients who have suffered from sexual abuse or some other trauma that has left them feeling disempowered, Lady's Mantle strengthens and tones their spirit and helps them to move beyond the shadow of past events. This results in a feeling of renewal and a readiness to move forward in order to make the most of their precious life. Lady's Mantle is protective of us, like a cloak wrapping us up against threatening influences. To benefit from the subtle healing properties of Lady's Mantle, it is worth knowing that the droplets that form on the leaves are said to have an energetic healing quality specific to those who have suffered sexual abuse. You can collect them and take them daily in drop doses if that calls to you.

In Tibetan medicine

Lady's Mantle primarily has an astringent taste, which means that the Earth and Air elements are predominant. It is a herb that is suitable in many situations, but prescribe with caution where there is constipation, a condition often associated with raised *rLung*.

In my dispensary

I prescribe Lady's Mantle in internal prescriptions as well as topical ones. It is a good choice for those who are suffering with heavy periods or menopausal flooding, especially when there is a history of sexual abuse or trauma.

The following is a case where Lady's Mantle was definitely called for. 'Josie' was in her 50s. She had experienced sexual abuse that had started from a very early age. I will not repeat the details, but it was shocking and heartbreaking to hear her story. Although she had done a lot of very brave and constructive work to process what had happened, the experience still seemed to dominate her life and caused her to sink regularly into episodes of depression and isolation. She admitted that she had an uncomfortable relationship with food and found swallowing difficult at times. She felt that she was sabotaging her health by eating irregularly and making poor dietary choices. Josie was a patient who was very insightful about her situation, recognizing that while her instinct was to do repeated drastic cleanses and 'detoxes', what she actually needed was to nourish her body better in order to finally process the trauma and move on.

I asked her to commit to eating regularly and establishing a steady daily routine. I also suggested that she reduced her sugar intake and increased the amount of protein she ate. For her herbal prescription we started with bitters, calming nervines, and grounding adaptogens. Although not normally placed into the above herbal categories, Lady's Mantle was also included at a rate of about one fifth of the blend for its emotional resonances and for its specificity to survivors of sexual abuse. Two weeks later Josie reported feeling profoundly calmer, and her sleep was improved. She was in a better routine of eating but had had some disturbing dreams, which had made her feel angry. She said she felt as though things were bubbling up. A month after starting treatment, she felt she had really turned a corner and was no longer craving sugary snacks. A further month after that she was feeling very different: she felt good and was much more comfortable in her body. She reported that the emotions and experiences that had felt 'stuck' in her

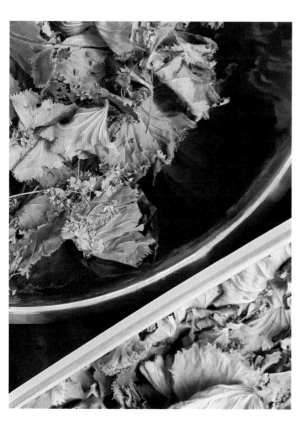

body were moving and shifting and being let go.

Although her prescription contained a blend of herbs to help with her digestion and to help her feel calmer, I feel that the Lady's Mantle had played a key role in helping her to better come to terms with her distressing childhood abuse. I should also emphasize that none of this would have worked if she had not grasped the importance of changing her diet and having a steadier routine around food.

Historical applications

Culpeper spoke highly of Lady's Mantle: '*It is one of the most singular wound-herbs that is, and therefore highly praised by the Germans, who use it in all wounds, inward and outward . . . [it] . . . wonderfully drieth up he humidity of the sores, and abateth Inflammation therein.*'

Magical

Lady's Mantle was considered the perfect treatment for 'elf shot', where it was believed that a person's failure to thrive was caused by a flint arrow shot by a malevolent elf. It is traditionally chosen for love spells.

Suggestion for the home apothecary

Sitz bath for post-partum recovery, inflammation, or incipient prolapse

Take two handfuls of fresh or dried Lady's Mantle leaves, place into a large pan or jug, and pour over 1 litre of boiling water. Leave it to steep for 20 minutes, then strain and pour into a sitz bath, adding more warm water if needed to get it to the right depth. Sit in the infusion for 10–20 minutes. Repeat daily.

Lavender 🌿 *Lavandula angustifolia*

'Lavender is a specific for nervous exhaustion and can reconnect us to our joyful state.'

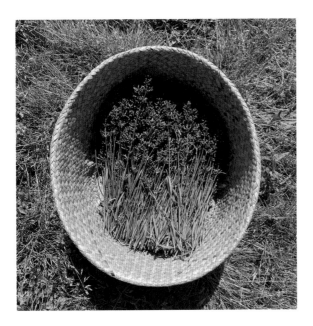

The name 'Lavender' originated from the Latin verb *lavare*, which means 'to wash'. For centuries laundry was rinsed in Lavender water, and in Elizabethan times washerwomen were called 'Lavenders'. As well as its widespread use in the beauty and fragrance world, Lavender is a wonderful medicinal herb and a specific for nervous exhaustion, whether that has been caused by years of overwork or through past trauma and anxiety.

Medicinal parts
- Flowers
- Upper leaves

Physiological actions
Summary
- Nervine
- Sedative
- Bitter
- Carminative
- Antidepressant
- Antispasmodic
- Analgesic
- Stimulant
- Diuretic
- Expectorant
- Antiseptic
- Antifungal
- Antibacterial
- Insect repellent

Physiological virtues

Lavender is a deeply restorative herb to the nervous system. It is a herb to consider for those who have forgotten what it is like to feel relaxed and spontaneously joyful. It is a specific for nervous exhaustion, calming the nerves while also supporting healthier digestion and therefore allowing the patient to digest and assimilate their past experiences. Its combination of liver and nervous system support makes it a good antidepressant herb.

Lavender gently encourages bile production, promoting more regular bowel action where that has been sluggish, as well as relieving wind and spasms in the digestive tract. It is not considered a primary cholagogue but can be a helpful herb in a blend where other factors call for it too.

It stimulates the circulation and acts as a diuretic. It also relaxes muscle spasms and is sedative and analgesic. Just to be totally clear, for internal use I am talking about whole herbal preparations. I do not recommend the taking of essential oils internally, apart from in very specific and highly controlled circumstances when prescribed by a medically trained professional.

Lavender has a wonderfully tranquillizing action that helps to dial down an over-stimulated nervous system, helping us to find a better balance in life, or at least to relax before bedtime. It can be worth considering in cases of hypertension, depending on the individual circumstances of the case. It is an expectorant, decongestant, and an anticatarrhal, so is helpful for colds and flu. It can also be good for alleviating asthma when it is exacerbated by nervous tension.

Its calming properties can be employed by sewing Lavender flowers into little sachets, which are placed under the pillow to aid restful sleep. I am also a big fan of Lavender foot baths for restless children before bedtime. Try it, and you will find bedtime a much smoother and calmer experience.

Topically, it is sedative and pain-relieving. It is a popular headache treatment, a balm or infused oil being applied to the temples and the back of the neck when a headache is starting. Its antiseptic, antibacterial, antifungal, and healing properties make it a very good first aid treatment for cuts, scrapes, infections, and burns. It can also be a good insect repellent. If you have head lice in the family, try a strong Lavender tea as a final rinse after nit combing. (Also see Wormwood for this.)

It is a uterine stimulant. Do not take during pregnancy.

Energetics
Lavender is bitter, dry, and cooling. It deeply heals the nervous system. It reconnects us with a sense of the joy and value of being alive.

In my dispensary
Since Lavender is a specific for nervous exhaustion, this is most often how I work with it in my clinic. It is a herb I consider for patients who have been running on adrenaline for a long time and feel as though life has 'knocked the stuffing out of them'. They may be struggling to get back onto an even keel after a long period of emotional stress combined with ongoing physical and mental demands. Circumstances may have meant that they have not had the time and space to pause and digest their experiences and emotions. Their nervous system is over-stretched and exhausted. They have 'emotional indigestion'. These patients need calming and nourishing herbs and a good diet, for sure, but they also need the penetrating and stimulating quality of Lavender to restore the nervous system and to help them digest their experiences and emotions.

I often recommend Lavender baths or footbaths to help soothe fractious children before bed and help them to sleep soundly. It can also be helpful for the parents of these sleepless children or any adults suffering with sleeplessness, especially those who feel unable to take additional herbs orally before bedtime. This is often the case with patients going through chemotherapy, for example. Lavender is also included as part of my favourite healing ointment blend.

The case of 'Alison' illustrates the sort of gradual deep nervous system healing that Lavender can support when a patient has forgotten what it is like to live without sadness and trauma. Alison was in her early 40s when she asked me for herbal support for her sadness, anxiety, and depression. While taking her case, I asked about any predisposing triggers. She explained that she had experienced a devastating bereavement some ten years earlier, but that she had done a lot of work on herself since then and had been able to process it. She did, however, feel anxious a lot of the time and had debilitating episodes of depression. She also had an ongoing tendency to vertigo. She frequently suffered with bloating, showing that her digestive system needed support, and she had poor circulation, having cold hands and feet, even in warm weather. On the plus side, she had a very healthy diet and was conscientious about sourcing great-quality natural foods and hydrating well. However, not so positive was the fact that she often skipped meals. She told me that she would get wrapped up in whatever it was she was doing and often could not be bothered to prepare something.

First, we had a talk about the importance of regular eating, especially in cases of anxiety, as this can be worsened by blood sugar highs and lows. Then I prescribed an individual tincture blend to support her nervous system, digestion, and circulation. Alison seemed to have forgotten what it was like to feel joyful and relaxed, and I felt that Lavender would be the best support for her on both a physiological and an emotional level. It would help her nervous system, digestion, and circulation so I made it a main herb, forming one fifth of her prescription. I also included other nervous system-, digestive, and circulation-supporting herbs such as Rosemary, Ginger, Caraway, and Wild Oat.

Within four weeks the dizziness had completely disappeared. She also said that she felt 'softer and more connected to the natural world'. She was experiencing significantly less bloating too. Although she still felt anxious, she noticed that she was sleeping a lot better. Over the next few months her anxiety steadily reduced, and her circulation improved dramatically. Although she had felt that she had completely processed her previous bereavement, she now realized that she had not really felt well since then and was now able to assimilate the bereavement in a calmer and more accepting way. Although she knew she would never 'get over it', she had been able to integrate it into her experience and no longer lived feeling as if she was under constant threat. She told me that she even felt spontaneously joyful sometimes:

this was something that had not happened for many years, and she was very happy to be able to experience it again.

'Izzy' was 21 years old and suffered with premenstrual dysphoric disorder, a very serious manifestation of premenstrual syndrome. Each month, two weeks before her period was due, she just shut down and withdrew from the world. At this time, she was hardly able to communicate with her family or to take any interest in food. She told me that she felt she had been living on adrenaline for many years, and she was feeling totally 'wrung out'. Her diet was not particularly good, as she was a student with a very demanding schedule, and she found it hard to create healthy meals while tired at the end of the day. She suffered with acid reflux and a tendency to a sluggish bowel. She also had quite poor circulation.

Together, we went through various quick and easy options for low-input, healthy meals, and she said she would try hard to improve her diet. I prescribed a tailor-made tincture to support liver and digestion as well as her circulation. I added Lavender, not only to support her digestion and circulation, but also because I felt that her nervous system was crying out for its deeply calming influence. Four weeks after her first appointment, she reported that her acid reflux was gone, her bowels were better, and her mood had been much improved over the previous menstrual cycle. She continued to improve over the next few months, though sometimes taking a step or two backwards when she went through periods of not eating as healthily as she should or when she did not take her tincture regularly. On the whole, though, she made steady improvements and felt much more able to interact with others normally during her premenstrual phase. She told me that she felt much calmer and more confident than she used to.

Historical applications

Lavender has a very long history of being considered a medicinal herb. It has been found in ancient Egyptian tombs and was often added to medicinal baths by the Romans.

Gerard wrote: '*The floures of Lavender picked from the knaps, I meane the blew part and not the husk, mixed with Cinnamon, Nutmegs, & Cloves, made into pouder, and given to drinke in the distilled water thereof, doth help the panting and passion of the heart, prevaileth against giddiness, turning, or swimming of the braine, and members subject to the palsie.*' . . . '*It profiteth them much that have the palsie, if they be washed with the distilled water of the floures, or anointed with the oile made of the floures, and oile olive.*'

Lavender was described by Parkinson as being of: '*especiall good use for all griefes and paines of the head and brain.*'

Culpeper wrote that '*a decoction made with the flowers of Lavender, Horehound, Fennel and Asparagus root, and a little Cinnamon, is very profitably used against the falling sickness and the giddiness or turning of the brain*'.

In the early 1900s, French chemist, René-Maurice Gattefossé, first discovered the antiseptic and skin-healing virtues of Lavender. He noted that it was especially helpful for burns. As a result, it later became a '*war herb*', helping to clean wounds and to ease suffering when stocks of allopathic medicines were scarce. During the Second World War, children were asked to gather Lavender flowers for the war effort.

Magical

Lavender brings happiness and encourages longevity. It is associated with love, protection, sleep, and purification. A cross made from Lavender sprigs and hung on the door would protect against the evil eye. It is said to help us to see ghosts, if that is what we desire. Place Lavender under the pillow and make a wish before going to sleep. If you have a dream relating to that wish, it will come true.

Whether worn, hung in the home, or placed in sachets among clothes, Lavender attracts love. When writing a love note, rub it with some Lavender to enhance its effects. It was known as 'Elf Leaf' in reference to its powers of enchantment, and 'Nardus' after a Syrian city called Naarda, where it was a favoured strewing herb.

Druids burnt branches of Lavender to help calm the mother and bless the baby during the birth.

Suggestions for the home apothecary

Lavender foot bath

Make a strong infusion of fresh or dried Lavender flowers and pour it into a shallow bowl or dish, large enough to bathe your feet in. Leave your feet in the infusion for 20 minutes and

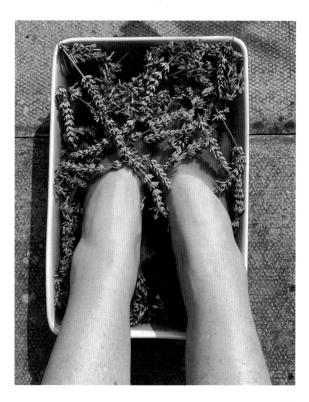

soak in its calming influence. A hand bath is also a very effective option if you are unable to make a foot bath. This is an ideal pre-bedtime routine for fractious children and their stressed parents.

Lavender flower tincture

To make a tincture, fill a jar with dried flowers or fresh flowers picked on a dry day. Cover them completely with alcohol, preferably 50% ABV (i.e. 100% proof). Most people who are making small batches choose vodka as their base. Lower-percentage vodka will be fine as long as the plant material is not high in water content, but it must exceed 25% ABV to keep well at room temperature. I choose a higher percentage in order to be sure that there is a good extraction of oil-soluble components in the tincture.

Put the jar away in a cool, dark place for 4 weeks or so. Check that the plant material is properly covered, and top up or give it a shake every so often. After it has macerated for the required time, drain, press, and bottle. Now you have a wonderful, calming nervous system

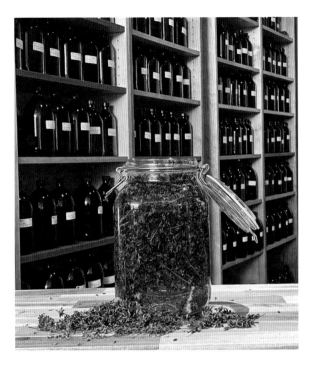

tonic. Add to your personalized blend or take a small dose, perhaps ¼ tsp, in hot water each day for a month or two.

Lemon Balm 🐝 *Melissa officinalis*

'Consider Lemon Balm when the nervous system is in a disordered state.'

The generic name, 'Melissa', refers to the Greek for honeybee, because it has a long association of being planted as a nectar plant for bees. It was also rubbed onto the hives to encourage the bees to return to them.

Lemon Balm is so easy to grow, you could say that it grows in spite of us. It spreads vigorously and self-seeds readily. If you are not careful, it will happily take over your entire herb garden. I think that as herb gardeners we are in danger of relegating this herb to just a flavoursome 'tea herb', but actually it is an excellent medicine and can hold its own in the dispensary against other more difficult to grow – and therefore perhaps more highly valued – herbs.

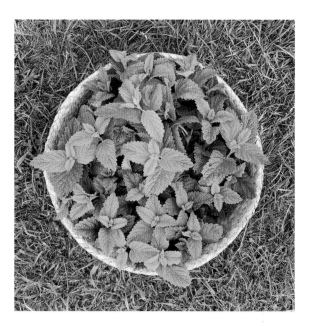

Medicinal parts
▷ Aerial parts

Physiological actions

Summary

▷ Nervine
▷ Antispasmodic
▷ Cardiovascular tonic
▷ Carminative
▷ Antiviral
▷ Diaphoretic
▷ Thyrostatic

Physiological virtues

Lemon Balm is a herb to relieve nervousness. Think of it for a nervous heart, a nervous stomach, or difficulties going to sleep. It has a particularly beneficial effect on the heart and cardiovascular system, soothing away tension and worry, calming the pulse, and creating a sense of relaxed acceptance. It is a specific for neurasthenia, also known as nervous exhaustion.

Traditionally, Lemon Balm is considered to be a remedy for disorders of the head and nerves, seeming to support memory, especially when this has been affected by stress. It also has a general antispasmodic action, gently relieving tension throughout the body and easing headaches caused by tension. Its delicious flavour makes it a good choice for tense and anxious children.

Its high level of volatile oils makes it a good carminative herb, easing digestive gripes and reducing tension in the digestive tract in general. It is the first herb to consider for patients whose digestive issues are made much worse by stress – for example, in cases of IBS, indigestion, nausea, bloating, or nervous upset tummies in children.

Lemon Balm is strongly antiviral. Research has shown that it has particularly good activity against the herpes family of viruses and is therefore a great home remedy to relieve cold sores, chickenpox, shingles, and mononucleosis. Influenza viruses are in a different family, but research has also indicated that Lemon Balm can prevent the ability of avian flu virus to replicate, so perhaps it may have activity against other influenza viruses. Regardless of whether or not it has a directly antiviral action on any particular influenza virus, it has a track record of reducing the unpleasant symptoms associated with the early onset of influenza.

When taken as a hot infusion, it is a gentle, relaxing diaphoretic, inducing a light sweat and helping to reduce fever without suppressing it. It is especially helpful where worry and tension are reducing the body's ability to relax the circulatory system and allow better blood flow to the surface. This, in turn, allows the heat of the fever to dissipate. It is rich in antioxidants and is a delicious way to keep fluid intake up while suffering from a feverish cold or influenza. As a bonus, Lemon Balm has a gently calming effect on the body, reducing anxiety and allowing us to sleep more soundly. This is especially important if we are fighting off a viral infection.

Lemon Balm is not often thought of as a topical treatment, but it works well as a compress for painful swellings such as gout. It can also be good as a topical treatment for cold sores or shingles, as well as insect bites or stings. Historically it was applied to 'green wounds' to seal them.

Lemon Balm inhibits thyroid function, so bear it in mind for some cases of hyperthyroidism. In general, if you have thyroid issues, it is best avoided in medicinal doses unless prescribed under careful professional supervision.

Energetics

Lemon Balm is sour and slightly bitter, as well as cooling. It holds us and lifts us when we feel we are at our limit and are too frazzled and exhausted to cope any more. It encourages us to relax and accept the situation instead of striving to overcome it head on. In creating acceptance, it brings space for us to see how a change of attitude or a different approach will make a big difference to how we feel.

In my dispensary

I work with Lemon Balm as tincture, a tea, and in capsules. I very often include it in my patient's prescriptions, especially for those whose digestive systems are affected by nerves and those with a tendency to anxiety or sleeplessness. Also, its value as an antiviral should not be underestimated.

The following case is a good example of where many of the virtues of Lemon Balm were called for. When I started treating her, 'Amanda', who was in her early 60s, had recently been widowed after many years as being the primary carer for her husband. She told me that she had been exhausted and stressed for a very long time. She knew that the reasons for this were multiple. She was processing a recent bereavement, she was unable to sleep well, and blood tests showed that she was low in iron. Since her energy levels were very low, she was often too tired to prepare herself healthy meals, and she had slipped out of the habit of eating regularly. She had a great many ongoing urgent responsibilities, and this made it very difficult for her to relax. As if all of this was not enough, for many years she had experienced cyclical flare-ups of the herpes virus coinciding with when she was stressed or run down.

Her poor appetite, acid reflux, and a significant after-lunch slump every day showed that her digestion was depleted. Her cold hands and feet showed that her circulation was not as it should be, and she told me that she often suffered with low mood, even though she tried hard to see the positives in life.

First off, I asked her to reduce caffeine, drink more water, and improve her diet and the regularity with which she ate. When thinking about which herbs to choose to support her, it was clear that her case called out for Lemon Balm on many levels. It would support her digestion, which was clearly affected by tension and stress, it would help to lift her mood, support her circulation, and act as an excellent antiviral. I therefore chose it as the lead herb in her prescription tincture blend, teaming it with other herbs such as Yarrow, Elderflower, St John's Wort, Vervain, Blessed Thistle, and Goat's Rue. She was to take 5 ml in hot water twice a day. I also prescribed two size '0' iron-rich blood-building capsules daily.

Amanda implemented my diet and lifestyle suggestions with gusto and took her herbal medicine consistently. Four weeks later she was already sleeping much better, her energy levels were greatly improved (going from 4/10 to 7/10), and, despite quite a stressful time, she had not succumbed to one of her 'usual' herpes flare-ups. Her digestion was much better, her appetite was improved, and her after-lunch slumps were greatly reduced or absent. While these early improvements were a result of all elements of her prescription including the lifestyle and dietary changes, there is no doubt that they were greatly assisted by the Lemon Balm. She continued to implement her lifestyle and dietary changes with the support of her herbal prescription over the next few months and felt more and more restored, telling me that she felt better than she had done for a long time.

Historical applications

We know that Lemon Balm has been a very important medicinal herb for many centuries. For example, in the year 789, the capitularies of Charlemagne ordered that it was to be planted in every monastery garden.

Paracelsus held it in very high esteem, believing that it would '*completely revivify a man*'.

The London Dispensary (1696) included the following entry for Lemon Balm: '*An essence of Balm, given in Canary wine, every morning will renew youth, strengthen the brain, relieve languishing nature and prevent baldness.*'

The seventeenth-century diarist, John Evelyn, wrote: '*Balm is sovereign for the brain, strengthening the memory and powerfully chasing away melancholy.*'

Gerard said: '*It comforteth the hart and driveth away all sadness*'. He added that '*the juice of Balm glueth together greene wounds . . . without any perill of inflammation.*'

Parkinson discussed it in the same section as Motherwort, as he felt that their properties are very similar. He wrote: '*The Arabian physicians have extolled the vertues of Baulme, for the passions of the heart. Serapio saith: it is the property of Baulme, to cause the mind and heart to become merry, to*

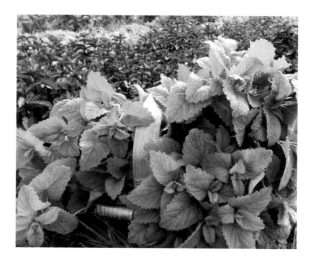

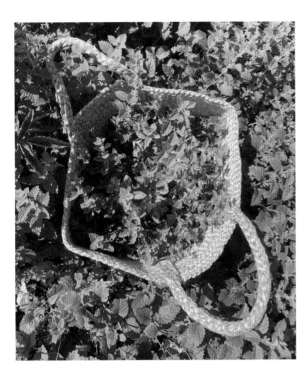

revive the fainting heart falling into swounings, to strengthen the weakness of the spirits and heart, and to comfort them, especially such who are overtaken in their sleepe, therewith taking away all motion of the pulse, to drive away all troublesome cares and thoughts out of the minde, whether those passions rise from melancholy or black choler, or burnt flegme.'

Lemon Balm is the chief ingredient in the preparation called '*Carmelite Water*'. The Emperor Charles V drank this daily. Daily Lemon Balm intake is associated with longevity. A John Hussey, of Sydenham, supposedly had Lemon Balm tea sweetened with honey every morning before breakfast and lived until he was 116.

Magical

In Arabian herb magic, Lemon Balm is considered to influence love. Pliny the Elder spoke of its powers to heal magically. If it was attached to a sword that had made a wound, the blood would be immediately staunched.

Suggestion for the home apothecary

Fresh Lemon Balm tea

Pick a 5–7-cm sprig of fresh herb, and place it into a cup; add boiling water, and leave it covered to infuse for 10 minutes before drinking. By covering the cup, you are preventing the aromatic compounds from escaping – an important measure as these are responsible for many of its medicinal qualities. If using dried herb, you should use 1 tsp, heaped, per cup in a tea ball or infuser.

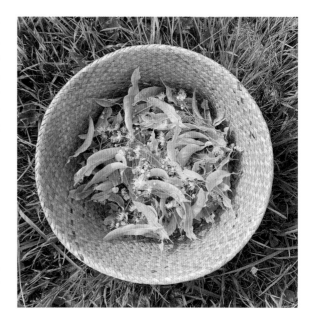
Lime – also known as Linden – 'calms the circulatory forces'. The flowers are calming and supportive, helping us to let go of our tendency to drive ourselves into an unbalanced state. They are especially wonderful at supporting patients who are tackling their tendency to hypertension. I would not want to be without them in my dispensary

Medicinal parts

▷ Flowers
▷ Bracts
▷ Bark
▷ Charcoal (sometimes)

The flowers should be picked before they turn to seed, as the seeds, if taken as tea, can produce symptoms of narcotic intoxication.

Physiological actions

Summary

▷ Nervine
▷ Relaxant
▷ Diaphoretic
▷ Hypotensive
▷ Antispasmodic
▷ Demulcent
▷ Expectorant
▷ Diuretic

Physiological virtues

Lime flowers are calming and relaxing; they are a good nervine to consider in cases of nervous exhaustion. They are also antispasmodic, which is why they are so helpful in cases of hypertension. They contain flavonoids that reduce inflammation in the circulatory system, further helping to lower high blood pressure. They can ease tension, reduce anxiety and palpitations, and encourage restful sleep. Their relaxing and demulcent properties help to encourage gentle expectoration when the lungs are congested. They are also diaphoretic, meaning they encourage sweating, especially when drunk as a tea. Drinking Lime flower tea, known as *Tilleul* in France, is a good choice when suffering from a feverish cold or influenza but is also popular as a fragrant and calming infusion to enjoy anytime.

Lime flowers are a gentle diuretic and demulcent, having a beneficial action on the urinary system. They soothe irritated tissues and help people to pass urine more easily.

The young bark has similar properties to the flowers, although it is perhaps a bit more astringent. It is worthwhile remembering the option of working with the bark, since the season for gathering Lime flowers is so transient and is easily sabotaged by inclement weather.

There is a tradition of prescribing powdered Lime charcoal for gastric or dyspeptic issues. This preparation can also be applied topically for burns or sores.

Energetics

Lime is sweet and warming. Lime flowers can help us to let go of pent-up tension or anger, helping us to feel 'softer' and more accepting. My herbal tutor, Ifanca, highlighted the frequent link between high blood pressure and anger. Sometimes the anger may be directed at a person or situation, and at other times it may be directed inwards. It may be held so deeply within our body that we may not even realise that it is there. Once the anger is resolved, the hypertension will reduce.

In Tibetan medicine

Lime flowers are not included within the Tibetan pharmacopoeia, but Tibetan medicine can shed further light on the matter of the link between hypertension and anger. In Tibetan medicine the 'mind poison' of anger is linked to all sorts of inflammatory diseases – including hypertension – and problems with the liver and gallbladder. We are taught that to transform anger into compassion is the best way to escape from its negative effects, both within our body and around us. If we can feel more 'at ease' in our body, then we are less 'dis-eased' and our circulatory system flows more freely and evenly. If you have high blood pressure, it may be worth checking in with yourself as to whether you have some long-term anger simmering away. Anger can become a habit if we are not careful. Lime flower tea would be a good support while changing things.

In my dispensary

I prescribe Lime flowers in tinctures, teas, and capsules, according to the case. Below are a couple of typical examples of where Lime flowers have calmed the circulatory forces.

'Jennifer' was in her late 70s and was full of energy and life. She preferred not to take allopathic medication, but a recent health check had flagged up that her blood pressure was too high. Her GP was insistent that she should start hypotensive medication as soon as possible. Jennifer was annoyed about this, because she felt that she had 'white coat syndrome', and she did not believe that her blood pressure was 'too bad'. I took it – not wearing a white coat – and her reading was 170/85. I told her that this definitely needed to come down, but I felt that with herbs and lifestyle changes we could shift things to a healthier level. During her consultation she told me that she was constantly annoyed by a complicated family situation and was especially angry with one of her relatives. She was also irritated by the way that allopathic medication was dispensed to so many people of her age, and she did not like attending her local exercise class because the instructor was patronizing and the other students were too 'doddery'. With all of this anger swirling around, it was pretty clear that Lime flowers were going to be helpful. She had an individually blended tea of Lime flowers with some other calming herbs, and we had a chat about the link between anger and hypertension. I also strongly encouraged her to go back to some regular exercise. She took it all on board and agreed to take her tea conscientiously. Four weeks later her blood pressure was coming down nicely and was at a level of 155/82. She had begun to feel much less 'tetchy'; a month later her reading was down to 135/85. She continues to follow her lifestyle and dietary guidelines and has her blood pressure regularly monitored by her GP.

Historical applications

Gerard wrote that '*The floures are commended by divers (people) against paine of the head. . . against dissinesse, the Apoplexie, and also falling sicknesse.*'

Maud Grieve recommended '*prolonged baths made with the infused flowers*' to treat hysteria.

Magical

According to Greek legend, the nymph Philrya was raped by the god Saturn, who was disguised in the form of a horse. As a result of this she gave birth to the centaur Chiron and was so horrified that she begged to gods to help her. They obliged by turning her into a Lime tree.

In folklore it is said that even sitting under a Lime tree will cure epilepsy.

Lime is associated with protection, branches being hung over the doorway of the home for this purpose. Carrying the bark is said to prevent intoxication, while leaves and blossom are used in love spells. It is a tree of immortality. Lithuanian women once made sacrifices to Lime trees as part of their religious observances.

Suggestion for the home apothecary

Dried Lime flowers for tea

Gather plenty of Lime flowers and lay them on trays in an airy place away from direct sunlight. You can also use a dehydrator if you live somewhere where the ambient humidity is high. Once they are thoroughly dry, store in an airtight container in the dark.

If you feel that your blood pressure is getting too high and you recognize that you are prone to feeling angry a lot of the time, you may find two cups of Lime flower tea a day helpful. Put

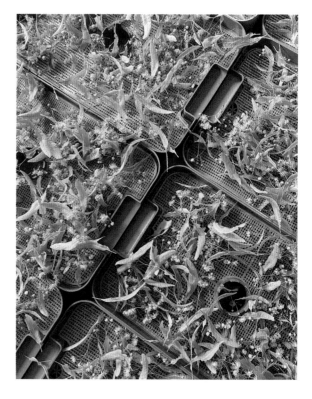

2–3 flowers into an infuser and pour on boiling water. Leave to infuse, covered, for 10 minutes before drinking. You will need to give it a hand though by committing to regular exercise and eating healthily, including plenty of fresh fruits and vegetables of as many different colours as possible in your meals each day. You should also take steps to change your habitual thought patterns away from anger to a more tolerant and compassionate outlook. If your blood pressure continues to rise or stays high, you should seek advice from your doctor. Sometimes being accountable to a real person is necessary to encourage the necessary changes.

Long Pepper 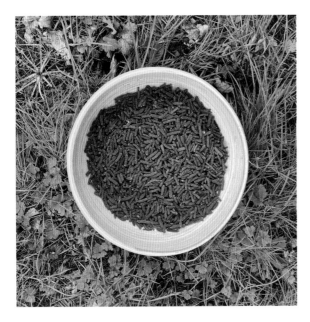 *Piper longum*

'Long Pepper restores digestive heat and encourages movement where there is stagnancy.'

Long Pepper brings the principles of heat and movement to cold stagnant conditions. This means that, as well as feeling better physically, patients taking Long Pepper often find that they feel more motivated to initiate new projects and to stick with new health regimes. As you can imagine this can be truly life-changing.

Medicinal parts
▹ Fruit

Physiological actions

Summary

▹ Stimulant
▹ Relaxant
▹ Antispasmodic
▹ Carminative
▹ Aperient
▹ Anti-inflammatory
▹ Decongestant
▹ Immune system tonic

Physiological virtues

Long Pepper is warming and stimulating while also being calming and relaxing. It has antispasmodic properties. With Long Pepper you have both stimulation and relaxation in one medicine. This is a powerful combination, because the warming aspects stimulate the circulation and the antispasmodic aspects relax the vessels, allowing the improved blood supply to move more freely through the tissues.

Long Pepper contains piperine, which stimulates the digestive system, enhancing absorption of amino acids from the gastrointestinal tract. It is a good herb to consider in cases of poor appetite, weak digestion, bloating, flatulence, and constipation.

Maud Grieve advises against combining Long Pepper with herbs primarily included in a prescription as astringents – for example, Raspberry leaf or Lady's Mantle – since piperine reduces the action of astringents. This is worth noting if, for example, your prescription aims to treat menorrhagia, and you wanted to include a warming circulatory stimulant and digestive support in the blend.

Long Pepper is a good anti-inflammatory in cases of arthritis and gout, where poor circulation is very often a contributory factor. It can also reduce the severity of allergic reactions in conditions such as hay fever.

It enhances our immune response, encouraging phagocytosis, which is the engulfing of foreign 'invaders', along with any of our own cells that have mutated and have become abnormal. Phagocytosis is a very important first line of defence against cancer.

Long Pepper gets things moving, improving the metabolism, and it can help to reduce fat tissue. It is a decongestant, easing the symptoms of colds and cutting through any build-up of bronchial catarrh. It reduces bronchospasm, which is why it is traditionally prescribed for asthma. Its antispasmodic action also makes it helpful for menstrual cramps and colic.

Topically, Long Pepper can be infused in oil to make a stimulating and warming massage oil. It can also be powdered and mixed with Ginger, Nutmeg, and Caraway and made into hormé packs. (See Nutmeg for details.)

Long Pepper is less harsh on the stomach than Black Pepper and is an excellent spice to have on hand in the kitchen.

Energetics

Long Pepper's taste is hot to sweet, with a warming, coarse, and sharp potency. It cuts through stagnation and apathy, promoting renewed energy and vitality. Taking Long Pepper can bring us new enthusiasm and motivation if this has been lacking. As well as being stimulating, it is also grounding and calming, reducing anxiety and insomnia.

In Tibetan medicine

Long Pepper is known as *Pipiling* [པི་པི་ལིང་] in Tibetan. It has a hot taste and a sharp potency, but this is transformed to a sweet taste after digestion. This means that Long Pepper does not increase the *Tripa* humour like Black Pepper does. Its potency is warm, rough, and fast-acting.

According to the Tibetan medicinal texts, Long Pepper treats loss of digestive heat and all cold ailments without exception. It is one of the herbs included in the digestion-supporting blend, 'Hot Pomegranate Five'. It is especially helpful for combined disorders of *Pekén* and *rLung*, as well as cold *rLung* spleen disorders. It is also viewed as a very good expectorant, reducing excessive formation of sputum as well as asthma. It is an aphrodisiac and is prescribed as a rejuvenation medicine.

In my dispensary

In my clinic I prescribe Long Pepper in capsule form in a Tibetan formula called Hot Pomegranate Five. It is specific for those with cold disorders of *Pekén*. A course of these usually results in increased motivation and a better ability to make lifestyle changes.

'Matthew' was 45 years old and suffering with a severe lack of motivation, as well as a poor digestion. He was very indecisive, so much so that he found it hard to decide on a response to many of the questions that I asked during his consultation. Each time I asked him a question – for example 'How would you describe your average energy level?' – he blew air out between his lips, shrugged his shoulders, and said he really did not know, it was hard to say. I prescribed 'Hot Pomegranate Five capsules, and he found that not only did his digestion and energy improve, he discovered a new-found decisiveness and made the decision to relocate and pursue a long-held dream.

Historical applications

Dodoens included an entry for Long Pepper in his herbal. He describes all the Peppers as '*hot and drie in the third degree . . .* [but that] *. . . Long Pepper is not so dry, because it is partaker of a certain moisture.*' He describes many virtues for Long Pepper and suggests it as a clearer of the eyesight, writing that '*Long Pepper is good to be mingled with eie medicines or colliries . . .* [gathered blends] *. . . made to clear and strengthen the sight.*'

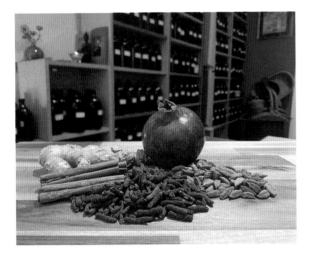

Suggestion for the home apothecary

Hot Pomegranate five

Blend the following powders:
  » *8 parts Pomegranate*
  » *1 part Cinnamon*
  » *1 part Green Cardamom*
  » *2 parts Long Pepper*
  » *4 parts Ginger*

Put into capsules and take 1–2 daily, preferably in the late morning.

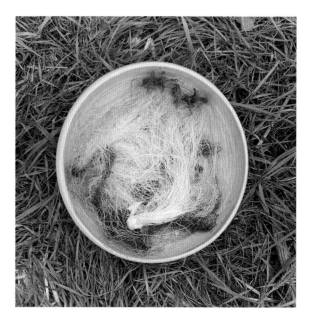

'Cornsilk soothes inflamed tissues in watery environments of the body.'

The Latin name of Maize reflects its enormously important role in supporting and nourishing us human beings. 'Zea' means 'cause of life' and 'mays' means 'our mother'. Cornsilk, the strands that form over the kernels, is a valuable remedy, most often prescribed in cases of urinary system inflammation, but also as a general diuretic.

Medicinal parts

▷ Cornsilk
▷ Seeds

The flower pistils are known as cornsilk.

Physiological actions

Summary

▷ Diuretic
▷ Demulcent
▷ Urinary system relaxant
▷ Anti-inflammatory

Physiological virtues

Maize Cornsilk is an ideal herb for supporting patients with urinary system infections, inflammation, or obstructions. It has a combination of helpful virtues that work together to achieve this aim. First, it is demulcent and excellent at soothing inflamed mucous membranes, especially in a moist environment. This makes it a very good choice for easing the discomfort of infections in the inner membranes of the urinary system. Second, it is a gentle diuretic. Third, it relaxes the kidney tubules and bladder. Together, these actions encourage the easier passage of urine and reduce discomfort where there is infection. Cornsilk is also very effective in reducing frequent urination where this is caused by bladder irritation or inflammation of the prostate. It can be also prescribed to help with the passage of urinary gravel and to reduce the formation of kidney stones.

It has a high potassium content, which may play a role in its diuretic action. Through improved diuresis it can play a role in reducing hypertension in some patients. It also contains allantoin, which is a tissue-healing substance also found in Comfrey. Cornsilk has a mild cholagogue action and may reduce blood clotting time.

Taste and energetics

Maize is sweet.

In Tibetan medicine

Zea mays is known as *A sho pa tra* [ཨ་ཤོ་པ་ཏྲ།]. The seed is the medicinal part, and it has a sweet taste, with a sweet post-digestive taste.

Its potency is cool and light. It is considered beneficial for oedema, dysuria, stones in the urethra, and other urinary system imbalances.

In my dispensary

As well as choosing Cornsilk in tailor-made prescriptions for patients with urinary issues, I also make a demulcent eye-drop blend with it. I discovered this when one of my patients could not tolerate over-the-counter moistening eye drops. I blended equal parts *Zea mays* and Calendula tinctures as an alternative to my usual astringent and antimicrobial eye-drop blend. Three drops are added to a clean eye bath containing distilled water or cooled boiled water. Bathe the eye thoroughly over a sink or basin up to three

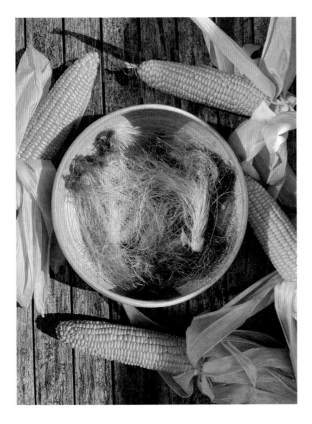

times a day if necessary, but once a day is usually sufficient. If treating both eyes, use a separate eye bath for each eye.

'Mary' had suffered from a persistent watering eye in the past and had been offered an operation to block or reduce the diameter of her tear duct. Unfortunately, this had resulted in the opposite problem: a very painful dry eye. She had been advised to use over-the-counter moistening eye drops, but she found that after a short time these did not agree with her, and her eyes became inflamed and swollen. I gave her a small dropper bottle of the Cornsilk and Calendula tincture to try, and I explained how to prepare and apply it. After two days she emailed me to say that the blend was 'absolutely miraculous', and she was overjoyed.

Historical applications

Corn has been cultivated in South America for at least 5,000 and possibly 7,000 years. It spread around the world after the Spanish conquest. It started to be cultivated in Europe from 1493 on, but it did not really thrive until hybrids were developed later. The Portuguese introduced it to Africa, where it grew well.

Maud Grieve mentions that in the past Cornsilk was prescribed in the treatment of gonorrhoea. She wrote that in its action it is like Holy Thistle.

Magical

Known as 'Sacred Mother' and 'Seed of Seeds', the Corn Mother represents plenty and fertility and is worshipped in many cultures. Corn as a medicine was included in Aztec herbals. In Mayan and Incan folk medicine Cornsilk and Corn cobs were employed as divinatory tools.

Suggestion for the home apothecary

Demulcent eye drops

Make a small batch of Cornsilk tincture and another of Calendula, both with 25% ABV if the herbs are dried; if the herbs are fresh, you will need 40–50% ABV. Blend 1 part of each tincture together to create your demulcent eye drops. Add 3 drops to an eye bath filled with cooled boiled water, and bathe the affected eye daily.

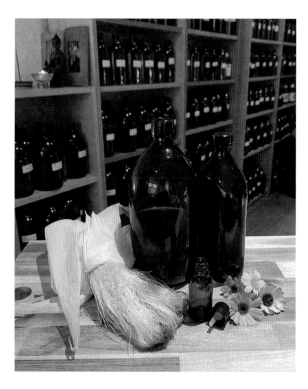

Marshmallow ✿ *Althaea officinalis*

'Marshmallow softens and soothes irritated tissues and jagged edges. It is a specific for preventing the spread of necrosis.'

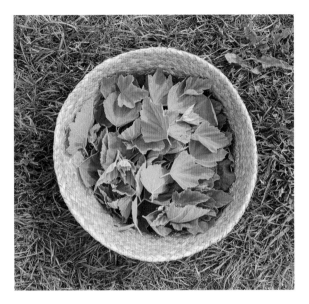

The name 'Althaea' comes from the Greek *altho*, which means 'to heal'. I harvest Marshmallow leaves each year to prescribe in teas, and once every four years I take a harvest of the roots. When you dig up a root, you immediately smell its characteristic sweetness and notice that its appearance is reminiscent of the trachea and bronchi of the respiratory system. You may also notice that the cut edges of the roots ooze a slimy, soothing liquid. The soft fuzzy leaves draw us in to stroke them and are beautifully comforting. With these attributes, Marshmallow is telling us how it can help us. You cannot help but to feel as though the plant is offering us a healing balm for our sore or jagged 'edges'.

Medicinal parts
- Leaves
- Flowers
- Roots

Physiological actions

Summary
- Demulcent
- Anti-inflammatory

Physiological virtues

Marshmallow, whether prescribed as a root, flowers, or leaves, is an excellent soothing demulcent. It can be very helpful for inflammatory conditions such as gastritis, oesophagitis, enteritis, diverticulitis, irritable bowel syndrome, tracheitis, irritable dry coughs, sore throats, and urinary system inflammation – for example, urethritis and cystitis. One extra special quality of Marshmallow leaves is their ability to stop the spread of necrosis and to heal the surrounding tissue. Stubborn leg ulcers or longstanding diverticular disease are two examples where Marshmallow leaf can be amazingly helpful as part of a holistic treatment strategy. I am not sure how this works exactly – perhaps it provides just the right balance of a nourishing anti-inflammatory influence while also being directly antimicrobial. Research has shown Marshmallow to be active against *Pseudomonas aeruginosa, Proteus vulgaris,* and *Staphylococcus aureus,* but it can probably inhibit many more bugs than these. If you suspect there may be hidden necrosis, for example in the gut, remember that Marshmallow can work wonders.

The root can be prepared as an overnight infusion to create a soothing drink, or it can be dried and powdered and administered as capsules. The dried or fresh leaves are also well suited to tea blends. In my clinic, I also have Marshmallow leaf available as a tincture, so I can add it to certain patient prescriptions when indicated. In general, though, an aqueous infusion is the best way to prepare Marshmallow.

Be aware that the mucilage in Marshmallow can reduce absorption from the gut, so if you want to avoid this, leave 2 hours between taking it and eating. However, in severe inflammatory conditions of the gut, the protective action of Marshmallow is a helpful starting point to heal the gut from the potentially irritating effects of food, so, as a short-term strategy, it is prescribed immediately before eating, and often afterwards too.

The leaves and root can be applied topically as an emollient to heal skin ulcers, wounds, burns, and boils and to draw out splinters or foreign bodies, as well as to treat necrosis affecting the surface of the body.

Energetics

Marshmallow is sweet, neutral, heavy, and a little warming. When you first taste it, it is overwhelmingly sweet, but there is also a little hint of a resinous warming influence.

As well as physically soothing and healing irritated tissues, Marshmallow can smooth the way for us to heal unresolved emotional issues from the past. My tutor, Ifanca, always used to emphasize that, in order to process past events and trauma, we need to be able to 'digest them' and assimilate the teaching that they bring us. If experiences are too 'indigestible', we are left with repeating patterns of projection and reactive behaviours, especially when faced with situations that remind our bodies of the original disturbing event. Marshmallow can be especially helpful when our inability to digest disturbing emotions and experiences is associated with a rawness or inflammatory state of our gut. In these cases, once we connect with Marshmallow, we find that it smooths the way for us to integrate disturbing emotions and move forward

with a new, more resilient attitude to the old triggers.

In Tibetan medicine

Marshmallow is sweet and is therefore well indicated for inflammatory states associated with excess *Tripa*. It was traditionally prescribed in cases of dysentery with blood loss, as it soothes the inflamed tissues and allows them to heal. Marshmallow can also be helpful in what may seem to be an opposing presentation. On a physiological level, Marshmallow can be helpful to relieve constipation associated with tension and dryness. On an emotional level, it helps patients to feel more grounded and accepting of past disturbing events. It is smooth, moistening, and nourishing, so we can look to Marshmallow as part of a prescription in order to counterbalance the airiness, dryness, and 'roughness' of disturbed '*rLung*'.

In my dispensary

The following case illustrates Marshmallow's moistening and softening influence. 'Alison' was in her mid-70s and had had Sjögren's disease for some time. As a result of this autoimmune condition, her tissues were very dry, and she had difficulty swallowing. She told me that she would have frequent mini choking episodes throughout the day, even when just swallowing her own saliva.

I asked her to remove both gluten and dairy from her diet, which, I felt, were contributing to her autoimmune tendencies. After my explanation, she committed to this dietary change wholeheartedly. Her herbal prescription was largely based on adaptogens such as Ashwagandha and Codonopsis, but I also included Marshmallow leaf as one fifth of the blend. She was to take 5 ml twice a day. She also had 2.5 ml a day of a double-extracted medicinal mushroom blend. After four weeks, she noticed that her mouth and eyes were feeling less dry, and four weeks after that she reported that the mini choking episodes were lessening. At the end of a year of treatment she was feeling much better, her digestion had improved, her eyes and mouth were more comfortable, and the mini choking episodes were only happening, at most, once a day.

The following case illustrates the ability of Marshmallow's to tackle necrosis. 'Charles' was a Type I diabetic in his 70s who had lost one of his legs to the disease ten years before I met him. His prosthetic leg caused him a great deal of discomfort where it fitted his stump, and he had been told that he was 'too old' to be fitted with a new one. He originally came to me for help in managing his blood sugar, as after many years of injecting insulin he was developing insulin resistance. He was quite the extrovert and used to regale me with funny stories and slightly bad-taste jokes. It was quite difficult to keep each consultation to the time slot allocated, but I could not take offense because he was such a lovely character.

After a year or so of treatment he was doing well, but, unfortunately, he had a fall and was admitted to hospital. The medical team told him he should not take any herbal medications while he was in hospital and so for several weeks he was inactive, in bed, eating hospital food. His circulation regressed, and a small cut on his toe became infected. Necrosis started to set in. He was familiar with the process after losing a leg ten years previously. He insisted on being discharged so that he could restart his herbal medicines, as he absolutely did not want to lose his remaining leg. Once home, he telephoned me straight away, and I saw him a couple of days later.

His foot and leg looked pretty bad. Three of the toes were already black, and his lower leg was quite cold and a dark red colour. We restarted his normal circulation-supporting herbs and added Marshmallow capsules and tea for its antinecrotic action. I provided him with plenty of dried Marshmallow leaves and explained to his wife how to make a fomentation that she was to apply twice daily. I prayed fervently that it was not going to be too late.

Charles's wife was the most devoted, determined, and amazing person. She had originally trained as a nurse, and she made sure that he took all of his various medications on time. Without fail she prepared and administered two Marshmallow leaf fomentations daily to his one remaining lower leg. The foot and leg started to improve almost straight away, and after a couple of weeks the lower leg was a much healthier colour and had begun to feel warm to the touch. Apparently, his doctors were quite surprised about this and delayed the amputation. With continued herbal treatment, things continued to improve, and I am delighted to report that in the end he kept his leg, only losing the two toes that had been the worst affected. Both Charles and his wife were extremely grateful for the 'miracle cure'. They used to tell me that 'my treatment' had saved his leg, but I know that it was actually the amazing herbs and the thorough nursing care administered by his wife.

Charles survived for another three years after this episode. When I heard that he had died, even though it was not a surprise, I was very sad. I had got to know him over the years and found his fighting spirit and determination to live very inspiring.

I want to share one more case about Marshmallow root's magic in a case of gut inflammation and possible hidden necrosis. 'Victoria' was in her late 70s and had long-standing severe diverticular disease. When she first asked me for herbal support, she was in extreme pain from an attack of diverticulitis that was not responding to antibiotic therapy. She was unable to tolerate any foods, and if she did try something simple, she had an explosively loose stool. Victoria had been told that she urgently needed a colostomy but that she needed to gain weight and strength in order to survive the surgery. She was losing weight and strength fast, and it was a frightening and serious situation.

I suspected that there may be necrosis in the gut and immediately prescribed capsules containing Marshmallow root. She was to take six each day, spread out in three doses of two capsules, one before and one after each 'meal'. I put the word meal in inverted commas because she was no longer able to eat proper meals by this stage. I told her that if no food was taken, she was still to take two capsules and drink some water at the normal mealtimes. Within two weeks she was feeling much better, her pain levels had significantly reduced, and her stool was more formed. Provided she was careful with her food choices, she was able to eat more normally again. She was delighted to see that she was gradually recovering her weight and strength. She recovered sufficiently to be able to go through the surgery and is doing well more than a decade later. She tells me that she is convinced that 'I saved her life', but of course I know it was the Marshmallow.

Historical applications

London apothecaries were supplied with the roots of Marshmallow by herb women who dug the roots from the salt marshes of the Thames Estuary. It was an essential herb in the household physic garden for '*Belly, Stone, Reins, Kidneys, Bladder, Coughs, Shortness of Breath, Wheesing, Excoriation of the Guts, Ruptures, Cramp, Convulsions, the King's Evil, Kernels, Chin-cough* [whooping cough], *Wounds, Bruises, Falls, Blows, Muscles, Morphew, Sun Burning*', as Culpeper wrote.

Gerard wrote of Marshmallow roots that they

are: '*thicke, tough, white within*' and containing '*a clammie and slimie juice*', and Culpeper said that laying this mucilaginous juice in water '*will thicken it . . . as if it were jelly*'. He described Marshmallow roots, when boiled in water '*help to open the body and are very convenient to the hot agues*'. Culpeper also described the application of boiled Marshmallow leaves as a poultice on the breasts of wet nurses to enhance lactation, and that this treatment could help to resolve '*inflammations or swellings*' in women's breasts. Marshmallow is clearly working on many levels here.

It is also fascinating to note that Pliny thought that Marshmallow was good for all diseases, but it was especially good for '*the falling sickness*' (seizures). We can see here how an historical source provides a tantalizing glimpse into a lost or forgotten action of a familiar herb.

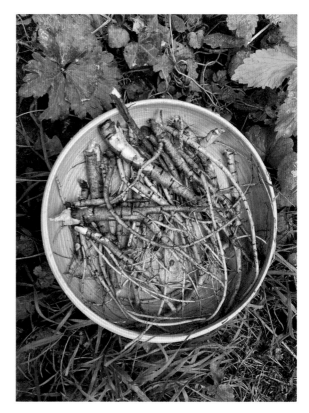

Magical

Marshmallow has long been used in protection rites. It is also considered to be a good stimulator of psychic power. It is burned as an incense or sewn into a sachet and carried.

Suggestions for the home apothecary

Marshmallow root cold infusion

Chop about 10 cm of a fresh Marshmallow root and add it to 570 ml/1 pint of water. Leave to infuse overnight at room temperature. In the morning strain and place the infusion in the fridge. Drink throughout the day to relieve inflammation in the digestive tract or to soothe a dry cough.

Marshmallow leaf fomentation

Infuse Marshmallow leaves in boiling water for at least 10 minutes. Strain and then soak clean muslin cloths in the tea. Gently wring out excess liquid, and apply warm moist cloths to the affected area. Repeat the process with fresh cloths as they cool, so that the warm fomenta-

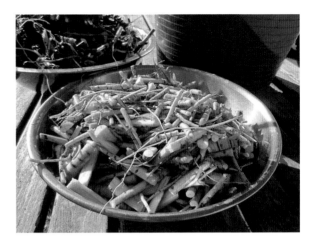

tion is in place for 30 minutes once or twice each day. You can also apply the leaves directly in place of the cloths if you have sufficient. In this case, cover the leaves with a cloth and leave in place for 30 minutes.

Marshmallow root drawing poultice

Mix the powdered root with water to make a paste and apply to the affected area.

'Meadowsweet is so much more than an alternative to aspirin.'

Meadowsweet was the first medicinal herb that I gathered from the wild, years before I formally studied herbal medicine. It was my 'gateway' herb, the one that drew me in, captivating me and encouraging me to explore other wild medicines. As such it holds a very special place in my heart. One of its main country names is 'Queen of the Meadow' – a fitting tribute to such a beautiful and valuable medicine. It has a very characteristic almond-like scent that is slightly reminiscent of the glue sticks my children used at nursery school. I absolutely love Meadowsweet's aroma, whether it is still on the growing plant or picked and placed into my harvesting basket, but not everyone does. Unfortunately, one of its other old country names is 'Courtship and Marriage', named because the flowers were considered to have a beautiful fragrance when fresh but, once plucked, the aroma became less sweet. I much prefer the name 'Meadowsweet' or 'Meadwort', the latter arising from its traditional role in the flavouring of mead.

Medicinal parts
▷ Aerial parts

I harvest the flowers only.

Physiological actions

Summary
▷ Astringent
▷ Anti-inflammatory
▷ Analgesic
▷ Diuretic
▷ Antispasmodic
▷ Diaphoretic
▷ Antimicrobial

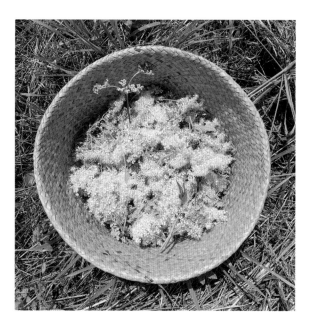

Physiological virtues

Meadowsweet is a member of the wider *Rosaceae* family, sharing those astringent, anti-inflammatory, and toning properties that we tend to think of when we consider Raspberry leaf or Agrimony. Unlike its relatives, though, Meadowsweet survives and thrives in poorly drained, wet soils. As such it seems to bring special much-needed healing qualities to our bodies when stagnancy, damp, acidity and inflammation are causing us problems. Think of Meadowsweet when faced with cases of gastric hyperacidity, attacks of gout (caused by a build-up of uric acid), or painful flare-ups of rheumatism after eating foods rich in oxalic acid. It reduces inflammation and dries out and tones 'soggy' tissues.

As well as being anti-inflammatory and astringent, Meadowsweet is analgesic, diuretic, and antispasmodic. It is therefore a herb to consider when there is joint pain, diarrhoea, stomach acidity, gastritis, and ulcers. It helps to flush out kidney stones and gravel and relieves the pain of urinary-tract infections. Meadowsweet is gently calming as well as able to soothe away pain, so it can be a good option to try in order to relieve a tension headache. It is diaphoretic when drunk as a hot tea, so can reduce fevers. As an additional benefit, it is antimicrobial.

Meadowsweet contains salicylates, which were first isolated from it in 1836 and led to the creation of the drug with the name 'Aspirin'. Inspiration for the patented name, 'Aspirin' comes from the old Latin name for Meadowsweet, which was *Spirea ulmaria*. Later on, it was discovered that Willow bark was a particularly good source of salicylates for drug production purposes, and nowadays everyone thinks that Willow, rather than Meadowsweet, was the plant that originally led to the creation of aspirin.

Meadowsweet beautifully demonstrates the difference between working with whole plants and isolated extracts. Aspirin is acetosalicylate, which is not exactly the same as the natural salicylates in Meadowsweet. Herbalists prescribe whole plants rather than isolated constituents, and herbal medicines provide a beautiful and sophisticated balance of natural compounds to the body, many of which have apparently 'opposing' actions to each other. This is quite different from manufactured pharmaceutical drugs, even if they did originally come from plants. Aspirin is highly irritant to the digestive tract, yet Meadowsweet is frequently prescribed successfully in cases where there is irritation and inflammation of the stomach lining. Additionally, Meadowsweet does not have the same blood-thinning action as aspirin. The whole plant delivers a balanced healing influence that moderates the potentially irritating effects of the salicylates that it contains.

Topically, Meadowsweet-infused oil can make an excellent analgesic rub for painful joints, or cloths soaked in a strong infusion can be applied as a fomentation. The tea can also be helpful as an astringent gargle and mouthwash for sore throats and bleeding gums. When cooled, it can be good as an eye wash for conjunctivitis.

Many people view Meadowsweet as a natural 'alternative to aspirin', but please remember that, like all herbs, it is far more than just a package of isolated 'active ingredients'. It is a beautiful medicinal plant with its own unique qualities. We should not define Meadowsweet by the chemicals that it contains – just as we cannot define our friends by the constituents that make up their bodies – but, having said that, we should prescribe it with caution to those who are sensitive to salicylates.

Energetics

Meadowsweet is astringent and bitter. It counteracts 'sogginess' and neutralizes excess acid in the body.

In my dispensary

Meadowsweet is a staple within my dispensary. I often reach for it when I need an anti-inflammatory or alkalizing influence in patients' prescriptions, whether that is in the digestive tract or in the musculo-skeletal system. I add it to Marshmallow root in demulcent capsule blends in order to support patients with IBS or chronic diarrhoea. I also make Meadowsweet and Celery seed capsules as an option for some patients going through treatment for arthritis and rheumatism. In a tea blend with Marshmallow leaf, Meadowsweet can be absolutely wonderful for patients suffering from heartburn or stomach ulcers. Mixed with Wood Avens leaf, it is a good choice to calm diarrhoea in children.

'Lizzie' was 60 years of age and determined to keep active, despite her worsening rheumatoid arthritis. She suffered with constant pain in her hands, feet, shoulders, and hips and took four paracetamol each day in order to be able to cope. She had long-standing diverticulitis and a frequent loose stool, as well as 'terrible' circulation. Despite all of this, she remained very positive and determined to live life to the full. She was involved in lots of charitable projects and was a very inspiring patient.

I prescribed capsules containing Meadowsweet and Marshmallow root as well as a personalized tincture blend that also included Meadowsweet alongside other anti-inflammatory and circulation-supporting herbs, such as Ginger, Prickly Ash bark, and Bayberry root bark. Within four weeks, her loose stool was much reduced, and her pain levels were reducing. Over time, her digestive system calmed down completely, and she was able to reduce her paracetamol intake. She remains very active and continues to manage her arthritis with a combination of allopathic medication and herbal medicine.

Historical applications

Meadowsweet was a traditional flavouring for mead, and its original name was probably Meadwort. Gerard wrote: '*It is reported, that the floures boiled in wine and drunke, do make the heart merrie . . . . The leaves and floures farre excel all other strewing herbes, for to decke up houses, to straw in chambers, halls, and banqueting houses in the Summer time; for the smell thereof makes the heart merrie, delighteth the senses: neither doth it cause head-ache, or lothsomenesse to meat, as some other sweet smelling herbes do. . . . The distilled water of the floures dropped into the eis, taketh away the burning and itching thereof, and cleareth the sight.*'

Parkinson said that it was a favourite strewing herb of Queen Elizabeth I, who '*did more desire it than any other sweet herbe to strew her Chambers withall*'.

Dodoens, in his *A New Herball* of 1586, wrote: '*Medewoort . . . doubtless drieth much, and is astringent, wherefore it restraineth and bindeth manifestly. The roots . . . boyled, or made into powder, and drunken, stoppeth . . . all issue of bloud. The floures boyled in white wine and drunken, cureth the fever Quartaine.*'

Magical

Meadowsweet is one of a trio of the most sacred Druidic herbs, the other two being Water Mint and Vervain.

In folk magic, fresh Meadowsweet has the capacity to cheer the heart. It was strewn about

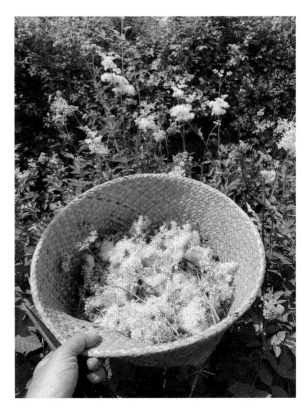

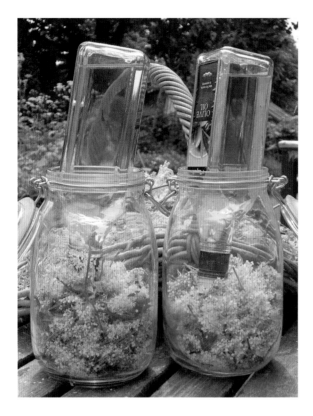

the house to make it smell good and lift the spirits, and it was considered to keep the peace. It is also traditionally used in love spells. If gathered at Midsummer, it can be used as a divination aid, giving information about those who may have taken something from you. A piece of Meadowsweet is placed on water. Apparently, if it sinks, the thief is a man, and if it floats, it is a woman.

Suggestion for the home apothecary

Meadowsweet-infused oil/rub for painful joints

Loosely fill a jar with either dried or fresh (but surface dry) Meadowsweet flowers, and cover completely with mild olive oil. Leave to infuse for a month, checking regularly that the flowers are completely covered. Once infused, you can use it as a muscle or joint rub.

Milk Thistle   🦋   *Silybum marianum*

'Protects the liver from toxins.'

Milk Thistle has a long-standing reputation as a liver herb. It is mostly about prevention – preventing liver damage caused by viruses, bacteria, fungi, and chemical toxins. It can also be very helpful as a cholagogue and biliary antispasmodic.

Medicinal parts
▷ Seeds

Physiological actions

Summary

▷ Cholagogue
▷ Hepato-protective
▷ Bitter
▷ Antidepressant
▷ Galactagogue
▷ Demulcent

Physiological virtues

The seeds contain flavonolignans, particularly silymarin, which protect the liver from toxins such as tetrachloromethane (carbon tetrachloride) and amanitin, while also offering antioxidant effects. In the case of poisoning from Death Cap mushrooms, if taken within 48 hours of ingestion, it can prevent severe liver damage. It can also protect the liver from the ill effects of some allopathic drug treatments, such as chemotherapy, but be aware that in some circumstances it may also reduce their efficacy. It is definitely a herb worth considering in cases of hepatitis, jaundice, and cirrhosis of the liver.

Milk Thistle is a popular self-prescribed choice to protect the liver from the ill effects of alcohol consumption, as it minimizes hangovers and reduces toxic fatty degeneration of the liver.

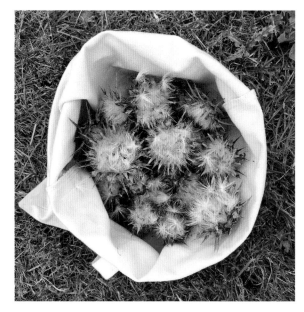

Of course, the best way to achieve these positive effects is to moderate or cease one's intake of alcohol.

It is a good antidepressant, which highlights the frequent link between poor liver health and depression. It is a specific for depression that comes on following hepatitis. It is also a galactagogue, indicated in its signature by the white veins in its leaves that are said to represent the Virgin Mary's milk.

Maud Grieve describes one of Milk Thistle's virtues as being a demulcent that is helpful in cases of catarrh and pleurisy. The tincture has a reputation of treating warts: Rudolf Weiss recommends taking 5 drops of the tincture three times a day for this purpose. A strong decoction of the seeds is said to have proved helpful as a topical treatment in some cancerous conditions.

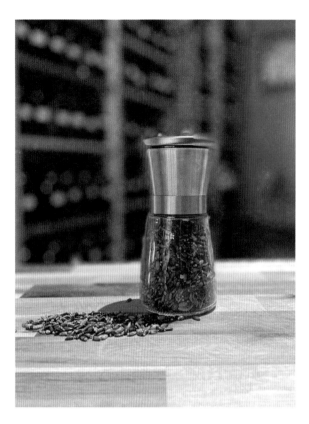

If taking Milk Thistle as a daily supplement, it should be freshly ground daily, as the seeds have a high level of fatty acids that quickly turn rancid once ground.

Energetics
Milk Thistle is bitter and oily.

In Tibetan medicine
Prescribe Milk Thistle extracts with caution in *rLung* conditions, due to their bitterness. If Milk Thistle seems like a good fit for a patient with a *rLung* imbalance, prescribe it as freshly ground seeds. That way, their oiliness can help to counteract the energetic ill effects of the bitterness.

In my dispensary
I do not often work with Milk Thistle in my practice, but am glad to have it available for certain cases in which it feels right. For me, the main indication is depression following liver disease. I prescribe it as a tincture, in decoctions, or in capsules. I often recommend patients to freshly grind some seeds onto their food daily.

Historical applications
Milk Thistle has been prescribed for centuries as a herb for depression and liver problems. Culpeper described the cooking and eating of the flower heads as a spring vegetable to cleanse the blood but advised: '*cut off the prickles unless you have a mind to choke yourself*'.

Gerard wrote: '*My opinion is that this is the best remedy that grows against melancholic diseases.*'

John Evelyn wrote: '*Disarmed of its prickles and boiled, it is worthy of esteem, and thought to be a great breeder of milk and proper diet for women who are nurses.*'

Suggestion for the home apothecary
Milk Thistle seed grinder

Fill a pepper grinder with dried Milk Thistle seeds and grind some onto your food every day as a helpful supplement if your liver needs support.

Mistletoe is a beautiful parasitic herb found frequently on old Apple trees and occasionally on Poplars, Limes, Ashes, Hawthorns, and Oaks. It is unusual, to say the least, growing as a parasitic plant without direct contact with the earth. It develops evergreen globes of tough twigs and leaves, only fruiting in the middle of winter. If you have ever walked through a landscape full of Mistletoe-bearing trees, you will know what I mean when I say that the leafy globes really stand out against the bare, leafless winter branches of their host trees. It seems magical that these perfect green globes should be so vibrant when all the plants around them are so dormant.

Mistletoe is in great demand as part of the greenery brought inside to celebrate Yule, kissing under the Mistletoe being the remnant of its application as a Druidical fertility-enhancing herb. The Celts believed that Mistletoe berries were drops of semen from the cosmic bull that impregnated the earth goddess. Mistletoe is still to this day associated with fertility and abundance. The sticky berries give rise to the generic name 'Viscum', which means 'sticky'.

For magical purposes, the Druids especially revered Mistletoe that was found growing on Oak trees. It had to be cut with a golden sickle and not be allowed to touch the ground when it fell. It is written that it should be cut on Midsummer's day or when the moon is six days old. In the South-West of England, you will still find keepers of old Mistletoe orchards who will not allow it to be cut unless it is the right time.

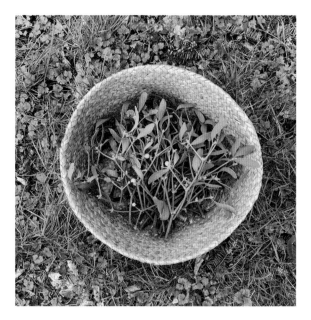

Medicinal parts

▹ Foliage
▹ Twigs

The berries are toxic.

Physiological actions

Summary

▹ Nervine
▹ Narcotic
▹ Hypotensive

Physiological virtues

Mistletoe is a nervine and a narcotic that has historically been prescribed to treat convulsions and epilepsy. Most often nowadays it is chosen to help treat hypertension and insomnia. Please be aware that although similar in appearance, this plant is quite different from

American Mistletoe (*Phoradendron leucarpum*), which is toxic.

In the past, Mistletoe was prescribed in a range of conditions, from St Vitus dance to typhoid. (See the section on historical applications, below, for more on these.)

Extract of Mistletoe has been found to play a positive role in cancer treatments. Research shows that it increases quality of life, improves the immune response, and protects healthy cells against the harmful effects of chemotherapy and radiotherapy. Fortunately, much work has been done to research ways of cultivating this plant to fulfil the demand. I would hate to see all the old West Country orchards be plundered of their leafy treasure globes.

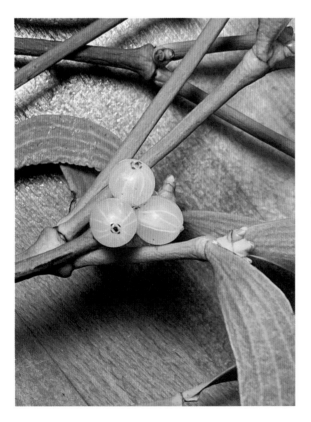

Energetics

Mistletoe is bitter and astringent. It has the very special energetic property of growing between Earth and Air, in that it grows on the solid foundation of its host tree and yet does not come into direct contact with the earth. It represents the sacred life force, the divine male principle, which is balanced by red-berried plants such as Holly (representing the divine feminine).

In my dispensary

I tend to prescribe Mistletoe tincture in mixes to support patients with insomnia. I blend it with other nervines like Hops, Wild Lettuce, California Poppy, Valerian, and Passionflower, depending on the individual case. The mix is considered a short-term support while the root cause of the insomnia is addressed.

Historical applications

In John Parkinson's time, Mistletoe was prescribed for patients suffering from '*the falling sicknesse*', that is, epilepsy and also '*Appoplexy, and Palsie very speedily, not onely to be inwardly taken, but to be hung about their necks.*' He did not appreciate the superstition and magical lore surrounding Mistletoe, though: '*it is fit to use it forty dayes together: and with this caution, that the wood after it is broken from the tree, doe not touch the ground which in my mind is too superstitious, as is their conceit also, that it hath power against Witchcraft, and the illusion of Sathan, and for that purpose, use to hang a peece thereof at their children's neckes.*'

In 1720 the apothecary Sir John Colbatch published a pamphlet entitled *The Treatment of Epilepsy by Mistletoe*. He regarded it as a specific for this and advised that '*the powdered leaves, as much as would lie on a sixpence, to be given in Black Cherry water each morning*'.

He also described how it is helpful in St Vitus dance, convulsions, hysteria, delirium, neuralgia, nervous debility, and even urinary disorders arising from a disordered nervous system.

In the past it was prescribed instead of Foxglove as a heart tonic in cases of typhoid fever. It lessens reflex irritability while strengthening the heartbeat and raising the rate of the pulse. The tincture or decoction was also often prescribed with Vervain and Valerian for all sorts of nervous disorders. Cayenne was added when there was digestive debility.

Magical

A sprig carried was believed to protect the bearer against lightning strike and other misfortunes. It is considered to encourage a state of immortality. It was believed that if placed in a baby's cradle, it would prevent the baby being stolen away by fairies and replaced by a changeling. Worn around one's neck, it would give the power of invisibility, and wearing a ring of Mistletoe wood is considered to protect the bearer from all sicknesses. For many years I have been on the hunt for a piece of Mistletoe wood large enough to make a ring from, and I'm excited to say that I have recently found one. We will see whether it will accept being made into a ring, though.

If you examine a Mistletoe berry closely, you will see four black semi-circular marks around a central dot. The Druids consider that these semi-circles represent the mystical cities of Sidhe (the fairy kingdom). In the North is Falias, and in the South is Finias. In the East is Gorias, and in the West is Murias. The central dot represents the all-encompassing etheric whole. The crescents and the dot really remind me of the Medicine Buddha mandala, in which four mountains at the cardinal directions support different types of healing compounds, and the Medicine Buddha sits in the centre, representing the space element (and much more). I love how different spiritual traditions have this understanding of the cardinal directions associated with different qualities. Often the theme is around the four elements and then a fifth element, which is ether or space, that encompasses everything.

If we contemplate Mistletoe, we can connect with something very deep. We are perhaps looking into our life's path and understand our elemental connection with both the Earth and the Spirit. So often, it is this connection that needs to be 'fixed' in order for us to be truly well.

Motherwort ❦ *Leonurus cardiaca*

'Like a mother protecting her children, Motherwort can be strong and fierce as well as nurturing and soft.'

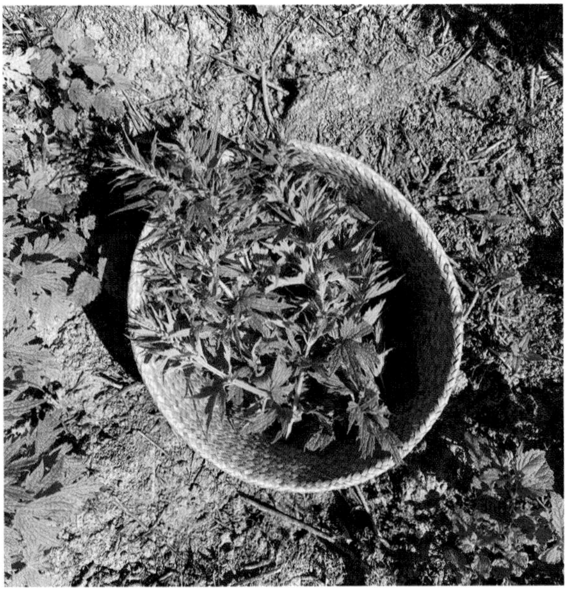

As its common name suggests, this is a herb that specializes in supporting and healing the mother energy. That may be on a physiological level, supporting the female reproductive system, or it can be more subtle, healing our idea of motherhood, whether that refers to ourselves or to the human who has borne or raised us. Motherwort's Latin generic name, 'Leonurus', refers to a lion, and its specific name, 'cardiaca', to its supportive action on the heart. You could say that this herb will help you to have a lion heart.

Before Motherwort flowers, it is gentle and fragrant and soft. At this growth stage it has an abundance of large five-lobed leaves just perfect to be harvested for calming herbal teas. The stems are green and supple and are easily snipped during harvest and processing. Once Motherwort flowers, it has quite a different character. It becomes a very fierce and powerful plant. Its leaves are much reduced in size and have only three lobes. Its flower heads are intensely prickly, and its stem is rigid and strong, not something that can be easily cut by hand for herbal teas. Once Motherwort goes into flowering and seeding mode, it is upright, determined, and confident in what it is doing. This is a plant that puts everything into ensuring that its offspring will be successful. Motherwort is a supremely abundant self-seeder and will happily take over your entire herb garden if you let it.

Medicinal parts

- Aerial parts

Physiological actions

Summary

- Nervine
- Bitter
- Emmenagogue
- Antispasmodic
- Cardiotonic
- Hypotensive
- Mildly thyrostatic
- Diaphoretic
- Astringent
- Antimicrobial

Physiological virtues

Motherwort is a bitter nervine. It is specific as a support to the female reproductive system, being an emmenagogue and allaying nervous irritability. It is a herb to consider when periods are scanty or when there is amenorrhoea. It can be helpful for period pain, as it relieves painful spasms, but it should be avoided in any quantity by those who have heavy periods, since it can worsen that symptom. I think of it for those who are anxious or nervous around their reproductive system, patients who worry about getting their periods, those anxious about whether they can ever become mothers, and those who struggle to cope with the demands of motherhood once they enter that portal. It can also help to soothe the worries of women entering menopause and perimenopause – although again, bear in mind the contraindication with heavy periods. It should be avoided in pregnancy and lactation.

Motherwort is antispasmodic, relaxing the circulation, including that of the heart, if this needs to be calmed in circulatory disorders. It contains cardiac glycosides, and so, while being relaxing, it is also mildly stimulating to the heart. This means that Motherwort can be very helpful where there are cardiovascular irregularities such as arrhythmia and tachycardia. It is especially good to calm palpitations when these are caused by nervousness. Motherwort works well in combination with Hawthorn to support healthy heart function, especially in elderly patients or in those with hypertension. Regular doses are needed to be effective. In old times the young tops were made into a sweet conserve in order to improve compliance, the tea being extremely bitter. Be careful to check for contraindications if the patient is already taking allopathic heart medications, especially digoxin.

As a bitter, it stimulates the digestive system, improving the absorption of minerals such as iron and therefore acting as an overall tonic. It can be worth considering as a support for mild cases of hyperthyroidism. As well as being mildly thyrostatic, it calms palpitations and tachycardia, symptoms that are frequently associated with hyperthyroid states.

Motherwort has a significant diaphoretic action and is a good choice to support someone with a fever who is suffering with nervousness and delirium. It is also directly antimicrobial and astringent. An infusion makes a good douche for vaginal infections and discharges.

Energetics

Motherwort is bitter and hot, with a cooling potency. It is a herb to consider if there is a need for healing in relation to the idea of motherhood, whether that is within ourselves or whether it relates to our own experience of being mothered. Sadly, many Westerners have 'issues' with their mothers, and this can have far-reaching implications for their outlook on life. My spiritual teacher, Akong Rinpoché, often used to talk about how different a baby's experience is growing up within traditional Tibetan culture, compared to those who grow up within modern Western society. He used to say that in Tibet all babies are constantly held and nurtured by mothers, fathers, aunts, uncles, siblings, and extended family throughout their early years. They are never placed into a cot, shut into a separate room, and left to cry. He believed that this experience of early separation in the West can lead to the development of deep insecurities, and it is one of the reasons he developed different approaches when teaching the dharma to Westerners and to Tibetans.

Within the West there are many who need support in healing their experience of being mothered and therefore their confidence in being able to be a good mother themselves. With Motherwort's influence we can develop flexibility and acceptance as well as a deep level of self-confidence. We understand that each of us is influenced by our own past experiences, or 'conditioning', according to Buddhism. Perhaps in our eyes our own mother did not do such a great job, but Motherwort helps us to see that she was doing her best according to her own causes and conditions. When we ourselves are mothering, Motherwort helps us to develop the selflessness required to transition and blossom into motherhood. We find it easier to combine softness and patience with the fierceness and heart of a lion when we need to stand up for our children or to create healthy boundaries as they are growing up.

In Tibetan medicine

In the Tibetan pharmacopoeia the species prescribed is *Leonurus heterophylla*, which is known as *Gurtik* (གུར་ཏིག in Tibetan script). It reduces febrile fever in the veins and treats diseases associated with blood and bile. It heals infected and inflamed sores.

Although a calming herb, long-term prescription is not recommended for patients experiencing an excess of *rLung*. Its bitterness will increase the *rLung*, unless other measures are taken to counteract it.

In my dispensary

I work with Motherwort in tinctures, teas, and capsules in my clinic. I tend to layer the intention with which I prescribe it, starting with physiological indications, for example nervousness and a tendency to palpitations. I then move on to emotional indications if I find that there is also a tension around mothering or being mothered.

'Janice' was in her late 60s and was suffering with hypertension and a slight arrhythmia. She had been assessed by her GP, who had recommended hypotensive drugs, but Janice was keen to try natural approaches before resorting to allopathic medication. When I went through her case, I discovered that she had multiple food intolerances and had a tendency to con-stipation, both signs that her digestion needed support. She also said that she often felt anxious and mentioned that she had had a very difficult relationship with her own mother. I decided to include Motherwort in her personalized tincture blend, and I also prescribed two capsules of Hawthorn and Motherwort per day. (For the proportions, see below.)

She responded very well to the herbal regime. Eight weeks later, at her next GP checkup, the arrhythmia was not detectable, and her blood pressure had come down well. To her relief it was decided that she would not need to start allopathic hypotensive drugs.

Historical applications

Parkinson wrote: '*Motherwort is held of later Writers, to bee of much use for the trembling of the heart, and in faintings and swoonings, from whence it tooke the name Cardiaca . . . a spoonefull of the powder drunke in wine, is a wonderfull helpe to women in their sore travels, as also for the suffocations or risings of the Mother, and from these effects it is likely it tooke the name of Motherwort with us. . . . It provoketh urine and procureth the feminine courses, clenseth the chest of cold flegme oppressing it, and killeth the worms of the belly. . . It is of good use to warme and dry up the cold humours, to digest and disperse them that are settled in the veines, joynts, and sinewes of the body, and to helpe crampes and convulsions.*'

Gerard wrote: '*Divers commend it against the infirmities of the heart. Moreover the same is commended for green wounds; it is also a remedy against certain diseases in cattell, as the cough and murreine, and for that cause divers husband-men oftentimes much desire it.*'

Culpeper said: '*There is no better herb to drive melancholy vapours from the heart, to strengthen it and make the mind cheerful, blithe and merry. May be kept in a syrup or conserve, therefore the Latins call it cardiaca. . . . It cleanseth the chest of cold phlegm, oppressing it and killeth worms in the belly. It is of good use to warm and dry up the cold humours, to digest and disperse them that are settled in the veins, joints and sinews of the body and to help cramps and convulsions.'*

Dodoens focused on Motherwort as a topical wound treatment: '*Motherwort bruised and laid upon wounds, keepeth the both from inflammation and apostumation or swelling, it stoppeth the bloud, and doth close, cure, and heale the same.'*

Magical

Having such a strong association with motherhood, Motherwort lends itself to talismans and incenses associated with healing maternal relationships, as well as with the development of inner trust and self-confidence. Motherwort is also associated with immortality.

Suggestion for the home apothecary

Dried Motherwort for tea or capsules

Harvest Motherwort before flowering, on a dry day. Cut into even-sized pieces and lay out on trays in an airy place away from direct light, or dry gently in a dehydrator. Alternatively, hang whole stalks complete with leaves upside down and passively dry in a place with good air flow. Once thoroughly dry, store in an airtight jar in a cool, dark place, and add to tea blends as needed. You can also powder and make into

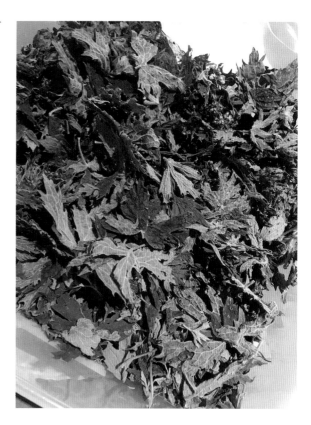

capsules mixed with Hawthorn. (See Hawthorn for instructions on powdering and sieving.) I recommend blending 3 parts Hawthorn and 1 part Motherwort for capsule blends.

Please seek professional advice regarding suitability if you are on cardiovascular medication or have a serious heart condition.

Mugwort 🌿 *Artemisia vulgaris*

'Mugwort is the 'Mother of Herbs', helping us to connect with our soft feminine aspect.'

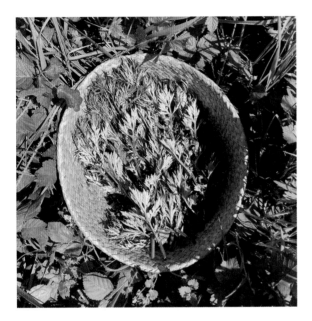

Mugwort has long been associated with femininity and supporting the female reproductive system. It is a warming, aromatic bitter herb, stimulating the liver and the digestion as well as being soothing to the nervous system. It commonly grows along country lanes, and if you find yourself travelling along those lanes by the light of the moon, you will notice that the silvery leaves of the Mugwort shine prominently. The pale undersides of its leaves seem to glow in those magical conditions. In this way, Mugwort is revealing itself as a herb of the moon. If you have never noticed the appearance of Mugwort on a moonlit night, you have missed something really special.

Medicinal parts
▷ Aerial parts

Physiological actions

Summary
▷ Bitter
▷ Cholagogue
▷ Carminative
▷ Nervine
▷ Emmenagogue
▷ Antispasmodic
▷ Anti-inflammatory
▷ Antifungal
▷ Anthelmintic

Physiological virtues

Mugwort is a warming bitter, stimulating the digestion while easing gas and griping. It helps the liver to be more efficient. When the liver is functioning at an optimal level, it is much more efficient at breaking down spent hormones, helping us to bring our menstrual periods into a healthier rhythm. Think of Mugwort for patients who suffer with premenstrual mood swings or headaches, for example. It can also reduce the bewildering emotional and physical symptoms that can accompany menopause and perimenopause in those who are out of balance. In cases of long-term stress or PCOS, Mugwort can play a very helpful role in reducing excessive androgens circulating around our systems.

I especially like to include Mugwort in prescriptions where patients seem to have become somewhat out of touch with their femininity. 'The Mother of Herbs' brings a soft, sensitive, and intuitive influence to whosoever will benefit from that, regardless of biological gender. This can happen where patients of either sex are working in high-pressure male-dominated environments and find that they have to take on more 'masculine' ways of relating in order to survive and be effective in their roles. While many cope well and even thrive under those conditions, others do find it tougher, with women often developing reproductive system irregularities and distressing symptoms, as well as difficulties around conceiving. Mugwort helps to bring the body into balance and allows all genders to feel stronger and more confident in their softer feminine aspects. Mugwort is a good herb to consider for those who have had to develop a hard shell in order to survive and for those who have lost touch with their intuition.

It is a relaxing herb, a calming nervine, less harsh and more nurturing than Wormwood. Think of it as encouraging a softer and more dreamy and relaxed state rather than an out-of-body experience. It soothes away the hardness that we develop when we have had to push ourselves over a long period to cope against all the odds. It is dreamy on one level, but through its ability to make us more comfortable in our own bodies, it is grounding and empowering.

It is a nervine stimulant, revitalizing a nervous system that has become disordered or dysfunctional through trauma, poor nutrition, or insufficient blood supply.

It is antimicrobial, antifungal, vermifuge, and anti-inflammatory. It is a good treatment for threadworms and can be prescribed topically as a wash or fomentation for fungal infections.

Mugwort can ease painful periods and bring the cycle into a steadier rhythm if it tends to vary in length. It stimulates menstruation by relaxing and improving the blood flow to the uterus. It can be made into an infused oil – sometimes with Ginger – to massage into the abdomen in order to alleviate menstrual cramps. Mugwort can be very helpful both at puberty, in order to establish a settled cycle, and in menopause, to help with the transition from having a regular cycle to no discernible cycle. It eases symptoms and helps us to feel feminine, empowered, and comfortable in our role as maiden, mother, or crone.

Mugwort can bring on menstruation, and it is not prescribed internally or topically during pregnancy in Western herbal medicinal traditions.

There is much knowledge of working with Mugwort – or at least its close relative, Sagebrush (*Artemisia tridentata*) – among the indigenous American community. I hope that many of my readers will have a living connection to this tradition and are safeguarding it for future generations. Sagebrush is the state flower of Nevada and an important herb for smudging. Its European relative, Mugwort, is naturalized in the United States and widespread. The indigenous community prescribe Mugwort as a tea for colds, colic, bronchitis, rheumatism, and fever, and combine it with Cramp bark, Mint, and Calendula to treat gynaecological disorders. There is a tradition of applying it topically as a strong infusion, or an ointment made with hog's grease, to resolve tumours and carbuncles after treatment with a drawing poultice made of Slippery Elm mixed with Cleavers and Bear's Foot (*Helleborus foetidus*).

Energetics

Mugwort has a bitter and hot taste. It helps us to get in touch with our softer feminine qualities, regardless of our gender. It is especially helpful for those who feel that they have had to create a hard exterior to cope with the pressures of their life or work.

In Tibetan medicine

In Tibet, there are two kinds of Artemisia. One, probably *A. absinthum,* is the white or pale version, known as *Ken kar* [མཁན་དཀར་]. The other, the dark or 'black' version, is called *Ken nak* [མཁན་ནག་པོ་]. It is also known as *Tshar bong mukpo* [ཚར་བོང་སྨུག་པོ་]. This is Mugwort. The medicinal part is the leaf, stem, and flower, which has a bitter and hot taste, a bitter post-digestive taste, and a potency that is cool and light. It is considered to stop bleeding and to reduce swelling in the limbs caused by *rLung* disorders and some hot disorders. It is considered especially good to cure the swelling of all lymph nodes. It treats pharyngitis and lung diseases. As well as being taken internally, it can be taken as a medicinal bath or via smoke inhalation. It is also made into moxibustion cones for the technique known as 'healing with fire'.

When I travelled to Amdo, in Tibet, I was completely bowled over by the scent of the Mugwort. It was growing everywhere. It was in the central reservation of roads in towns, around buildings in monastery complexes, on grazing lands, and perhaps, most beautifully, in the mountains. The scent of Mugwort and Yak dung pervaded everything while we were camping at high altitude. It was totally wonderful.

In my dispensary

I am a big fan of Mugwort. I generally prescribe it in tincture form where it is indicated, but also sometimes as part of a tea blend. I always prescribe it as part of an individually tailored blend rather than as a simple. I also infuse it into oil as a topical treatment for period pain.

Here are a couple of examples where prescribing Mugwort has made a big difference in my patients' lives:

'Carrie' had a demanding job in a competitive industry. She was very stressed by her professional lifestyle, and her menstrual periods had become quite irregular and painful. She did not sleep well and had a sluggish digestion that manifested as frequent bloating and a long-term tendency to constipation. She struck me as someone who had had to develop a hard exterior in order to survive her job. She was not comfortable with her more intuitive and soft side, yet she yearned to connect with it. I prescribed Mugwort in a personalized prescription blend that included Cramp bark, Caraway seed, Skullcap, and Agrimony. Over the following months she began to feel a lot more confident and settled in her own skin. Her digestion and menstrual periods improved, and she became more flexible in her outlook. In her time off, she started to explore esoteric subjects, such as spiritual and shamanic journeying, while learning to be solidly grounded and to implement better boundaries with her work colleagues. As she felt better and truer to herself, she began to make big plans to change her work–life balance.

'Sally' was in her early 50s and loved her job but admitted it was quite pressurized, and she had to be very organized in order to cope with it. She was pretty organized in her personal life, too, going to the gym before work most days and batch-cooking healthy meals at the weekends. She was always on the go and pushed herself hard, but she said that she enjoyed her life and felt positive about it. She was perimenopausal, and, despite her efforts to have a healthy lifestyle and a healthy diet, she was experiencing 'raging hot flushes', but did not want to resort to allopathic medication.

I felt that in order for her to get her health back into balance, she would need to introduce a little more relaxation into her life, and perhaps a bit less coffee. Her case called out for the softening and relaxing virtues of Mugwort, along with its liver-supporting qualities, so I prescribed an individual blend with it as the lead herb, backed up by Cramp Bark, Rosemary, Shatavari, and Goji berry. Four weeks later she reported feeling calmer despite work being particularly stressful, but she said that she found it impossible to switch off from it. Her hot flushes continued to be intense but were fewer in number. Four weeks after that, her hot flushes had further reduced. She was only having one each night, and her daytime ones had disappeared completely. She told me that her body felt 'more regulated'. She also noticed that her hair was feeling in very good condition, and she felt calmer than she had done for many years. She was better able to switch off from work and was enjoying a better work–life balance.

Historical applications

Gerard wrote: '*Pliny saith, That traveller or wayfaring man that hath the herbe tied about him feeleth no wearisomenesse at all: and that he who hath it about him an be hurt by no poysonsome medicines, nor by any wilde beast, neither yet by the Sun it selfe; and also that it is drunke against Opium, or the juyce of blacke Poppy. Many other fantasticall devices invented by Poëts are to be seene in the Works of the Antient Writers, tending to witchcraft and sorcerie, and the great dishonour of God: wherefore I do of purpose omit them, as things unworthy of my recording, to your reviewing.*'

Parkinson advised that Mugwort should be mixed with other herbs as a hot decoction for women to sit over – something that would

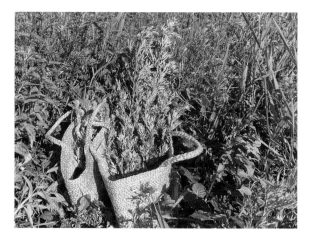

nowadays be called a '*yoni steam*'. He said that it was '*to draw down their courses, to helpe the delivery of the birth, and to expel the secondine or afterbirth, as also for the obstructions and inflammations of the mother*'. He also described it as a diuretic and treatment for kidney stones: '*it breaketh the stone, and causeth one to make water where it has stopped: the juyce thereof made up with Myrrhe, and also put under as a pessary, worketh the same effect, and so doth the roote also*'. The fresh juice was also considered to be an antidote to Opium overdose, and '*three drammes of the powder of the dryed leaves taken in wine, is a speedy, and the best certaine help for the Sciatica*'. It was also prescribed, with Chamomile and Agrimony, as a warm fomentation to apply to areas affected by '*the crampe*'.

Culpeper said: '*A very slight infusion is excellent for all disorders of the stomach, prevents sickness after meals and creates an appetite, but if made too strong, it disgusts the taste. The tops with the flowers on them, dried and powdered, are good against agues, and have the same virtues with wormseed in killing worms.*'

Magical

In the Middle Ages Mugwort was known as '*Mater Herbarum*' – Mother of Herbs. It has always been associated with magic and dreaming.

It is one of the nine sacred Druidic herbs believed to protect against evil and poisons. This is the incantation to Mugwort from the Anglo-Saxon 'Nine Herbs Charm':

> '*Have in mind, Mugwort, what you made known,*
> *What you laid down, at the great denouncing.*
> *Una your name is, oldest of herbs,*
> *Of might against thirty, and against three,*
> *Of might against venom and the onflying,*
> *Of might against the vile She who fares through the land.*'

[quoted from Geoffrey Grigson, *The Englishman's Flora*]

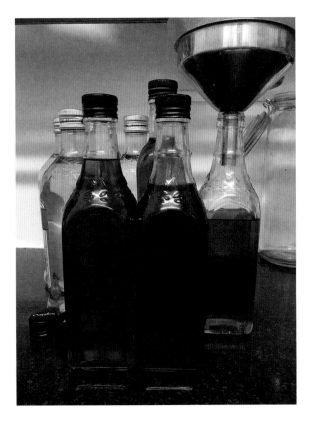

Mugwort has a long, unbroken history of being considered a highly protective herb. Wearing it as a girdle, garland, or crown while travelling was believed to preserve the wearer from fatigue, sunstroke, wild beasts, and evil spirits. Hanging garlands or wreaths of Mugwort in the house prevents elves and 'evil thynges' from entering. If the girdle or garland was thrown into the fire after use, it was believed to continue to provide protection for the following year. In fact, the throwing of Mugwort garlands into the fire is a tradition still maintained on the Isle of Man on 5 July each year. Attending the Mugwort ceremony on the Isle of Man is most definitely on my 'bucket list'.

In Japan, bunches of Mugwort are used by the Ainus to exorcise spirits of disease who are thought to hate the odour. In China it is hung over doors to keep evil spirits from entering.

As well as being protective, Mugwort helps us to see more clearly and to be more sensitive to subtle influences. Mugwort infusion drunk before bed helps us to remember our dreams, and stuffing Mugwort into a pillow encourages prophetic dreams.

In both Chinese and Tibetan medicine, it is the basis of moxa, which is used in moxibustion treatments. Moxibustion is 'healing with fire'.

Suggestions for the home apothecary

Mugwort-infused oil

Take dried Mugwort and loosely fill a jar with it. Pour over mild and light olive oil until the herb is thoroughly covered. Leave the jar in a dark place for at least four weeks, checking regularly to make sure that the herb is not poking up above the level of the oil. You can speed up the process by sitting the jar in a gentle warm water bath every so often but never apply direct heat to the oil.

Once the oil is ready, strain it and filter it into bottles. Store in a cool, dark place. Massage the abdomen with it to relieve period pains.

Calming digestive tea blend

This is a great tea blend for those who are finding that stress is affecting their ability to enjoy and digest their food. All of the herbs are calming, Mugwort and Chamomile stimulate the digestion, and Catnip and Chamomile are good carminatives, easing griping and wind in the digestive tract. Simply combine equal parts of the herbs. Make a tea and sip after a meal.

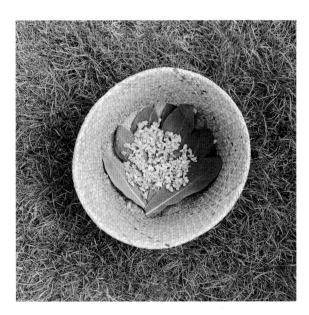

'Mullein is softening, moistening, and soothing, counteracting lack of inspiration.'

Mullein is a biennial herb, forming a rosette of woolly leaves in the first year and a towering flower spike of beautiful little yellow flowers in the second year. Its leaf arrangement catches rainwater and funnels it directly to the roots, moistening the soil where it is needed.

It is primarily thought of as a herb to help with respiratory issues, especially dry coughs and catarrh. Its virtues of being softening, moistening, and soothing reveal themselves instantly when you reach out and touch the leaves. Mullein is a little diaphoretic in action, making it perfect for acute feverish chills with hard coughs, while also being excellent for chronic respiratory complaints where dryness is a factor. The leaves have been prescribed as a cough remedy for centuries and were, at one time, smoked as a treatment for asthma and tuberculosis.

Medicinal parts

▷ Leaves
▷ Flowers
▷ Roots

Physiological actions

Summary

▷ Expectorant
▷ Demulcent
▷ Anticatarrhal
▷ Antitussive
▷ Astringent
▷ Diuretic
▷ Sedative
▷ Diaphoretic

Physiological virtues

Mullein is expectorant, demulcent, sedative, astringent, and a mild diuretic, helpful for dry inflammatory conditions in either the respiratory or digestive tracts. It is most often considered to be specific for deep, tickly coughs. It moistens and soothes the airways as well as loosening and resolving long-standing sticky catarrh. It is prescribed in cases of acute feverish coughs as well as in chronic conditions such as asthma and tuberculosis. Its astringent properties make it a good choice for when there is bleeding from the lungs or bowels. It also means that it is a good first aid herb for diarrhoea.

Mullein is slightly sedative and very mildly narcotic, further explaining its antitussive properties. It has a strong reputation for being able to calm spasmodic coughs, even the hacking dry cough associated with tuberculosis.

It is most often prescribed internally as a tea or tincture. As a simple, a long-steeped tea drunk freely is considered best for a dry irritating cough. The hot tea of Mullein is a little diaphoretic in action, making it especially suitable for coughs combined with fever. The cooled tea can also be taken as a gargle for sore throats. A tincture is usually more convenient for making up personalized blends, especially when one wants to include roots or seeds less suited to passive infusion. For example, Mullein combines very well with stimulating expectorants such as Elecampane and Thyme, yet if extracting Elecampane root in water, it is best done as a decoction rather than a passive infusion. In tincture form these different herbal preparations can be combined straight away, making the prescribing of tinctures quickest

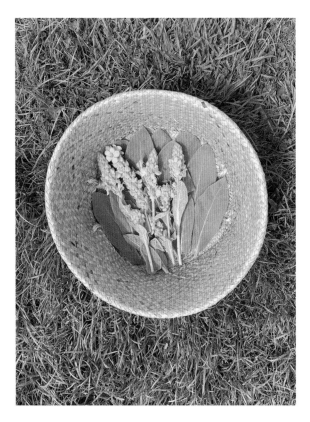

and simplest in a busy herbal practice, as well as being easiest for patients to prepare and take. However, if alcoholic extractions are to be avoided, one just needs to decoct the roots first and then add the Mullein and other leafy herbs to the hot decoction once it has been removed from the heat.

Mullein has diuretic properties. According to Native American tradition, a decoction of equal parts Horsemint (*Monarda punctata*) and Mullein is excellent for kidney diseases.

It can also be made into topical preparations. The flowers are traditionally infused in oil as a preparation for ear troubles, including itchy ears, earache, or blocked ears. Apply 3 drops into the ear as needed (but do not do this if the ear drum has perforated). The infused flower oil is also a good treatment for itchy eyelids. For ear infections, make an oil with equal parts Mullein flowers and chopped Garlic. Fresh leaves can be bruised and applied directly to boils and carbuncles, while a fomentation is a traditional treatment for haemorrhoids.

Mullein delivered as steam is helpful for both respiratory conditions and throat inflammation. The leaves are simmered in water with a little vinegar added, and the steam is inhaled. This is appropriate for respiratory infections, chronic coughs, acute tonsillitis, sore throats, and mumps. Mullein steam can also be helpful for joint pain and ulcers if you are able to direct the steam to the affected part.

The dried leaves were traditionally smoked to relieve lung congestion and asthma.

Energetics

Mullein is bitter, astringent, and sweet. I have noticed that when patients have dryness and congestion in their respiratory tracts, their lack of 'physiological inspiration' – that is, the in-breath – is often mirrored by a lack of inspiration in their wider life. Mullein soothes the airways and encourages easier and deeper breathing, helping us to feel more inspired to pursue our dreams.

In Tibetan medicine

Verbascum thapsus is included in the Tibetan pharmacopoeia. It is known as *Yug pae ser jye* [གཡུག་པའི་གསེར་བྱེ་], and the plant is considered to be a substitute for a mineral medicine found in large and small rivers with granite rocks and sand. It has a lustrous yellow and white colour.

The plant has a taste that is bitter-to-astringent and a post-digestive taste that is bitter. Its potency is cooling. It is considered especially helpful for hot disorders of the lungs, and it cures toxicosis associated with hot disorders including inflammatory pimples and dropsy. It is chosen to treat injuries and sprains, acting as a styptic when there is haemorrhage.

In my dispensary

I prescribe Mullein as tincture and in infusions, and it is also included in a respiratory-system-supporting capsule blend. The infused flower oil is also included in my ear drops. Mullein is a very important herb for those experiencing dry coughs and lack 'of inspiration', both physiologically and energetically. The case of 'Jenny' illustrates this.

Jenny was 65 years old and had been suffering with asthma and a chronic dry cough for over twenty years. She regularly woke up in the night with a very dry throat, feeling that she could not get her breath. These episodes would leave her feeling vulnerable and panicky. She had experienced significant worsening of her symptoms after a recent bad bout of influenza and was now quite breathless when walking up hills as well. She had been through a number of medical assessments and had been diagnosed with COPD (chronic obstructive pulmonary disease). When she first contacted me, she was feeling quite lost and low. Her energy was at rock bottom, and, in addition to her respiratory congestion, she did not have much of an appetite and experienced bloating a lot of the time. She felt she had to let go of her hopes and dreams because her health was deteriorating and she did not have the energy to pursue them.

We started by looking at her lifestyle, and I suggested that she needed to try to establish a better routine in terms of eating and drinking. Her diet was quite high in carbohydrates, and she admitted that she was not hydrating properly. She was also eating a lot of mucus-forming foods, in particular dairy products. I asked her to reduce her carbohydrate intake, to increase fresh fruits and vegetables, and to include more foods that are high in protein. I also asked her to completely give up dairy during the period of treatment, and to aim to drink more water, with a target of 2 litres each day.

I prescribed her a tailor-made tincture that contained Mullein as the main herb, with other respiratory herbs in a supporting role, including St John's Wort, Red Clover, and Thyme. She was to take her tincture twice a day in hot water and to take two of my respiratory blend capsules per day. Four weeks later she was feeling much better. She had more energy, her cough had considerably lessened, and she had far fewer night-time panicky episodes. Her appetite was improving and her bloating had reduced. She had noticed that her breathlessness was less than it had been, and I noticed that her voice had changed in quality and was much less croaky. Overall, she was feeling very happy that there was some improvement so soon after starting herbal treatment. She was already feeling more motivated to actively pursue her dream of relocating to another area.

Jenny continued to improve steadily and after four months reported feeling 'really good', saying she had a zest for life that she had not felt since she had been in her 20s. Her night time panics had completely ceased, and her cough and breathlessness had gone. She realized that she missed being sociable, so she had taken up new interests and was enjoying meeting more people, as well as moving forward with her dreams of relocating. Although Mullein did not act alone in this prescription, I can see its influence very clearly.

Historical applications

Hildegard of Bingen recommends Mullein for sore throat with hoarseness and sore lungs: '*Those who have a sore throat and hoarseness with pain in their chest cook mullein and Fennel in equal parts in pure wine, strain it through a linen cloth, and drink it often, and their lost voice will return again.*'

Gerard wrote of Mullein's ability to heal cattle: '*The country people, especially the husbandmen in Kent, do give their cattel the leaves to drink against the cough of the lungs, being an excellent approved medicine for the same, whereupon they call it Bullocks Lungwort.*'

He also mentions its preservative abilities: '*The report goeth (saith Pliny) that figs do not putrifie at all that are wrapped in the leaves of Mullein.*' In sixteenth-century Britain, Mullein was carried to prevent '*the falling sickness*', but this practice was later debunked by Gerard.

Parkinson had a lot to say about Mullein. He tells us how Dioscorides prescribed it: '*It is commended by Dioscorides against the laskes and fluxes of the belly, if a small quantity of the root be given in wine: the decoction therof drunke is profitable for those that are bursten, and for those that have crampes and convulsions; and likewise for those that are troubled with an old cough: the decoction thereof gargled, easeth the paines of the toothache.*' Parkinson also mentions that an infusion of the flowers in '*oyle*' is beneficial for piles, but he does not mention

it for earache. He describes how Mullein can be helpful for intermittent fevers: '*The juice from the roots taken before it beare stalke* [i.e. in the first year of growth]', is recommended to be '*taken in a draught of Muscadine every time, for three or four times one after another, an houre before a fit of the quartane ague commeth upon any, it shall surely helpe them*'. For gout he advised drinking three ounces of the distilled water of the flowers '*every morning and evening for some days together*' for the '*hot gowt*', saying '*there is not a better remedy*'. The powdered dried flowers were prescribed for '*belly aches, or the paines and torments of the collick*' and a decoction of the root of the leaves was '*of great effect to dissolve the tumors or swellings, as also the inflammations of the throat*'.

Apart from medicinal virtues, Mullein has offered us other helpful and practical qualities for centuries. The leaves were wrapped around fruit, especially figs, in order to act as a preservative. The flower spikes were dipped in tallow to make candles, and the leaves were put inside stockings to keep the feet warm in winter.

Magical

Mullein is magically associated with courage and protection. It is said that if one wears it, it will protect one from wild animals when walking in wild places. According to Homer, Ulysses took Mullein with him on his travels to protect him from evil. He called it 'moly'. When he landed on the island of Aeaea, where the enchantress Circe lived, he avoided being turned into a pig, unlike his unfortunate men. He was able to force her to restore them to human form with the help of Mullein.

In India, Mullein is still considered to be the most potent protection against evil spirits and magic. It is hung over doors and carried in sachets for this purpose.

Mullein is also associated with health promotion and love. A few leaves placed into the shoes

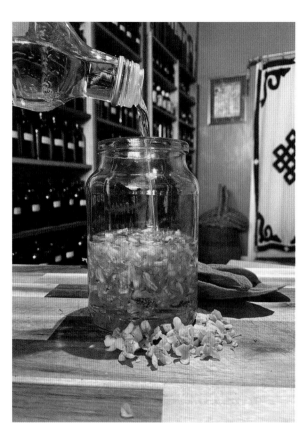

were considered to prevent one from catching a cold, and carrying it would help to attract love. Stuff it into a pillow to guard against nightmares.

Mullein stems have been used to perform love divinations. Men in the Ozarks would bend a Mullein stem towards the house where their love lived. If the Mullein grew upright again, their love would flourish. If it died, it meant that she loved another.

Suggestion for the home apothecary

Mullein flower ear oil

Take individual fresh Mullein flowers picked on a dry day and put them into a jar. Cover with mild olive oil and leave in a dark place for around four weeks, or until the flowers have become transparent. Strain and decant the oil into a clean, dry bottle, being sure to leave any watery layer at the bottom of the jar. Apply 3 drops into the ear twice a day if there is earache or if the ear is blocked. This is not suitable if the eardrum is perforated.

Nettle 🍃 *Urtica dioica*

'Nettle is a powerhouse herb, restoring vital energy where it is lacking.'

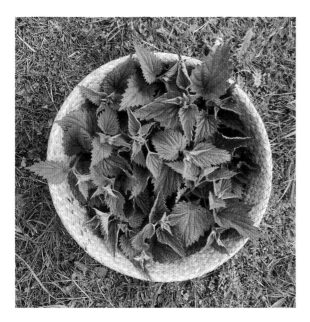

Herbs with many different virtues are often described as a medicine chest on their own. Nettle has a myriad virtues, but to describe it as a 'medicine chest' seems much too passive. Nettle is full of potency and movement. It is a herb that gets things done. It is a 'powerhouse' herb.

Nettle is a very common wild plant, in my corner of the world at least, and is widely looked down on as a nuisance and a weed. Here is a classic example of familiarity breeding contempt. Luckily, as herbal folk, we see that this is an enormously valuable and powerful medicine that is 'hidden in plain sight'.

Nettle may appear inconspicuous, but it definitely gets us to notice it. The name 'Nettle' is derived from the Anglo-Saxon word 'noedl', which means needle, a reference to its sting. It has a reputation of growing best near human habitation, seeking out muck heaps and fertile ground. It has a particular affinity with nitrogen, and is very rich in protein and minerals, often being thought of as a nutritive support. It is not purely nutritive, though, it also encourages enhanced elimination of waste products, particularly urates, from the body. This is a herb that cleanses our body while nourishing and restoring it.

When I was studying Tibetan medicine, we were taught about a Tibetan Yogi called Jetson Milarepa. He lived and meditated in a cave high in the Himalayas and existed almost solely on Nettle soup. It sustained him for many years while he was dedicated to spiritual practice as well as writing beautiful and very insightful spiritual songs. I often think about Milarepa when I think about Nettle.

Medicinal parts

> Leaves
> Seeds
> Roots

The leaves should be harvested early in the year, before flowering. Leaves harvested later in the season are potentially irritating to the kidneys as they contain cystoliths. These are tiny rods of calcium carbonate that can be absorbed by the body and interfere with kidney function. If you wish to extend your leaf harvest, cut back a patch and wait to harvest the new young growth.

Physiological actions

Summary

> Tonic
> Nutritive
> Diuretic

- ▷ Stimulant
- ▷ Astringent
- ▷ Anti-inflammatory
- ▷ Kidney tonic
- ▷ Adrenal tonic
- ▷ Adaptogen
- ▷ Prostate tonic

Physiological virtues

As a protein and iron-rich blood builder, Nettle leaves are an excellent tonic for those who need extra nourishment, during pregnancy and lactation, convalescence, and in cases of anaemia, for example. Nettle's ability to assist with the removal of urates from the body makes it a good choice for gout, arthritis, and kidney disease. By supporting the kidneys, it can resolve long-standing oedema.

Nettle is a stimulating tonic, having a long history of restoring function to parts of the body that are paralysed or atrophied. My teacher, Barbara Howe, told a story about a patient who was losing the feeling in his feet and lower legs. She prescribed daily barefoot walking through a Nettle patch, until the feeling was fully restored. The patient followed her advice religiously, and a complete cure was obtained within one growing season. Nettle leaf also has the reputation of restoring the function of internal organs and glands. Its action on reviving the kidneys, thyroid, nerves, and muscles is well documented by other herbalists.

Nettle has an affinity with the circulatory system, being helpful in cases of low blood pressure and postural hypotension when the pulse feels sunken and slow. It also encourages circulation to the head, supporting hair growth and counteracting mental dullness and forgetfulness. A hair tonic can be made by simmering a handful of Nettle leaves in a litre of water for 2 hours, then cooling, straining, and bottling. The hair should be saturated with it every other night.

Alternatively, you can extract fresh Nettle juice and comb it through the hair daily.

Nettle leaves are astringent and anti-inflammatory and reduce the sensitivity of tissues to allergens. They are one of the first herbal choices for hay fever, and they are often prescribed in asthma support. As a herb that helps to eliminate toxins via the kidneys, Nettle is well indicated for skin conditions such as eczema and psoriasis, particularly when it is most prominent in the periphery of the body, such as in the fingers, or in the scalp. Nettle's astringency gives it a helpful role to play to resolve bleeding from the digestive tract or the respiratory system. It is also traditionally considered to be a superlative topical application for first- and second-degree burns. An infusion is prepared and the cooled infusion applied to the burned areas as a fomentation.

David Hoffman famously said: 'When in doubt give Nettles', advice which has helped many a newly qualified herbal practitioner as well as plenty of more seasoned ones.

The ripe seed has amazing medicinal properties, being capable of restoring kidney function when it is failing. I first learnt of this action from herbalist Matthew Wood, and I have since seen it multiple times in my own practice. To hear patients reporting improved kidney function when they were told that this would be impossible never fails to fill me with awe.

It is also an adrenal support, excellent for adrenal burnout, adrenal fatigue, adrenal exhaustion, or whatever label you want to use. Nettle seed is an adaptogen and helps us deal more effectively with stress. It can be quite stimulating, so it is best not to take it last thing at night.

The Romans favoured Nettle seed and Rosemary as a topical treatment for arthritis, something I discovered when researching ancient ointment recipes to bring to a primitive archery event years ago. Since making that first trial batch of ointment, it has become a much admired staple of my 'off-the-shelf' range, helping hundreds of people reduce the pain and discomfort of arthritis.

The roots of Nettle are considered specific for the treatment of benign prostatic hyperplasia (BPH). I was taught this virtue of Nettle root by my mentor and tutor Edith Barlow, who based her understanding on years of empirical knowledge and experience. Nettle root is well known to be anti-inflammatory and diuretic, providing relief for symptoms of difficulty in urination and a tendency for urinary retention.

Looking at Nettle root through the lens of biochemical analysis, it is interesting to discover that the extract is able to reduce the capacity of 'sex hormone binding globulin' (SHBG) in the prostate gland. SHBG build-up is a major factor in the development of BPH as men age. While allopathic hormone treatments can disrupt the normal endocrine balance within men's reproductive systems, Nettle root effectively supports BPH patients without influencing the concentrations of testosterone in their blood plasma. My patients taking Nettle root for BPH tell me that their herbal medicine has reduced their symptoms and restored their zest for life.

Energetics
Nettle is astringent, salty, a little bitter, and sweet.

In Tibetan medicine
Urtica tibetica is known in Tibetan as *Zva phyi a ya* [ཟྭ་ཕྱི་ཨ་ཡ།] or *Zva tsoe* [ཟྭ་ཚོད།]. It has a taste that is sweet, hot, and bitter and a post-digestive taste that is bitter. It is warm and oily in potency. It treats *rLung* disorders and increases body heat. It is helpful in both chronic hot and cold disorders. It is suitable to treat *Pekén* and *Tripa*

combinational disorders as well as blood disorders. It is beneficial for third-stage oedema and wounds. *Urtica triangularis* is known as *Zva brum* [ཟྭ་འབྲུམ]. It generates heat and cures chronic fever accompanied by *rLung*. The leaves are pungent, bitter, and heating. Made into a soup, they are good for *rLung* disorders. Taken as a tea, they are cleansing and diuretic.

In my dispensary
I most frequently prescribe Nettle leaf in capsule form for those who are suffering from debility, anaemia, and hair loss. I reach for the seed when patients are experiencing a long-term adrenalized state accompanied by exhaustion, and I also choose the seed when there is reduced kidney function or if the patient has had one kidney removed in the past. I prescribe the root, either in a tincture or a capsule blend, for men experiencing BPH.

This case illustrates the effectiveness of Nettle root in supporting the prostate: 'Alistair' was a fit and active 57-year-old who was suffering from nocturnal urinary frequency due to BPH. When he did get up to pee, he found it difficult to start and stop the stream of urine. He told me that he had a tendency to be tense and anx-

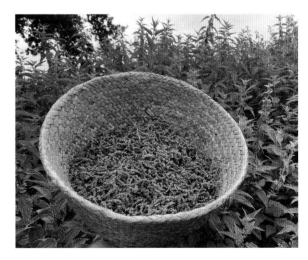

ious, especially about his health, and he asked for herbal support for both his prostate and his mood. His prescription contained nervines such as Lemon Balm, Vervain, and Cramp Bark, as well as prostate- and urinary-system-supporting herbs, including Nettle root, Cornsilk, and Couch. Within four weeks his nocturnal urinary frequency had much reduced, with starting and stopping the stream of urine being much easier. Four weeks after that he reported that he often slept through the night without needing to get up at all.

The following case shows the value of Nettle seed and Rosemary topical preparation. 'Lydia' was 60 years old and had longstanding rheumatoid arthritis. She relied on allopathic medication to be able to manage the condition but wanted herbal support to help her avoid increasing her allopathic protocol. Her hands were especially badly affected, and she had noticed that, despite the medication, she was gradually losing strength and mobility. She also had digestive issues and recognized that in order to be as well as possible, she needed to try to address these too. We started with an individually formulated herbal regime to improve digestion and encourage better elimination through the kidneys. She also had a blend of medicinal mushrooms in double-extracted tincture form predominantly for their immunomodulating properties. Alongside her internal herbal medicine, she had my Nettle-seed ointment, which she massaged into her fingers and hands daily. She reported an immediate positive effect in terms of reduced pain and stiffness. She continues to do well with her blend of herbal and allopathic support.

Historical applications

Hildegard of Bingen recommended an external application of Nettles in a 'Memory Oil for people who are becoming forgetful: '*Persons who are forgetful against their wishes should take stinging nettles and pulverize them, add olive oil, and rub their chest and temples energetically when going to bed; this they should repeat and their forgetfulness will decrease. The pungent warmth of the stinging nettles and the warmth of the olive oil stimulate the constricted vessels of the chest and temples which sleep a little, by waking consciousness.*'

In Native American medicine, Nettle root is used traditionally as a decoction for dysentery, to reduce bleeding, and to relieve asthma, bronchitis, and other respiratory ailments.

Sir John Harington, in *The English Man's Doctor*, was very impressed with the medicinal virtues of Nettle:

> *'The Nettles stinke, yet they make recompense,*
> *If your belly by the Collicke paine endures,*
> *Against the Collicke Nettle-seed and honey*
> *Is Physicke: better none is had for money.*
> *It breedeth sleepe, staies vomit, fleams doth soften,*
> *It helps him of the Gowte that eates it often.*'

Gerard described Nettle as: '*of temperature dry, a little hot, scares in the first degree: it is of thin and subtil parts; for it doth not therefore burne and sting by reason of its extreme hot, but because the downe of it is stiffe and hard, piercing like fine little prickles or stings, and entring into the skin: for if it be withered or boiled it stingeth not at all, by reason that the stiffness of the down is fallen away.*' He also wrote: '*Nicander affirmeth, that it is a remedie against the venomous qualitie of Hemlocke, Mushrooms, and Quicksilver. And Apollodorus saith that it is a counterpoison for Henbane, Serpents, and Scorpions. Pliny saith, the same author writeth, that the oile of it takes away the sting that the Nettle it selfe maketh.*'

Parkinson wrote: '*The leaves boyled in wine and drunke, is said to open the belly and make it soluble: the rootes or leaves boyled, or the juice of either of them, or both made into an electuary with Honey or Sugar, is a safe or sure medicine to open the pipes and*

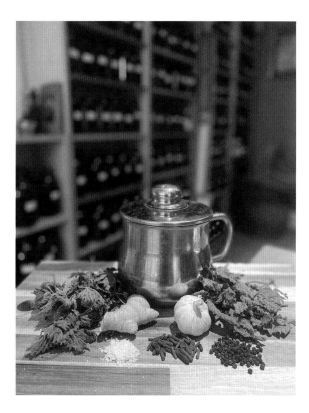

passages of the Lungs which is the cause of wheesings and shortnesse of breath, and helpeth to expectorate tough cold flegme sticking in them, or in the chest or stomacke, as also to raise impostumated Pluresie, and spend it by spitting.' He also suggests Nettle electuary can be used as a gargle for tonsillitis, saying that it: '*helpeth the Almonds of the throate when they are swelled*'. He mentions the seed, saying that it can be prescribed as a diuretic – it '*provoketh urine, and expelleth gravel and the stone in the reines or bladder. . . . The seed being drunke is a remedy against the stinging of venomous creatures, the bitings of madde dogs, the poysonfull qualities of Hemlocke, Henbane, Nightshade, mandrake or other such like herbes, that stupefy and dull the senses, as also the Lethargy*'. He recommends applying a handful of fresh Nettle leaves mixed with '*Wall-*

wort [Danewort or Dwarf Elder]' to '*the Gout, Sciatica, or joynt aches*'.

Magical

Nettle is associated with fieriness and a warrior spirit. It is traditionally associated with exorcism, protection, healing, and provoking lust. It is said that Nettle can be used to remove a curse and send it back to the originator. To do this, Nettle is sprinkled around the house, where it will repel evil influences. It can be thrown into the fire to avert danger, and it is held in the hand to ward off ghosts. Carried with Yarrow, it will allay fear, and it is worn as an amulet to repel negativity.

It is said that placing a pot of freshly cut Nettles beneath a person's sickbed will aid their recovery. If you want to dispel a fever, you should pull up a Nettle plant by its roots while reciting not only the sick person's name but also those of his parents.

Suggestion for the home apothecary

Tibetan Nettle soup

This is a good alternative to bone broth for people who do not eat meat.

» *about 4 cups fresh or 2 cups dried Nettle leaves*
» *3 cups cold water*
» *about 1–2 tsp sea salt*
» *about 2 tsp Ginger (chopped)*
» *about 1 tsp Long Pepper (crushed)*
» *about 1 tsp Black Pepper (crushed)*
» *about 1 tsp Garlic (chopped)*
» *3–4 tsp ghee or Coconut oil*

Place all the ingredients into a pan and add the water. Stir, then leave to soak for 10–15 minutes. Place onto the heat and bring to the boil, then turn down the heat and simmer until it reduces to approximately two cups of liquid.

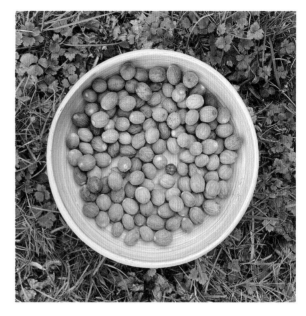

'Nutmeg is calming, with an affinity to the heart.'

Nutmeg is a well-known culinary spice, but it is also a very valuable and effective medicine, with a special affinity to the heart. It is a calming tonic to the nervous system and a good physiological support to the reproductive system. It allays nausea and griping and is an excellent treatment for shock and insomnia.

Medicinal parts

▷ Kernel (seed)

The kernel is covered with a brilliant red arillus, called Mace, which is also medicinal.

Physiological actions

Summary

▷ Nervine
▷ Sedative
▷ Cardiotonic
▷ Analgesic
▷ Carminative
▷ Antiemetic
▷ Astringent
▷ Vermifuge
▷ Reproductive tonic

Physiological virtues

Nutmeg is a calming nervine that reduces mental agitation and promotes restful sleep. It has a particular affinity to the heart and can reduce symptoms of angina and treat palpitations. It is analgesic and can be helpful in cases of painful periods, arthritis, and muscle pain, and as a relaxant it can reduce symptoms of incontinence or frequent urination when this is worsened by stress and worry.

Nutmeg relaxes the digestive tract, reducing flatulence and bloating, particularly when these issues are linked to stress and tension. Maud Grieve describes the primary medicinal virtue of Nutmeg (and Mace), to be as a carminative and antiemetic, especially when nausea and vomiting are caused by allopathic medication. Its astringency makes it a good first aid treatment for diarrhoea, especially nervous diarrhoea. Another of Nutmeg's virtues is that it is a vermifuge.

As well as its action on the nervous system and the digestive tract, Nutmeg is a tonic to the reproductive system. It is worth considering for low libido, premature ejaculation, prostatitis, and erectile dysfunction. It can reduce period pain and help to improve the regularity of the menstrual cycle. This is especially the case when the irregularity is linked to stress or shock.

Nutmeg also has expectorant properties, easing coughs, reducing phlegm, and getting rid of catarrh.

It is excellent grated into warm milk as a home remedy for insomnia, but be aware that large doses are narcotic and can cause hallucinations. Each person's tolerance of Nutmeg is different, so, if trying it, it is important to start with small doses taken at least one hour before bed, and then work up gradually to ½ tsp. Once you get to more than ½ tsp of grated Nutmeg or Nutmeg powder per night, proceed very cautiously. A dosage of 7.5 g could produce convulsions.

In cases of insomnia, palpitations, and nervous agitation, a very good alternative to internal prescribing is applying it in the form of hot packs dipped in warmed sesame oil. This technique is known as 'hormé' or 'Mongolian moxibustion'. (It is described under 'In Tibetan medicine' below.) Grated Nutmeg mixed with lard is recommended by Maud Grieve as an excellent ointment for haemorrhoids.

Energetics
Nutmeg is warming and oily. It is also a little bitter and astringent.

In Tibetan medicine
In Tibetan, Nutmeg is called *Dzati* [ཛཱ་ཏི]. It has a hot and sweet taste, with a bitter post-digestive taste. Its potency is oily, heavy, warming, drying, and fast-acting. It is calming and grounding and is considered to be a very effective treatment for excess *rLung*. It has a particular affinity to the heart and is therefore a good choice for patients with symptoms where the action of the heart is affected by *rLung* disorders – for example, heart palpitations caused by anxiety, as well as other symptoms of anxiety or grief held in the heart area. Since its post-digestive power is cooling,

it is considered to be unsuitable for people with kidney disorders.

Nutmeg can be applied topically using a technique called hormé (Mongolian moxibustion). In this process, carefully chosen herbs and spices are powdered, then made into a pack by wrapping them in muslin cloth and tying it into a little bundle with thread, leaving a cloth 'tail' that acts as a handle. The pack is dipped into warm oil and applied to special points on the body.

In my dispensary
I frequently work with Nutmeg in my dispensary, including it in a tincture blend to support patients suffering with palpitations, panic attacks, anxiety, and insomnia. The tincture is a blend of warming, oily, and nutritious herbs that counteract *rLung*. Another way of benefitting from Nutmeg is to make hormé packs dipped in oil as a topical application. (See 'Suggestions for the home apothecary' below for more information.)

Historical applications
Pliny, writing in the first century AD, described a tree bearing a nut that had two separate flavours. It was first imported to the Western world by Arabic traders in the Middle Ages, and they soon became highly sought after and extremely expensive.

Dodoens described Nutmeg as: '*hot and dry in the second degree: and of the same nature and complexion is Macis: moreover they be somewhat astringent*'. Of its virtues he wrote: '*The nutmegge doth heat and strengthen the stomacke which is cold and weake, especially the orifice or mouth of the stomacke, it maketh a sweete breath, it withstandeth vomiting, and taketh away the hicket or yeox, in what sort soever it be taken. . . . It is also good against the paine and windiness of the bellie, and against the stoppings of the liver and milt* [ejaculation].'

Suggestions for the home apothecary

Nutmeg hormé

Powder Nutmeg and place 2 tsp, heaped, of the powder into a little square of muslin. Gather up the edges and tie securely with red thread. It is a good idea to make several hormé packs at one time, so you can rotate them in and out of the warm oil while doing a treatment. Place some Sesame oil or butter in a room diffuser that is warmed by a tea light. Once the oil is warm, dip the herbal pack into the oil. Test it on your hand before applying it to the patient. It should be warm to hot, but it should not burn the skin. Apply very gently in a calm and mindful dabbing action to the mid-sternal point, which is in the centre of the chest midway between the nipples. Start with brief dabs. It will feel quite hot, and the application point will look a little redder than the rest of the skin, but it should not result in a burn. Once the temperature is tolerated, hold the pack in place for up to a minute before lifting it off. Be guided by the patient as to when it feels too hot and when the pack needs to be lifted, since the skin there is much more sensitive than on one's hand. Packs can also be applied to points in the centre of the patient's palms of the hands and soles of the feet. You may wish to re-dip the packs and re-apply several times, depending on the situation. Hormé is a lovely treatment for patients

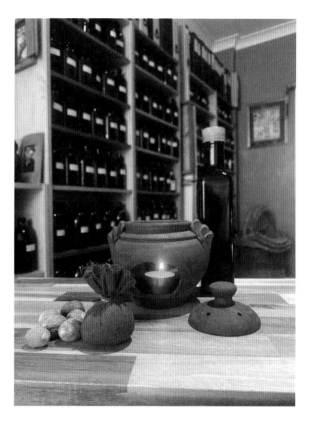

suffering with *rLung* disorders. There are many different hormé herbal combinations, chosen oils, and points to which they are applied. These are chosen according to the circumstances of each case. This method is a simple version shared with the aim of helping those with acute anxiety.

Old Man's Beard 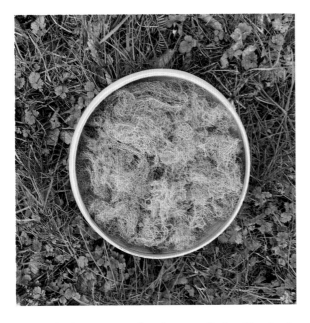 *Usnea barbata*

'Usnea, the lungs of the Earth, helps us to repel infection and stimulates our immune systems.'

Usnea is known as the lungs of the Earth. It is best gathered from recently fallen branches rather than from living trees, as it is very slow-growing and is a precious part of the ecosystem. It grows in tufts that look beard-like and is distinguished from look-alikes by a white elastic fungal thread in the centre of each thallus, which can be seen when it is pulled apart.

It has a significant antibiotic action, being particularly effective against gram-positive bacteria such as *Streptococcus*, *Staphylococcus*, *Mycobacterium tuberculosis*, and other bugs that tend to present a rapid challenge to our bodies. It is also antiviral, inhibiting Epstein-Barr virus activation and *Herpes simplex* virus. Its antifungal properties mean that it can play a part in supporting patients with Candida overgrowth, athlete's foot, ringworm, etc.

Medicinal parts
> Thalli

Physiological actions

Summary
> Antimicrobial
> Antiviral
> Antifungal

Physiological virtues

Usnea contains polysaccharides that are immuno-stimulatory and have antitumoural activity. It also contains lichen acids, such as usnic acid, which are directly antibiotic, disrupting bacterial cell membrane function as well as inhibiting ATP formation and oxidative phosphorylation. It only targets bacterial cells, so is not at all harmful to human cells. As well as being directly antimicrobial, Usnea supports our tissues with soothing mucilage and has pain-relieving properties.

Usnea has a particular affinity with the lungs and urinary system and is a really good medicine to consider in cases of sinusitis, acute/chronic lung infections, and cystitis, for example. I would add a note of caution here. If reaching for Usnea, or any natural antibiotic herb, it is very important to understand the underlying reasons why the infection has occurred and address those as well. If we do not investigate, understand, and treat the root cause, we are at risk of the infection becoming a regular and worsening challenge.

It can be prescribed in short-term acute situations but is also suitable for longer-term prescribing in order to support patients with depressed immune systems – for example those suffering with HIV, herpes, and other chronic conditions. If prescribed over a longer time frame, it is not accompanied by the same contraindications as long-term prescribing of antibiotics.

Topically, it is a good first aid treatment for wounds. Apply the powder directly to the wound. For impetigo and cellulitis, apply some tincture diluted in water as a wash. This can also be prescribed as a gargle for sore throats.

Energetics
Old Man's Beard is bitter, sweet, and neutral, cooling, and drying.

In my dispensary
Usnea is not extracted very efficiently in water or as an ordinary short-steep tincture. Some people use heat to help the extraction while tincturing, but I prefer to carry out a double extraction process similar to the one that I use to prepare medicinal mushroom extracts.

In my clinic my Usnea tincture is always prescribed in tailor-made formulae for my patients, since I am always conscious of treating the reason for the infection as well as the infection itself.

Historical applications
In the traditions of the indigenous peoples of North America, Usnea represents the lungs of the Earth and is associated with the direction North. It is considered to have a sacred relationship with trees, strengthening them and protecting them from infections.

Usnea was probably the inspiration for tinsel as a decoration on Christmas trees in Northern Europe.

Oregon Grape 🍇 *Mahonia aquifolium*

'Oregon Grape cuts through obstacles and stagnation.'

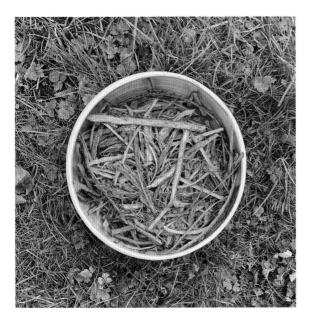

Although not native to the United Kingdom, Oregon Grape is widely chosen as a landscaping plant in urban developments. It tolerates shade and is very hardy, its prickly foliage helping to discourage unwanted access to off-limits areas. Its medicinal virtues were taught to us by the indigenous people of the west coast of North America, who chose it to treat fevers, indigestion, gout, and gallbladder insufficiency.

Medicinal parts
- Stem bark
- Flowers
- Roots

Physiological actions

Summary
- Cholagogue
- Bitter
- Tonic
- Alterative
- Antilithic
- Anti-inflammatory
- Febrifuge
- Expectorant
- Decongestant
- Antimicrobial
- Antifungal
- Anthelmintic

Physiological virtues

The intense yellow colour of Oregon Grape's inner bark and roots gives away the fact that it contains the alkaloid berberine. Berberine is a strong bitter that is a cholagogue, stimulating bile production by the liver and encouraging more vibrant digestion in general. This means that Oregon Grape can be a good choice for those with sluggish bowels or who suffer with indigestion. In stimulating the liver, it also encourages the release of stored iron and can play a helpful part in treating anaemia.

It has powerful antimicrobial, anthelmintic, and antifungal properties, and it supports a healthy immune response by the body. Its antibiotic action means that it can be a good short-term choice for various infections, especially those of the digestive tract, such as amoebic dysentery or Shigella infection. However, be aware that long-term treatment with large doses over a long period of time could reduce the diversity and abundance of our healthy gut flora. We need to weigh that risk up against the need for an antibiotic.

Berberine has been shown to have the ability to inhibit the growth of abnormal skin cells. This is one of the reasons that Oregon Grape is popular as a herb for patients with psoriasis and eczema. It acts as an alterative, cleaning the blood and resolving skin conditions such as acne, boils, and herpes. It is anti-inflammatory, playing a helpful role in alleviating joint pain as well as inflammation elsewhere in the body such as in the cardiovascular system. This may be one of the reasons that it acts as a hypotensive.

Its medicinal virtues are numerous and wide-ranging. It is a decongestant and an expectorant, and it reduces the formation of stones in the body. It should be prescribed with caution in cases of large asymptomatic gallstones, because it could move them out of the gallbladder, and they could become lodged in the bile duct, where they would most certainly no longer be asymptomatic.

Oregon Grape is also a thyroid stimulant and can be helpful in cases where there is irregularity and pain associated with the menstrual cycle. In acute fevers it is a valuable febrifuge.

Topically, a decoction of Oregon Grape bark is an excellent wound wash to tackle infection. Alternatively, you can sprinkle powder of the dried bark directly into the wound.

Energetics

Oregon Grape is bitter, astringent, and cooling. It is full of contradictions. It is prickly and powerful but has beautiful, gentle, fragrant flowers. It is a protector and a harmonizer, a gentle healer, as well as a formidable antimicrobial. It will remove obstacles in the body, but take it for granted or treat it like an allopathic drug, and it will start to cause obstacles. It shows us that herbs are to be respected as individuals, not considered as natural substitutes for chemical drugs.

We need to digest our experiences before we can learn from them. Oregon Grape can help us to become 'unstuck' if 'stuck' digestion has compromised our ability to assimilate and digest experiences and move on. Consider this herb for people who suffer with poor digestive function and who often mention old resentments and past slights.

In Tibetan medicine

This is a herb that calms excess *Tripa* and is especially one to consider for fiery, irritable perfectionists who suffer with indigestion.

In my dispensary

Oregon Grape addresses digestive insufficiency so quickly that it is my herb of choice to prescribe to patients who suffer with very poor digestion after having had their gallbladder removed. Three drops of the tincture on the tongue before eating stimulates the liver to increase the production of bile and immediately improves compromised digestion. My post-cholecystectomy patients tell me that this strategy is 'miraculous'. I provide them with a small dropper bottle that they can take with them wherever they go and advise them to stick to the very small dose suggested. This is so that their gut flora is not adversely affected over time.

This case shows how small doses of Oregon Grape root can make a big difference: 'Emma' was in her mid-60s and had chronic constipation. She would regularly go for several days without a bowel movement. She was prone to anxiety and cloudy thinking, so I did not want to prescribe too many bitter herbs. She did need them, though, to support her bowels. We went through the dietary changes that would be needed: more water, more fresh fruit and vegetables, and the removal of refined carbohydrates. She was a meat-eater, so I asked her to drink bone broth regularly (one mug each day) to help counteract her *rLung*. She was also to take 3 drops of Oregon Grape root tincture on the tongue before meals.

After four weeks her bowel habit was much better, and she felt less anxious. She told me that her thinking was clearer: it was like 'a fog had lifted'. Over time these health improvements continued. She felt energized and mentally on the ball, and she had lost the excess weight she had been carrying.

'Jennifer' was in her late 70s and complained of constant belching and bloating, which had been worsening recently. She had had her gallbladder removed six years earlier, and her digestive problems had started after that. When I went through her case, I discovered that, despite the original dietary advice she had been given by her doctor, she had gradually gone back to eating foods that were quite high in fat. For example, she enjoyed going for a cup of tea and a pastry at her local bakery. Along with the recommendation to be careful about eating fatty foods, I prescribed her 3 drops of Oregon Grape tincture on the tongue before meals. Within four weeks the belching had gone and the bloating was considerably reduced.

Historical applications

Indigenous peoples of the west coast of North America are the knowledge holders for this herb as both medicine and food. It was only introduced into the European *materia medica* in 1822, and I would not claim to be in a position to accurately describe its historical applications. I have described its medicinal virtues to the best of my ability, but I am sure there is a great deal more that could be added by those who have lived with it for generations and know its stories.

Magical

Oregon Grape is considered to act as a protective herb: three branches are placed over the doorway to keep out those who would do us harm. A small piece can be carried as a talisman to provide a defence against negative energies as well as to encourage the flow of popularity and wealth towards us.

Suggestion for the home apothecary

Oregon Grape bark tincture as a digestive support

Loosely fill a jar with fresh Oregon Grape bark and cover with 50% ABV. Leave in a cool, dark place for four weeks, then drain and bottle. Take 3 drops on the tongue before meals if suffering from digestive insufficiency or if you have had your gallbladder removed and your digestion has never been right since.

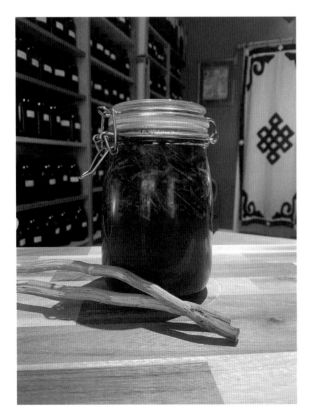

Passionflower 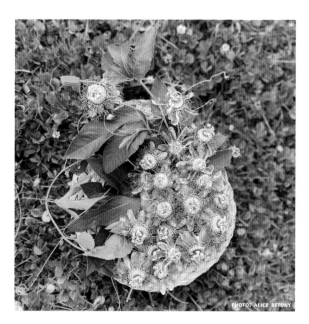 *Passiflora incarnata*

'Passionflower helps us to see the bigger picture and induces sound sleep.'

Passionflower was so named because its flower structure can be linked with the crucifixion of Christ. Each flower has five stamens, which represent the five wounds, it has three styles that represent the three nails, the radial filaments suggest the crown of thorns, and its flower colour – white and purple – represent purity and heaven. Beyond its purely Christianized associations, it also has a resonance with higher levels of spiritual awareness, such as the cultivation of empathy, the ability to see the bigger picture, and a reduction in our attachment to worldly distractions. When you study the beautiful flower, you can see that it looks 'other-worldly' and is reminiscent of visual depictions of the bodily energy centres or chakras. Each flower only lasts one day, so it is a potent reminder of the value of appreciating the present moment.

This vine is also known as 'Maypop'. The name is probably derived from the Powhatan name 'Maracock', but it has widely become known as Maypop. This is said to be because the seed pods form on the rambling vines in late May, and when people step on them, they make a loud popping sound. Another of its names is Wild Apricot.

Medicinal parts
- Leaves
- Small stems
- Flowers

Physiological actions
Summary
- Nervine
- Sedative
- Anticonvulsant
- Antispasmodic
- Analgesic
- Hypnotic
- Vasodilator

Physiological virtues
Passionflower is sedative, anticonvulsant, pain-relieving, and sleep-inducing. Its key constituents are alkaloids, including harmine, harman, harmol, and passiflorine, as well as flavone glycosides and sterols. They work synergistically in the whole plant, making it sedative, hypnotic, antispasmodic, anodyne, and nervine.

It is excellent for insomnia and is non-addictive. However, it is contraindicated for patients suffering from clinical depression and those whose insomnia is characterized by early morning waking rather than difficulty getting off to sleep at first. It is a remedy that is well indicated to relieve tension headaches, anxiety, panic attacks, mood swings, and irritability, as well as chronic fatigue.

Passionflower is a good antispasmodic and has vasodilatory properties, so is worth considering in a prescription for hypertension where that is linked to long-standing tension. It is also a bronchodilator and can be a good choice when treating asthma. It can be prescribed as an anticonvulsant and to alleviate the symptoms of Parkinson's disease. It is helpful to ease menstrual cramping and has pain-relieving properties, so it can be prescribed as a remedy against neuralgia, shingles, and other nerve pain. Some cases of migraine respond well to

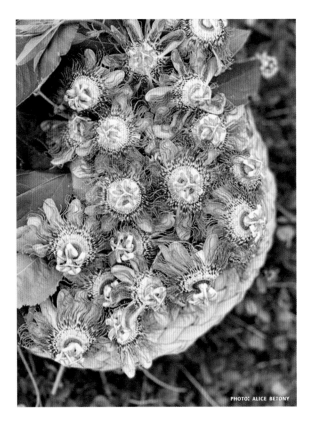

PHOTO: ALICE BETONY

Passionflower if it is taken at the first sign of an attack.

A topical compress can relieve toothache, earache, and inflamed eyes.

Passionflower can cause the uterus to contract, so should be avoided in pregnancy.

Energetics

Passionflower is bitter. It is linked to the higher realms of existence, whatever that means to you within your own beliefs and traditions. It helps us to distance ourselves from our day-to-day concerns, allowing churning repetitive worries to loosen their grip on us, making it easier for us to relax and to sleep more soundly.

In my dispensary

Passionflower is a staple within my dispensary, and I work with either *P. incarnata* or *P. caerulea*. I especially like to include this herb in prescriptions for people who are filled with worries and find it very hard to let go of their worldly concerns. Including Passionflower helps them to see the bigger, more interconnected picture and can start them on the process of cultivating a new, more balanced, perspective on life.

Historical applications

The Houma tribe of Louisiana took an infusion of the roots as a general tonic. It was described by a visiting European doctor in 1783 as a cure for epilepsy.

Magical

Passionflower is associated with peace and spirituality. If it is brought into the house, it will not only encourage a peaceful atmosphere to prevail, but it will also be a potent reminder of impermanence and the value of appreciating the present moment. Place a sprig under your pillow to promote sound sleep.

Suggestion for the home apothecary

Passionflower tea

Dry Passionflower for year-round calming tea blends. Blend with herbs such as Lemon Balm, Lime flower, Hops, Wild Oat, Lavender, and Skullcap. Infuse covered and drink before bed. If you are prone to waking up in the night and not being able to get back to sleep, try taking a small flask of it to bed and have it available near your bed to sip if needed.

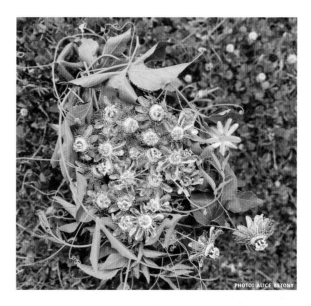

PHOTO: ALICE BETONY

Pellitory-of-the-Wall *Parietaria diffusa*

'Pellitory-of-the-Wall opens the channels and clears obstructions to the flow of liquids.'

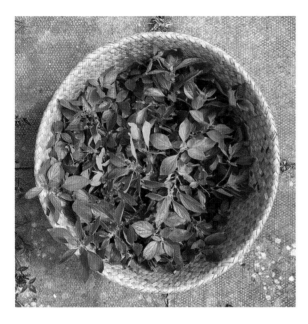

Pellitory-of-the-Wall has the distinction of removing obstacles to the flow of liquids in the body, usually urine. It is restorative rather than 'just' diuretic and so is very well indicated for chronic conditions rather than purely being an acute treatment option for cystitis, for example.

Its generic name, 'Parietaria', is from the Latin *paries*, which means a wall. Parietaria grows in old walls so is adapted to grabbing any available moisture and channelling it into its vessels. It makes a lot of sense energetically that Pellitory-of-the-Wall is an excellent kidney tonic. As a kidney tonic, it has the special and valuable property of being demulcent at the same time as being astringent.

Medicinal parts
- Aerial parts

Aerial parts should preferably be harvested before flowering.

Physiological actions

Summary
- Diuretic
- Anti-inflammatory
- Demulcent
- Urinary system tonic
- Expectorant
- Aperient
- Astringent

Physiological virtues

Pellitory-of-the-Wall is most often thought of as a urinary system herb. It is a specialist at overcoming the obstacles to the movement of water. You can contrast this with the ability of Cleavers to move water through long distances. Cleavers has an ability to get water from A to B and to encourage invigoration and movement in tissues that have become sluggish, but Pellitory-of-the-Wall is a remover of obstacles to the flow of water.

It has long been considered to have a long-term restorative action on the kidneys, gently strengthening and supporting them as well as helping to dissolve stones and remove calculus. It is a herb to be considered in cases of nephritis, pyelitis, renal colic, and oedema. It is most often prescribed as an infusion but can also be prescribed as a tincture or even topically as a poultice on the back over the kidney area.

Pellitory-of-the-Wall has an anti-inflammatory and slightly demulcent action that soothes the passages and helps in the process of resolving obstacles to flow. Since prostate inflammation and enlargement is linked closely with difficulties in passing urine and in urinary retention, Pellitory-of-the-Wall can be very helpful in the relief of prostate-related discomfort. These days, Pellitory-of-the-Wall is mostly taught as a kidney herb, and its affinity with prostate action is rarely mentioned.

Pellitory-of-the-Wall has other qualities too. It is also a respiratory herb, specific for chronic dry coughs, and it is a gentle laxative. As a topical application, it can be helpful for burns and wounds. The pollen can be an allergy trigger, so it is best avoided by those with significant hay fever, although potential problems can be minimized by harvesting the plant early in the season, before flowering.

Energetics

Pellitory-of-the-Wall is bitter and astringent. It is a remover of obstacles that block flow. This applies to both the physiological and the emotional realms. It makes a lot of sense when you consider the link between our emotions and the element of water. If you are experiencing blocks in your life and you cannot sense, or intuit, the best way to respond or flow around these obstacles, try connecting with Pellitory-of-the-Wall. You may find it helpful to visualize your life as a flowing river and see the current obstacle as a large rock. You know that the water in the river will easily flow around the rock, it just needs to adjust its direction temporarily.

In my dispensary

I prescribe Pellitory-of-the-Wall in individual blends for my patients. I choose between tea, tincture, or as part of a capsule blend depending on each case. I probably most often prescribe it for patients who have urinary system symptoms or prostate enlargement. I used to worry that prescribing diuretics to patients suffering with urinary frequency would make matters worse, but at the right dose and in a well-balanced blend, I find that the opposite applies.

The case of 'Kevin' is typical of how Pellitory-of-the-Wall can act as a remover of obstacles and encourage smoother flow, beyond just the physiological level. Kevin was in his mid-70s, ate a very healthy diet, and had a regular exercise regime. Despite his apparently healthy lifestyle, he suffered from prostate enlargement, which caused him to need to pee quite frequently during the day and at least three times during each night. Whenever he peed, he found that it was hard to start the stream of urine, and it did not always stop 'cleanly', both being common symptoms of prostate issues. He was under the care of a consultant and had been offered surgical treatment, but he wished to avoid this, if possible. Kevin also suffered with dry eyes and arthritic thumb joints, and I suspected that he was not drinking enough water – a common trait in those who are frustrated by having to pee frequently. As well as his physiological symptoms, he described how he was experiencing obstacles that felt like 'brick walls' in several areas of his life. This made him feel angry and frustrated.

I prescribed him a tailor-made tincture prescription designed to support his prostate health, circulation, and liver, also asking him to increase his hydration levels and level of activity. I included Pellitory-of-the-Wall in his tincture prescription, alongside other herbs, including Nettle root, Rosemary, Lemon Balm, and Artichoke leaf. It was hard at first to persuade him to increase his hydration levels, but when he did, he found that his urinary frequency did not increase. If anything, there was a reduction in frequency, particularly in the night. He also found that starting and stopping the stream of urine was easier too. As his prostate symptoms resolved, he noticed that he had developed a less angry and more flexible approach to the obstacles he had been experiencing in his life. He found

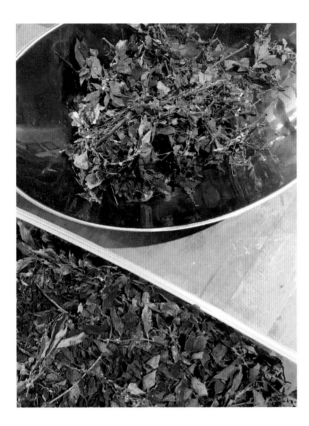

pose. Historically, though, it was not just viewed as a diuretic herb, Parkinson describing it as a singular remedy for '*any old continuall or dry cough, the shortnesse of breath and wheezings in the throate*'. For this purpose it was to be made into an electuary or a decoction '*with Sugar or Hony*'. He also recommended it for tinnitus: '*the jouce dropped into the eares easeth the noise and hummings in them, and taketh away the prickings and shooting paines in them*'.

Gerard wrote: '*The juice held awhile in the mouth easeth pains in the teeth; the distilled water of the herb drank with sugar worketh the same effect and cleanseth the skin from spots, freckles, pimples, wheals, sunburn etc.*' He also recommended it as an ointment for piles, gout, and fistula.

Magical

If you are experiencing obstacles to the flow of your life or your intuition, consider Pellitory-of-the-Wall.

Suggestion for the home apothecary

Dried Pellitory-of-the-Wall for year-round teas

Harvest Pellitory-of-the-Wall on a dry day before it flowers, when there is lush growth. Cut the stems into roughly 5-cm-long pieces and lay them out evenly on trays. Dry passively in a warm, dark, airy place, or use a dehydrator on a low heat. Once the stems are completely brittle, store in an airtight container in a cool, dark place.

Drink two cups of infusion per day in the event of a urinary-tract infection. If you are suffering with these regularly, please remember to address the root cause, which often, but not always, is a lack of sufficient hydration, combined with a diet high in refined sugars.

a less confrontational way of dealing with things, and as a result his life became much 'smoother' and more relaxing.

Historical applications

Parkinson said that '*the juyce thereof taken to the quantitie of three ounces at a time doth wonderfully ease those that are troubled with the suppression of their urine, causing them very speedily to make water, and to expel both the stone and gravell that are engendred in the kidnies and bladder. . . .*' It is interesting to note that he also recommended it as a topical application to the back in order to '*mitigate the pain of passing gravell or stone*' or used as a decoction in a bath for the same pur-

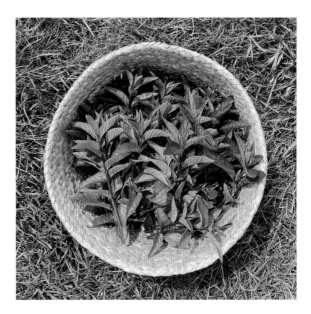
'Peppermint is cooling at first but then warms the system and encourages sweating.'

Peppermint is beloved of all cultures and much relied upon for medicine, cosmetics, confectionary, and culinary purposes. It is usually thought to be a hybrid of Water Mint (*Mentha aquatica*) and Spearmint (*Mentha spicata*). Although a very popular herbal tea, it is significantly medicinal and should not be underestimated. If you are drinking several cups of Peppermint tea per day, you are taking a medicinal dose. That may or may not be positive, depending on your circumstances.

Medicinal parts
> Aerial parts

Physiological actions

Summary

> Carminative
> Bitter
> Antispasmodic
> Antibacterial
> Antiparasitic
> Decongestant
> Analgesic
> Diaphoretic
> Nervine

Physiological virtues

Peppermint's best-known medicinal virtue is its action as a carminative, due to the high level of volatile oils that it contains. It is helpful for digestive discomfort, easing gripes and wind, as well as stimulating the production of digestive enzymes and bile. It can be helpful in cases of chronic diseases of the pancreas or the biliary ducts. It is a popular tea choice for after meals because of its digestive properties but it should be avoided by those who are prone to heart-

burn, acid reflux, or hiatus hernia. It relaxes the stomach and the oesophageal valve, potentially exacerbating these conditions.

Within allopathic medicine, Peppermint is often prescribed to relieve the discomfort of IBS symptoms. This is sometimes heralded as some sort of victory for herbal medicine, because it means that a herb has been 'accepted' by the allopathic community. Unfortunately, unless the underlying causes for the IBS are identified and addressed, the Peppermint is fighting a losing battle. This is a herb that can do so much more than to temporarily prop up an unsustainable lifestyle and diet.

As a pleasant-tasting digestive stimulant, it can help to encourage the appetite in those who are off their food. It relieves nausea and reduces vomiting through a mild anaesthetizing effect on the mucous membranes of the stomach. It eases colic and wind due to its ability to relax the muscles of the entire digestive tract. This virtue makes it helpful in diarrhoea caused by tension and stress, while it also relieves constipation caused by a spastic colon.

Peppermint is antibacterial and antiparasitic. This makes it a good choice for infections of the gastrointestinal tract. It can also be helpful when patients have digestive discomfort originating from abnormal fermentation processes in the intestine, often caused by a disrupted intestinal flora.

Since it is a general antispasmodic, Peppermint relaxes the muscles of the uterus and is worth considering for period pain. This does make it unsuitable in large doses during pregnancy though. It also reduces breast milk production so it should be avoided while lactating.

Its menthol content also makes it a great ingredient in decongestant preparations and teas, as well as in topical rubs. If made into a balm or oil and rubbed onto the chest and throat, it relieves respiratory congestion. When applied to the skin in general, it is analgesic and cooling, relieving sensitivity and directly fighting infection. Choose a strong cooled infusion and apply to hot, itchy, or painful skin disorders. It can also be applied as a compress to inflamed joints or for areas affected by neuralgia.

When applied as a balm to the forehead and temples, it can be helpful to relieve headaches and migraines. Sip some tea at the same time to tackle the headache from two angles. This latter is especially indicated for headaches caused by digestive disturbances.

Although cooling in action superficially, Peppermint raises the internal heat of the body and encourages sweating but less strongly than some of the other diaphoretic herbs. A really good tea blend for the first onset of colds and influenza is equal parts of Peppermint, Yarrow, and Elderflower. Inhale the aromatic steam as you drink this tea.

Peppermint has a calming action and can be helpful in cases of palpitations. Where there is hysteria or '*nervous disorders*', Maud Grieve describes how adding Wood Betony to an infusion of Peppermint '*augments its action well*'.

Peppermint is a very popular herbal tea and is consumed widely and frequently by people who consider it innocuous. However, it is significantly medicinal and is really best drunk when needed, rather than as a daily habitual choice. If treating patients who drink large amounts of Peppermint tea, it will be important to take its effects into account and preferably persuade them to widen their herbal tea repertoire.

I do not recommend the ingestion of the essential oil of Peppermint (or of any other essential oils, for that matter). Be careful if taking the herb in pregnancy and lactation and do not exceed the therapeutic dose of 2–3 cups of infusion per day. Peppermint is not suited to infants. Choose Catmint (*Nepeta mussinii*) instead.

Energetics
Peppermint is hot, dry, and cooling. It gently reduces discomfort caused by excessive tension. It helps us to let go of what does not serve us and encourages us to move on afresh after a health challenge.

In Tibetan medicine
Mentha arvensis and *Mentha piperita* are included in the Tibetan pharmacopoeia. *M. arvensis* is called *Gur tig* [གུར་ཏིག]. It has a sweet-to-bitter taste, with a post-digestive taste that is sweet and a potency that is neutral to cooling. It is considered to cure hot disorders present in the nerves, blood disorders associated with *Tripa*, and spreading hot disorders associated with inflamed wounds. *M. piperita* is called *Gogza*

phowari [ཕོ་བ་རི་]. It has a sweet-to-astringent taste and a sweet post-digestive taste. Its potency is warming. It is considered to cure *rLung* disorders and to ease stomach discomfort.

In my dispensary

Peppermint is a lovely ingredient in my dispensary. I am especially fond of prescribing it in teas, particularly those for acute colds and influenza, but I also prescribe it regularly in tincture form.

This case illustrates how Peppermint can help with easing griping and nervousness in a case of IBS: 'Jason' was 24 years old and worked in the building trade. He had suffered with IBS for several years and tended to have two or three loose stools daily. They often contained mucus, and he experienced regular painful cramps on the left of his abdomen below the ribs. As well as his digestive symptoms, he had skin flare-ups in the form of raised itchy rashes on his forehead and torso. He knew that he was better when he avoided dairy and gluten, but he did not stick to this and often had whey-based protein shakes and take-out pizzas. As a result, he experienced regular flare-ups of both gut and skin symptoms, each of which lasted around four weeks. He often felt tired and was sluggish on waking and had a persistently stuffed-up nose. He also admitted that he was someone who was quite prone to anxiety. When I examined his tongue, I could see that it had a thick, greasy coating towards its rear half.

I had a chat with him about looking after himself better and avoiding the foods and supplements that he knew would cause a flare-up. In the meantime, I prescribed a personalized tincture blend to ease his gripes and support his digestion. I chose Peppermint, Agrimony, Vervain, and Blessed Thistle, together with some Cleavers to support the clearing of his lymphatic system. Four weeks later, things were very different. His skin rashes had disappeared, and he was no longer having any painful gripes. His stools were less frequent and much firmer in consistency, and his nose no longer felt stuffed up. He was happy to report that his energy levels had improved, and he was now bouncing out of bed in the morning. He also said that he felt much calmer. When I examined his tongue, I was not surprised to see that it was now clear.

Historical applications

Peppermint has a very long history as a medicinal herb. Dried leaves were found in Egyptian pyramids dating from around 1000 BC. It was very popular with the Greeks and the Romans, who used to wear crowns of it at their feasts. It was mentioned in the Icelandic pharmacopoeias of the thirteenth century but did not reach the herbal *materia medica* of Western Europe until the eighteenth century. In England it was widely cultivated around Mitcham in Surrey from 1750 onwards.

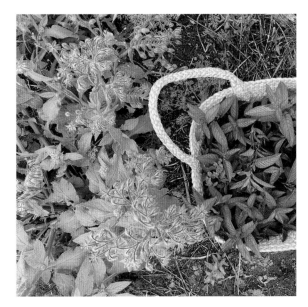

Parkinson wrote that Mint roots are '*so plentifull, that being planted in a garden, they are hardly rid out againe, every small piece therof being left in the ground increasing far enough*'.

Culpeper summed it up: '*Briefly, it is very profitable to the stomach.*'

Magical

Peppermint is associated with purification, protection, sleep, love, and psychic powers. A sprig is placed under the pillow in order to encourage prophetic dreams. Wear it on the wrist to guard against illness, and rub it on furniture and floorboards to banish negativity. It is also considered to attract prosperity: if you want to try this, place a few leaves in your wallet.

Suggestion for the home apothecary

Peppermint liquor

> » *350 ml brandy*
> » *½ cup fresh Peppermint*
> » *½ tbsp fresh Lemon Balm*
> » *¼ tsp Fennel seeds*
> » *¼ tsp Cinnamon*

Add the ingredients to a jar, and cover with the brandy. Place in a cool, dark place for 4 weeks

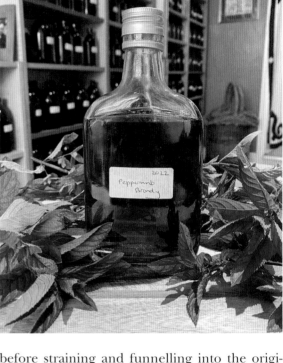

before straining and funnelling into the original bottle, with an appropriate label. Take 1 tsp to ease bloating or digestive discomfort. Avoid in cases of acid reflux.

Pilewort/Lesser Celandine 🦋 *Ranunculus ficaria*

The beautiful, shining stars of Pilewort were poet William Wordsworth's favourite flower and are depicted on his gravestone. The Celtic name for this plant is *Grian* (the sun), not only because of the appearance of the flowers but also because they only open when light levels are high enough, closing again in the late afternoon. The petals are green on the underside, so when they close, the flowers are quite inconspicuous. Below ground, the plant forms little tubers that are reminiscent of the shape of haemorrhoids and so, according to the Doctrine of Signatures, they signal its special virtues. This is a herb loved by herbal practitioners because it lives up to its name so well. It is truly a great astringent for toning and shrinking piles (haemorrhoids).

Medicinal parts

▷ Whole plant

Physiological actions

Summary

▷ Astringent
▷ Anti-inflammatory

Physiological virtues

Lesser Celandine is astringent and is specific for tightening and toning lax veins, whether they are haemorrhoids or varicose veins. Piles are an annoying fact of life for many patients: they may pop up during pregnancy, when the body is under more strain than usual, or they can develop as a messenger from a liver complaining of congestion. Not only does a congested liver create venous 'back pressure', but it is also likely to bring with it a tendency to constipation,

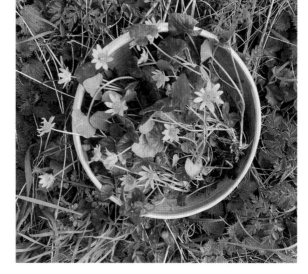

and the resulting straining does not help matters if you are prone to piles.

If you are suffering from haemorrhoids, you really need to get to the bottom of the problem (if you will pardon the pun).

Energetics

Lesser Celandine is astringent.

In my dispensary

When patients tell me that they have piles, I want to establish the root cause of the problem, so that a lasting solution is obtained. Each case is different, because each person I see is unique. A person may need herbs such as Agrimony to help blood circulation in the liver, or they may need herbs to help increase the flow of bile, such as Dandelion and Blessed Thistle. Where venous integrity is a problem, herbs such as Witch Hazel and Horse Chestnut will play

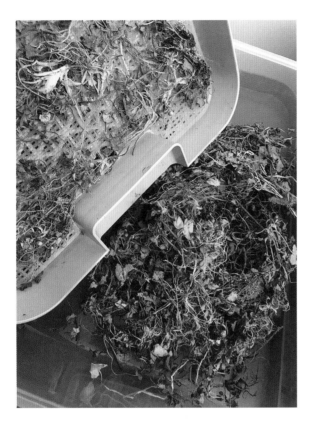

their part, and sometimes the circulation in general needs support with herbs such as Ginger and Prickly Ash. There is no 'one-size-fits-all' approach, but, having said that, Pilewort is a very valuable part of the treatment, because it is so effective at shrinking piles quickly. I mostly work with Pilewort in external preparations, but it can also be prescribed internally as a tincture or capsule formula, combined with other circulatory supportive and liver-clearing herbs.

'Carrie' was in her 40s and came to see me asking for help with a distressingly large haemorrhoid. She was not comfortable sitting down for a consultation, as the offending pile was the size of a duck egg. I sent her away with a pot of Pilewort ointment and told her to apply it liberally and to lie down and rest as much as possible. Within one week, it had shrunk to the size of a pea; a couple of weeks later it was com-

pletely gone. Once she was more comfortable, we were able to go through her case properly and start to tackle the underlying causes, so that it did not happen again.

Historical applications

Parkinson wrote that it is by *'good experience, that the decoction of the leaves and rootes doth wonderfully helpe the piles or hemorrhoides, as also kernels by the eares and throate, called the King's Evil, or any other hard wennes or tumors.'*

Culpeper said: *'The herb, on account of its signature, is accounted to be good for the haemorrhoids or piles, to ease their pain and swelling, and stop their bleeding.'*

Suggestion for the home apothecary

Pilewort ointment

Harvest whole Pilewort plants in spring: include flowers, leaves, stalks, and tubers. Wash them thoroughly after harvest. Do not leave them soaking in water, just wash them and then lay them out on a tray to dry immediately. Leave in an airy place or use a dehydrator to make sure they are completely dried. Loosely fill a jar with the dried whole Pilewort plants, and cover to the top with mild and light olive oil. Leave to infuse for at least 4 weeks, then strain through a coffee filter in a conical colander or sieve. Measure the volume of oil you are left with; pour it into a double boiler, and start to gently warm it, ensuring that the oil itself is not placed directly on the heat source. Weigh out 1 g of beeswax granules (or grated beeswax) for each 7 ml of oil that you have. For example, if you have 140 ml of infused oil, you will need 20 g of beeswax. Add the beeswax to the warm oil, and stir until melted. Immediately pour the oil and wax mixture into a jug, and then pour it into clean, dry jars. Leave them to set before picking them up to lid them. Apply liberally to haemorrhoids, if needed.

Plantain 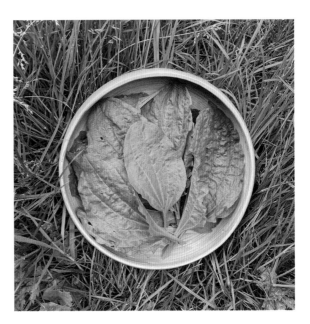 *Plantago major/P. lanceolata*

'Plantain helps us to recognize and repel harmful influences.'

I think that Plantain is one of those herbs that can quite easily be taken for granted, because it is so widely available. It is ubiquitous, growing pretty much everywhere in the temperate world. But do not be fooled by this: Plantain is a very valuable and precious herbal medicine. It especially grows on compacted ground, on paths, tracks, roads, and byways. You often see it in meadows by gateways or cattle feeders, where the cows have trodden down the vegetation. It is a medicine of the road and for travellers. It is resilient, tough, and elastic. It bounces back when pressed down into the mud. It may not be showy, but it is always there and can be relied upon. Plantain is known as a snake-bite medicine, and the leaves of both Plantains have a snakeskin-like appearance. This is especially noticeable in *Plantago lanceolata*. The seed head is also reminiscent of a snake's head in the way that it is carried on its stalk.

Plantain was known as 'Waybread' in Anglo-Saxon times, as travellers would grind the seeds to form flour and make it into rough flat breads.

Medicinal parts
- Leaves
- Root

I gather the leaves of both Broadleaved Plantain (*P. major*) and Ribwort Plantain (*P. lanceolata*) for medicine, although the root is sometimes also prescribed, and the nutritious seeds can be gathered for food.

Physiological actions

Summary
- Demulcent
- Anti-inflammatory
- Astringent
- Expectorant
- Urinary system demulcent
- Immune system support/antiallergenic
- Vulnerary

Physiological virtues

I consider the different species of Plantain to be interchangeable medicinally but some people feel that *P. major* has more of an affinity with the urinary system than *P. lanceolata*. The physiological actions of Plantain leaves centre around soothing and healing irritated tissues as well as drawing out poisons or pus. Topically, Plantain can be applied to bites, infected wounds, abscesses, haemorrhoids, and boils. It is a perfect blister treatment for walkers: simply chew or crush a leaf and apply it to the affected area. In times gone by, pilgrims used to line their shoes with leaves to ease their walking sores.

As a demulcent and anti-inflammatory herb that is mildly astringent, it can calm irritation in the respiratory, digestive, and urinary tracts. It eases dry, irritated coughs, sore throats, tracheitis, and allergic rhinitis, and it can be a good choice for patients with very long-standing respiratory infections, including in cases of tuberculosis and emphysema. Plantain is also especially good to draw out foreign bodies that have entered the lungs and damaged them – for example, through chemical or smoke inhalation. Plantain removes particles and expels them. The patient will usually start to cough up pus or thick mucus, as the Plantain supports the expulsion of the foreign material. As a related note, it can be very helpful for those going through the process of giving up smoking. It helps to repair and clear the lungs, as well shifting their relationship with cigarettes, making the next one seem like a much less attractive prospect. Plantain also has the very useful attribute of reducing fibrosities in the lungs – a quality that is rarely mentioned in herbals. All these examples share the presence of an invading influence: a pathogen, allergen, or foreign body causing the inflammation and irritation. This is the specific territory of Plantain as a medicinal herb.

In the same vein, Plantain can be very helpful for 'hot diarrhoea' when that is caused by inflamed mucous membranes in the digestive tract. This is diarrhoea that has been triggered by irritation or infection, the influence of some sort of foreign body that has upset the balance of the digestion.

We can also look to Plantain to be part of the approach for other cases where there is an invading influence. This may be bites, stings, infections, or even growths that should not be present, such as cancers or, according to Maud Grieve, '*malignant ulcers*'. It is described as a snake-bite medicine because it can help us to deal with venom, foreign bodies, stings, pus, dirt, and infection. In the ancient Welsh herbal lineage of Myddfai, Plantain is placed in the forefront for snake-bite treatment. '*For the bite of an adder: Take the juice of plantain, ground ivy and olive oil, an equal quantity of each. Give the patient a good draught of it, and anoint the wound with the same. It will destroy the poison and cure the patient.*'

In the urinary tract, Plantain offers itself up as a treatment for cystitis or kidney inflammation, especially when there is blood in the urine. It is considered to be a specific for urinary incontinence, whichever age group the patient falls into. I believe this action to be largely due to its ability to help the body to deal with irritation and infection. Plantain can also be a good choice to help relieve vaginitis and vaginal discharge, either as a douche or taken internally as tea or tincture.

Energetics

Plantain is sweet, cold, moist. It is good at resisting being trodden down or overrun. It bounces back. If you are feeling downtrodden, you might find Plantain helpful. It seems to strengthen the body's ability to react to invasion or 'being overcome'. You could say that Plantain helps us to strengthen boundaries, but this is in a completely different way from the physical-boundary-strengthening action of, say, Hawthorn. Plantain shows our body that we can mount an appropriate reaction to something that we may have been passive to. It helps us to recognize and respond to what is alien, fixing situations where the body has been invaded, and its capacity to recognize what is not supposed to be present has been overrun. Plantain is also very helpful when the body overreacts to a challenge, producing a more extreme reaction than is really needed.

In Tibetan medicine

Plantago major is known as *Tha Ram* [ཐ་རམ] and *Plantago lanceolata* as *Na Ram* [ན་རམ].

Both have a sweet-to-astringent taste, with a sweet post-digestive taste. Their potency is light and cooling. *Plantago depressa* is also part of the Tibetan pharmacopoeia, having the same taste profile as the other two Plantains mentioned. *P. depressa* is described as having a small singular stalk with a tip that looks like the tail of a monkey.

In Tibetan medicine, *P. major*, *P. lanceolata*, and *P. depressa* are considered to be '*like nectar for curing diarrhoea*'. It is important to note that this refers to 'hot diarrhoea' caused by inflammation and infection, rather than 'cold diarrhoea', which occurs when the digestive system is too weak and is unable to process food properly. The treatment for this latter involves stimulating and strengthening the digestive system rather than focusing on calming inflamed and irritated mucous membranes.

As well as treating dysentery (hot diarrhoea), the Plantains treat burns and severe wounds accompanied by an accumulation of lymphatic fluid. They are taught as herbs to help stem bleeding and to heal chronic sores. They are also prescribed for 'lung fever' and kidney disorders, including cases where there is difficulty in passing urine.

In my dispensary

In my clinic I prescribe Plantain in teas and tinctures, always in individually formulated blends. The following is a case that illustrates Plantain's ability to moderate an excessive reaction to bites and stings:

'Greta' was 14 years old and attended my clinic, accompanied by her mother, because she had inflammatory digestive issues. During the consultation she mentioned that she had always reacted very badly to horsefly bites, and I made a note to include Plantain in her prescription. Horsefly bites tend to be quite challenging for most people, but Greta had an extreme reaction, with swelling and pain that lasted twice as long as horsefly bites on her siblings. I prescribed her a tailor-made herbal tincture that included a significant amount of Plantain, both as an anti-inflammatory and demulcent for her gut but also for its ability to moderate excessive reactions to bites and stings. Four weeks into treatment she was bitten by a horsefly and was amazed that, very unusually for her, the bite had hardly swelled up at all and was much less painful and itchy than usual. This is a typical Plantain influence.

Another indication for Plantain is when patients have 'never been well since' reacting to a bad bite or sting, often when travelling

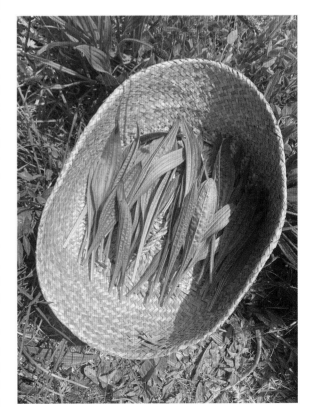

abroad. I have treated many patients who share this general aetiology. They often report that they developed fatigue and joint pains that persisted for years after the bite itself had resolved. Blood tests had not revealed any lingering infection, but the patients knew instinctively that the bite or sting was a turning point for their health. Their herbal prescriptions call for the addition of Plantain within a personalized blend that supports them holistically. After a few weeks of treatment, it is lovely to see them bouncing back to full health, free of fatigue and joint pain.

Historical applications

Dioscorides wrote that Plantain is a vulnerary and good against ulcers, sores and much else. Hildegard of Bingen recommended Plantain for insect bites. '*Plantain is warm and dry . . . if a spider or another worm touches or stings a person, then this person should immediately rub the spot with plantain juice and he or she will be better.*'

Culpeper wrote that '*The juice clarified and drank for days together by itself, or with other drink, helps excoriations or pains in the bowels, the distillations of rheum from the head, and it stays all manner of fluxes, even women's courses when too abundant.*'

Plantain has long been passed down as a folk remedy to heal varicose ulcers. In Tudor times Plantain was a key ingredient in a recipe to heal a sore mouth. '*Take the juice of plantain and rose water mixed with the same, and frequently wash your mouth; and if your gums are sore, take gun-powder, roche alum, bole ammoniac and honey, of each an equal quantity; mix them well together, and when you rub your gums with the same, let the rheum run out of your mouth.*'

Magical

Plantain is revered as a herb with special magical powers. It is one of the nine sacred herbs

that make up the Anglo-Saxon 'Nine Herbs Charm' recorded in the tenth-century medical manuscript the *Lacnunga*. Each of the nine herbs has an address that is read as it is being added to the blend. This is the one for Plantain:

> '*And you, Waybread, mother of worts,*
> *Open from eastward, powerful within,*
> *Over you chariots rolled, over you queens rode,*
> *Over you brides cried, over you bulls belled:*
> *All these you withstood, and these you*
>   *confounded,*
> *So withstand now the venom that flies through*
>   *the air,*
> *And the loathed thing which through the land*
>   *roves.*'

The nine sacred herbs/worts: were:

- Mugwort
- Waybread (Plantain)
- Stime (Watercress)
- Atterlothe (this may have been Viper's Bugloss)
- Maythen (Chamomile)
- Wergulu (Nettle)
- Crab Apple
- Chervil
- Fennel

Plantain can be used for divination, and British folklore carries this knowledge. On Shetland, flowering stems (scapes) were picked by boys and girls to see if they would marry. In Berwickshire the anthers were removed, and the two stems were wrapped in a dock leaf and placed under a stone until the next day. When examined again, if new anthers had grown, the match would be true love.

The leaves of *P. lanceolata* were known as 'fire leaves' and used for perhaps a more down-to-earth version of divination. Farmers would twist the leaves in order to estimate how much moisture was in their hay and therefore the chances of their hay rick catching fire. (Moist hay can naturally reach high temperatures and can spontaneously catch fire.)

P. major root has long been incorporated in amulet necklaces according to magic numbers. People put 3, 7, 9, or 99 roots in amulets around the neck in order to ward off worms, fevers, and evil spirits, to protect against love charms, or to win a lawsuit. It was considered important that the Plantain root was dug up with a tool made from a material other than iron. The amulet tradition continued for generations, and from the seventeenth century onwards the root was commonly worn in an amulet around the neck to guard against King's Evil (scrofula). Sufferers would also queue to receive the 'royal touch', in which the reigning monarch was believed to be able to cure the disease by touching the sufferer.

Carrying a piece of Plantain root in one's pocket was considered to protect against snake bites. Its capacity to protect from 'evil influences' features in a prescription for headache from the *Leech Book*. You must '*dig up* [Waybread] *without iron before sunrise, binding round the head with a red filet* [red wool]'. Binding with red wool was a widespread custom in Britain and Europe during those times, as red was a colour sacred to Thor and abhorred by witches and all evil beings.

Suggestion for the home apothecary

A Plantain and Lavender ointment for insect bites and stings

Loosely fill a jar with dried Plantain leaves and Lavender flowers, and cover to the top with mild and light olive oil. Leave to infuse for at least 4 weeks, then strain through a coffee filter

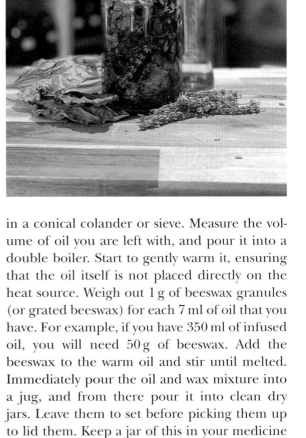

in a conical colander or sieve. Measure the volume of oil you are left with, and pour it into a double boiler. Start to gently warm it, ensuring that the oil itself is not placed directly on the heat source. Weigh out 1 g of beeswax granules (or grated beeswax) for each 7 ml of oil that you have. For example, if you have 350 ml of infused oil, you will need 50 g of beeswax. Add the beeswax to the warm oil and stir until melted. Immediately pour the oil and wax mixture into a jug, and from there pour it into clean dry jars. Leave them to set before picking them up to lid them. Keep a jar of this in your medicine cabinet, and apply as needed to bites and stings.

Pomegranate 🍂 *Punica granatum*

'Pomegranate is the king of increasing digestive heat.'

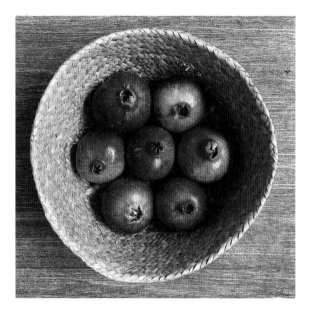

Pomegranate is a fabulous digestive support. It is sour and sweet and so it encourages the digestion without increasing the *rLung*, as bitter herbs can do. It is a symbol of abundance and fertility – quite rightly, because when our digestive systems are in good shape, we feel vibrant, energetic, and balanced, ready to create and enjoy abundance in our lives. If you feel that you want more abundance in your life, you would do well to connect regularly with Pomegranate.

Medicinal part
  ▷ Fruit (including rind and seeds)

Physiological actions
Summary
  ▷ Digestive tonic
  ▷ Vermifuge
  ▷ Astringent

Physiological virtues
Both Pomegranate rind and fruit are sour and are the best herbal medicine to steadily and sustainably encourage a more vibrant digestion. The rind contains strong alkaloids that can act as a potent vermifuge that is especially effective against tapeworms. In more moderate doses the rind is an astringent helpful to relieve diarrhoea.

It is worth noting that this fertility symbol has seeds that are a source of oestrone. The oestrone contained in Pomegranate seeds is considered to be bioidentical to the genuine human hormone.

Energetics
Pomegranate is sour, astringent, and sweet, warm, and dry. It supports abundance in our life through supporting our digestion and metabolism. As well as being a very important aspect of our health, digestion is a highly symbolic and spiritual process. When we eat, we are taking in substances that are 'of the Earth' and are transforming them to temporarily become part of our physicality. To have a weak digestion – or an unhealthy relationship with food – is to create a block on the flow of this beautiful interconnectedness between human being and the wider environment. When our digestion is vibrant, we feel in harmony with the world and ready to embrace the opportunities and abundance that it has to offer us, whether that is spiritual, material, or a healthy mixture of both.

In Tibetan medicine
Pomegranate is known as *Se'dru* [སེ་འབྲུ]. Its taste is sour and sweet, and it has a post-digestive

taste that is sour. Its potency is warming and oily as well as dry and a little rough. The dried seeds and the flesh are usually the medicinal part. It has a special affinity with supporting the digestive system. It cures loss of stomach and liver heat. It increases blood and drives away 'animalcules'. Its entry in the *Gyudzhi* can be translated as: 'It treats all stomach ailments without exception. It increases the digestive heat and overcomes phlegm/cold ailments.'

The 'Pomegranate Five' formula is perfect for general digestive support. It has a balance of warming herbs and Saffron, which is cooling. This makes the formula widely suitable as a long-term digestive support. Khenpo Troru Tsenam felt that most people could benefit from this formula.

In my dispensary
I work with Pomegranate mostly for its positive digestion-supporting actions. Occasionally I add it to a vermifuge blend. I have never prescribed it for its oestrone content, so cannot report first-hand on that.

Historical applications
The 'Apple' that played such a leading role in the Adam and Eve story was, most likely, actually a Pomegranate. It has been a potent symbol of fertility and abundance since the earliest times, especially in the Jewish tradition. It represented the future in the Temple of Solomon, and it featured in ancient Egyptian tomb paintings. The Pomegranate found its way to China in 126 BC and was immediately adopted as a popular item at festivals and celebrations due to its auspicious bright red colour.

Magical
Pomegranate is associated with wealth, luck, protection, and fertility. It is known as 'Love Apple'. This may at first seem like a fruitful

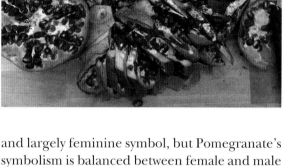

and largely feminine symbol, but Pomegranate's symbolism is balanced between female and male aspects. Take a look at the bud before it opens: you will see the form of a penis.

Pomegranate is also associated with divination and making wishes. It is said that if you carry the seeds or the skin with you, it will increase fertility and wealth. Since it can manifest wishes, it is a good idea to always make a wish before eating one. Traditionally, there is a special type of fertility divination associated with Pomegranate. If a woman throws a Pomegranate hard onto the ground, it is said that the number of seeds that fall out show the number of children she will have. Branches of Pomegranate hung over doorways also guard against evil, and the juice can be used as magical ink.

Suggestion for the home apothecary
Sendru Dangné Tincture for digestive support

You will need:
- » *8 parts dried Pomegranate*
- » *1 part Long Pepper*
- » *1 part Cinnamon Bark*
- » *2 parts Cardamom pods*
- » *4 parts Saffron*

Pound the ingredients in a pestle and mortar to break them into smaller pieces. It is a good idea at this point to repeat mantras or do positive visualisations – whatever feels right within your own spiritual tradition. If you are feeling unwell or negative, please make this tincture on another, more positive day. Add the herbs to a jar and cover completely with 45% ABV alcohol. Place in a cool, dark place for at least 4 weeks before straining, pressing, and bottling.

Take 5 ml daily in hot water if you feel that your digestion needs support and that you have been lacking in vibrancy and motivation.

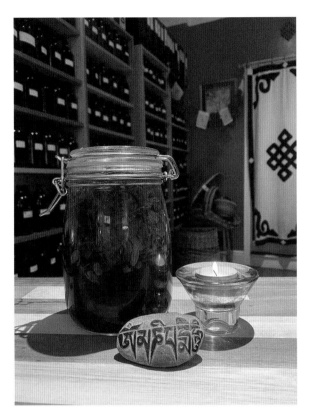

Poplar 🍃 *Populus x gileadensis / Populus x candicans / Populus tremuloides*

'Poplar helps us to breathe freely and let go of fear.'

Here in the United Kingdom, we have *Populus x gileadensis* – or *P. x candicans*, which is the same species. It is planted as an ornamental and is known as 'Balm of Gilead'. This can lead to some confusion if you are relying only on the common name, as other completely unrelated plants are also known as Balm of Gilead. Here is a good reminder to always be aware of Latin nomenclature. Those who live in the United States may have access to Cottonwood, a native Poplar with very large, fragrant, medicinal, sticky buds. Aspen, *Populus tremuloides*, is also medicinal, but it is the bark that is harvested from this tree.

Poplars love to grow in moist areas. They are high in salicylates, like their damp land fellows, the Willows and Meadowsweet. These damp land, salicylate-containing herbs can be thought of as balancing 'soggy states' in the body. They help to relieve inflammation and resolve stagnation that can be causing pain.

Medicinal parts

- Buds
- Bark
- Leaves (sometimes)

Physiological actions

Summary

- Anti-inflammatory
- Antiseptic
- Expectorant
- Analgesic
- Vulnerary

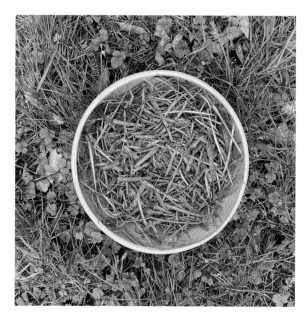

- Febrifuge
- Tonic

Physiological virtues

Balm of Gilead buds have been prescribed for several thousand years to soothe inflamed or irritated skin and to fight infections. They contain chemical constituents that are very similar to propolis. This is not surprising, as the resin secreted by the tree to protect its buds is gathered by bees in order to create propolis. I think that Balm of Gilead or Cottonwood bud resins are good local alternatives to imported resins, such as Myrrh. In a world where we cannot take long-distance supply chains for granted, it is very good to have local alternatives to consider.

Preparations made from the buds can be applied topically to treat cuts and grazes, chapped and itchy skin, sunburn, and chilblains. In the 1970s Soviet doctors had great success in healing bedsores, resistant infections, and post-operative abscesses with topical treatments made from the buds. Extracts of these resinous buds can also be made into suppositories that are excellent for internal haemorrhoids. They make a good massage oil to relieve the pain of rheumatic joints and strained muscles.

The buds have expectorant, antiseptic, and analgesic properties and are a common ingredient in cough mixtures. They are a very good remedy for sore throats, dry irritable coughs, bronchitis, and other respiratory ailments.

The bark is rich in salicylates, so, like the buds, it is pain-relieving, fever reducing, and anti-inflammatory. It was always considered a safe alternative to 'Peruvian Bark' for fever-

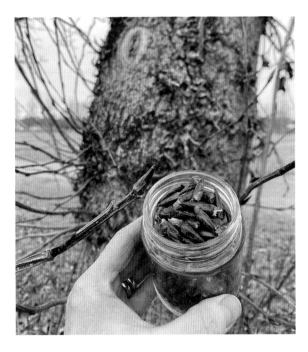

ish states. My dear tutor, Edith Barlow, taught me that Poplar bark is also a valuable general tonic. It stimulates the digestion and supports the urinary and reproductive tracts in both male and female bodies. She used to include Poplar bark in prescriptions for people suffering with urinary-tract, prostate, or menstrual disorders, as well as for those with nervous debility or burnout. It can be a helpful anti-inflammatory astringent in cases of IBS.

Avoid if sensitive to salicylates.

Energetics

On an energetic level, Poplar is associated with moving through fear. It has an affinity with the kidneys – organs that are traditionally associated with processing fear. As human beings, if we are not careful, we can fill our lives with fear. All the 'what ifs' playing through our consciousness can be totally exhausting.

If you look at Poplar in the summer, you can see that its leaves tremble naturally, but this is just a way of dissipating the energy of the wind. Poplar teaches us not to solidify our fears – to be more flexible and accepting. We can try to deal with what actually presents itself to us at the time rather than worrying about all the many things that might happen. Everything may work out just fine. If it does not, we know exactly what we are dealing with, and we can take comfort from knowing that all things will pass.

Dr Edward Bach saw *Populus tremuloides* as a support for people who are seized by sudden fears or worries for no specific reason. They have inexplicable anxiety that may be accompanied by trembling.

Poplar is also strongly associated with community. It spreads by throwing up suckers around the base of the tree and spreading further into surrounding spaces. Poplar stands are actually one large, beautiful, interconnected community. When we are fearful, Poplar reminds us that we are part of something much bigger that can support us through our challenges. No wonder Poplar's medicine is a very good tonic.

In Tibetan medicine

Populus spp. in general is called *Yarpa* [ད་བྱར་པ་]. It has a bitter taste and a post-digestive taste that is also bitter. It has a cooling potency. The medicinal part is the bark. It is considered to restrict the spread of toxicosis in the body, and it treats gout and arthritis.

The species, *Populus davidana*, is known as *Ma gal* [མ་གལ་]. Its bark is considered beneficial for lung diseases and smallpox.

In my dispensary

A tincture of sticky Balm of Gilead Poplar buds, made with high-strength alcohol, results in a dark, resinous, and powerful preparation, with the fragrance and astringency of propolis. A little goes a long way.

My tutor and mentor, Edith, often included the bark of *P. tremuloides* at a low level in prescriptions for people suffering with urinary-tract, prostate, or menstrual disorders, as well as for those with nervous debility or burnout. She said that it was like a tonic that made the medicine work better. It would form perhaps just 5%–10% of a blend. I follow this way of working with it, especially when making capsule blends.

Historical applications

Culpeper referred to the '*Ointment of Populeon*', which Dioscorides described: '*The oyntment called "populeon" which is much of this poplar, is singular for all heat and inflammation in any part of the body and tempereth the heat of wounds. It is much used to dry up the milk in women's breasts.*' It consisted of Poplar buds, Poppy, Blackberry tips, Black nightshade (Henbane), Wild Lettuce, and Violet. The herbs would be infused in lard and applied as needed.

Peasant women in China used to add Poplar buds to butter, which was left to melt in the sun. This oil-based infusion was used to add a sheen to their hair.

The Cottonwood tree is still sacred to many indigenous Americans. Historically it was considered to be a symbol of the sun by the Apache tribes, and northern Mexican tribes associated it with the afterlife, using Cottonwood branches in funeral rites. The Hopi, Pueblo, and Navajo tribes carved ceremonial objects out of Cottonwood roots. Many of the Plains Indian tribes thought of Cottonwood as a medicine tree and chose the trunks and branches for sacred poles and sundance artefacts. The leaves and bark were gathered to treat wounds and swellings, and aqueous extracts were made as an eye-wash. The Objiwa people treated earache with extracts of *Populus tremuloides* bark in bear fat.

Magical

Poplar is associated with manifestation of personal dreams, overcoming personal fears, and enduring hardships. It is also associated with attracting wealth. It is said that if you carry the buds and leaves, you will attract money to you.

Suggestions for the home apothecary

Poplar bud/Cottonwood bud tincture

Place fresh Balm of Gilead or Cottonwood buds into a clean, dry jar. Cover with high-strength alcohol, preferably at least 80% ABV (160% proof). Leave in a cool, dark place for at least 4 weeks, but up to 12 months is fine. Strain and bottle. Dilute at a rate of 5 ml : 25 ml of cooled herbal infusions for mouthwashes or

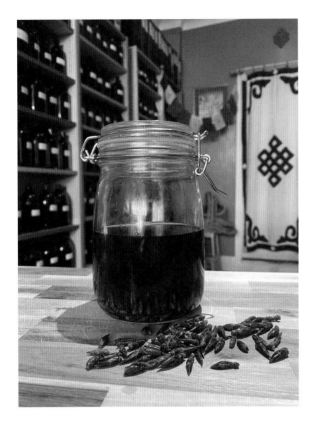

wound-cleaning water, as needed. Apply neat to infected cuts or slow-healing wounds.

If you do not have access to high-strength alcohol, make an infused oil for topical application. Do not take infused oils internally.

Infused Poplar bud oil

Fill a jar about a third full with the buds, and cover with mild olive oil. If working with fresh buds, do not lid tightly, as the moisture will need to escape. Alternatively, open the lid daily and wipe away condensation from the inside. Leave it in a warm place for 6 weeks, then strain, filter, and bottle.

Pot Marigold 🌱 *Calendula officinalis*

'Calendula enlivens the tissues. It brings movement and clarity, clears away debris, and encourages healing.'

I think that Calendula is probably the sunniest of all herbal medicines. It never fails to bring a smile to my face as I reach for it in my herb store. According to the Doctrine of Signatures, the Calendula flower was considered to represent the iris of the eye. Calendula has indeed long been used in physical eye treatments, and traditionally it helps us to see more clearly beyond the earthly realms. To me, the signature of this beautiful herb is all about its ability to bring the enlivening energy of the sun into stagnant areas of the body. The bright fiery oranges, yellows, and magentas of Calendula flowers are like a mass of mini suns that track the passage of the sun through the sky. Sunshine is very healing: it can help to clear up infections and skin disorders as well as lifting the spirits. Its French name, '*soucie*', means 'one who follows the sun', referring to the opening and closing of the flowers with the sun. Calendula flowers close at low light levels or when it rains, and it is said that you can forecast the weather by observing them.

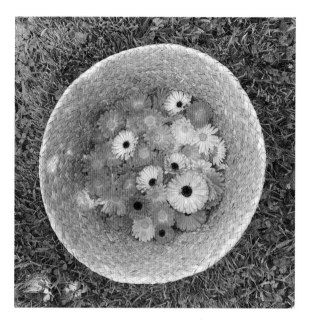

Medicinal parts
  ▷ Flowers

I gather the whole flowers, including the green calyces. To work only with the petals may look very pretty and make a lighter herbal tea, but it is not making the most of its healing properties. Calendula calyces are an important source of medicinal bitter compounds.

Physiological actions
Summary

  ▷ Lymphatic tonic
  ▷ Vulnerary
  ▷ Bitter
  ▷ Anti-inflammatory
  ▷ Diaphoretic
  ▷ Bacteriostatic
  ▷ Antifungal

Physiological virtues

The topical application of Calendula as a wound healer is well known. It is especially indicated for scratches, such as cat scratches, where the edges become raised and red quickly. Calendula quickly reduces inflammation and encourages speedy healing. We need to pause, though, before we categorize Calendula as simply 'being good for wound-healing'. It is a herb that offers far more than that to our bodies.

Calendula enlivens the lymphatic system either when applied topically or when prescribed internally. Beyond direct mucous membrane support, it seems to encourage more efficient movement in the lymphatic vessels in the body as a whole. I see it as thinning the lymph and improving the ability of the vessels to clear away infection and debris. Enhanced movement in the lymphatic vessels helps to encourage better circulation. It is all very well prescribing peripheral circulatory stimulants, but you also need effective lymphatic movement to assist with providing a 'pull' factor to the blood at the very ends of the capillaries. I have noticed that patients with a tendency to cold hands and feet often have more lasting relief when treated with lymphatic tonics like Calendula rather than just with traditional circulatory stimulants like Chilli and Ginger. By encouraging the circulation, Calendula is a good diaphoretic, especially in cases of deep fever.

Calendula's special healing attributes encourage faster healing of wounds and less tendency to form pus or scar tissue. Its ability to bring movement to stagnant areas means that it is an excellent choice for slow-healing ulcers of all kinds – for example, varicose ulcers. Calendula stimulates and restores the venous and capillary circulation and is bacteriostatic, slowing the growth of bacteria rather than being directly antiseptic. In 1880 the homoeopath Dr Richard Hughes pre-empted modern research by saying '*no suppuration seems able to live in its presence*'. It is also an excellent antifungal, and I prescribe it as a topical wash or soak for athlete's foot and other fungal issues.

I always include Calendula in my general healing ointment, along with Comfrey, Agrimony, and Lavender. It is a staple of the first aid cupboard of many of my patients. It is a very good choice for post-partum healing, especially where there has been tearing or epi-

siotomy. I prescribe Calendula in sitz baths for this, but you could also choose a fomentation or a spray.

I add Calendula tincture to my Myrrh-based mouthwash blend, which I find excellent for bleeding gums, tooth infections, or gingivitis. The Calendula brings a gentle soft healing influence to the tissues, and this seems to moderate the power and intense astringency of the Myrrh.

Calendula's mucous membrane support extends to internal use for gastritis, stomach ulcers, and inflammatory states within the digestive tract in general. By including the bitter calyces, you get the beautiful alchemy of an effective mucous membrane healer along with a gentle digestive stimulant, helping to resolve the sluggish digestion that probably contributed to the inflammation in the first place. Calendula's bitterness means that it is a great herb to choose as part of the prescription where you have lymphatic congestion combined with sluggish digestion – for example, when there is a history of tonsillitis or persistent oedema. In these cases I find it is usually helpful to remove dairy from the diet, at least temporarily, until the digestion has had a chance to pick up.

Calendula can be a very good herb in the support of women with menstrual symptoms, such as dysmenorrhea, as it enlivens the pelvic circulation due to its positive influence on the lymphatic system. This means that Calendula can play a positive role in the treatment of menorrhagia and fibroids.

Energetics
In traditional Greek medicine, Calendula is described as '*warm in the first degree*'. It is a diaphoretic and enlivens the body when it is sluggish. Peter Holmes describes it as bitter, sweet, salty and pungent, neutral with a cooling potential, dry, calming, decongesting, astringing, stimulating, softening, dissolving.

In Tibetan medicine

Calendula's name in Tibetan is *Le gan menpa* [ལེ་བཀན་དམན་པ།]. It is also known as *Metok gurgum* [མེ་ཏོག་གུར་གུམ།], which means 'flower Saffron', because it is sometimes chosen as a substitute for Saffron in formulae. Its taste is bitter and a little sweet with a post-digestive taste that is bitter. It has a cooling potency. The *Gyudzhi* teaches us that Calendula helps in joining ruptured channels, heals wounds, and removes abscesses in the lungs.

Think of Calendula for patients with oedema and sluggish circulation, combined with weak digestion – symptoms largely associated with *Pekén* disorders. In these cases, if inflammation arises, it is difficult for the body to resolve it due to stagnation in the lymphatic and circulatory system. Calendula is generally a very good choice, as it helps to resolve 'heat trapped under cold'.

In My Dispensary

I see Calendula primarily as a lymphatic support. Very many patients present with a congested lymphatic system leading to fatigue, foggy thinking, sluggish peripheral circulation, low mood, poor immunity, and slow-healing wounds. They have swollen tongues with tooth indentations and suffer from enlarged cervical glands, benign breast cysts, or infections in areas where there is a concentration of lymphatic tissue, such as the underarms, tonsils, groin, or breasts. This latter observation means that I really resonate with the insight that Calendula is a herb for 'where the sun doesn't shine'. This phrase originally came from Minneapolis-based acupuncturist Chris Hafner and was reported by Matthew Wood in his excellent *Earthwise Herbal* (2008, 2009).

I had a patient – let us call her 'Sara' – who was suffering from 'hidradenitis suppurativa': a so-called incurable skin condition characterized by deep-seated abscesses and boils in the underarm and groin areas – definitely areas where the 'sun doesn't shine'. She had been prescribed long and repeated courses of antibiotics without any lasting relief, and she was very ready for a new, more holistic approach. She needed general digestive and circulatory support, but, alongside that, her case really called for Calendula. She bathed the affected areas twice daily with a combination of Myrrh and Calendula tinctures in a wash, and I gave her an internal blend that included Calendula. I encouraged her to clean up her diet and to introduce more regular exercise: Calendula will get the lymphatic system moving, but exercise will help it to carry out its work. She worked hard at her new regime and was rewarded by being clear of all lesions within eighteen months – not bad for a condition that had been going on for very many years. She has remained clear of the disease for seven years and is now a firm advocate of herbal medicine. I am sure that Calendula played an enormous part in this transformation.

Another patient, 'Melissa', presented with very long-standing chronic fatigue, multiple

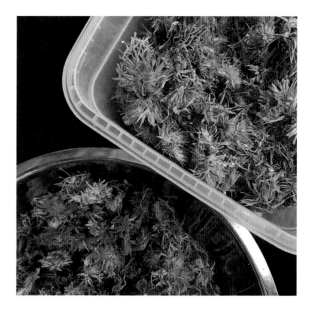

digestive issues, repeated respiratory infections, and low mood. I started by supporting her digestion and strengthening her immune system. She made steady improvement in energy levels and digestive power, but in the beginning there were repeated acute infections that diverted treatment away from the underlying key issues. It felt like two steps forward and one back, but over time her symptoms reduced, and her acute illnesses happened much further apart. I began to see more clearly what was going on and realized that what she really needed was Calendula alongside more warming foods and behaviour patterns. Calendula would counteract her lymphatic congestion and her tendency to 'sogginess', as well as bringing much-needed sunshine into her system, as she always experienced a real dip in mood during the winter months. Add to that the persistent raised cervical glands under her chin, lymph nodes 'where the sun doesn't shine', and her poor peripheral circulation, and there was no doubt that Calendula was the herb for her. I prescribed it on its own as a tea, and the transformation was immediate and huge. She felt a significant increase in energy and a welcome uplift in mood. Her persistently puffy fingers shrank, and she felt slimmer and more herself. I have always given myself a hard time over not spotting this sooner.

Overall Calendula brings sunshine and clarity. People with clogged lymphatic systems often reflect inner stagnation in their external environment and find themselves living in clutter. They may hate the clutter but feel helpless and lack the energy and will to start to tackle it. I have lost count of the number of patients who report that they suddenly experience a huge urge to declutter when they start taking Calendula. As well as feeling much better in themselves, they end up living in tidy and organized surroundings, which, in turn, makes them feel even better.

Historical applications

In early Indian and Arabic cultures, Calendula flowers were considered to be a protective talisman, as well as medicine, food, dye, and an ingredient for cosmetics. In ancient Greece and Rome, Calendulas were also popular for their protective and healing properties.

The original Anglo-Saxon name for Calendula was '*marso-mear-gealla*' – that is, the Marsh Marigold. In the Middle Ages the flowers were dedicated to the Virgin Mary; the name 'Marigold' is said to be derived from Mary's Gold. The name Calendula comes from the Roman word '*kalends*': it is said to be in bloom on the first of every month throughout the year. Gerard wrote: '*It is to be seen in floure in the Calends almost of everie moneth.*'

In his eleventh-century herbal, *Floridus De viribus Herbarum*, Macer recommended that simply looking at a Calendula plant will '*improve eyesight, clear the head and encourage cheerfulness*'. King Henry VIII, a keen amateur herbalist, believed that Calendula could combat the plague.

Culpeper extolled the virtues of Marigold for measles: '*Marigolds are very expulsive and little less effective in smallpox and measles than saffron.*' Calendula is still known as 'measles wort' in some areas. It was cultivated in kitchen gardens, and the flowers were added as a tonic to winter stews and soups, which were known as 'pottage', hence its common name of 'Pot Marigold'.

According to Maud Grieve, Fuller wrote: '*We know the many and sovereign virtues in your leaves, the Herbe Generalle in all pottage*' (*Antheologie*, 1655).

In 1658, Coles wrote: '*The distilled water helpeth red and watery eyes.*'

Charles Stevens, in *L' agriculture et maison rustique* (1580), mentions the Marigold as a specific for headache, jaundice, red eyes, toothache, and ague. The dried flowers are still used among the peasantry '*to strengthen and comfort the hart*' (from Maud Grieve).

In the nineteenth century the Shakers, who traded on a very large scale in herbs and herbal remedies, promoted Calendula as an effective treatment for gangrene. Dr William J. Clary, of Monroeville, Ohio, wrote in 1854: '*As a local remedy after surgical operations, it has no equal in Materia Medica. Its forte is in its influence on lacerated wounds, without regard to the general health of the patient, or the weather. If applied constantly, gangrene will not follow, and I might say there will be but little, if any, danger of tetanus. When applied to a wound. it is seldom that any suppuration follows, the wound healing by replacement or first intention. It has been tested by several practitioners, and by one, it is used after every surgical operation with the happiest effect. You need not fear to use it in wounds, and I would not be without it for a hundred times its cost.*'

During the Second World War large quanti-

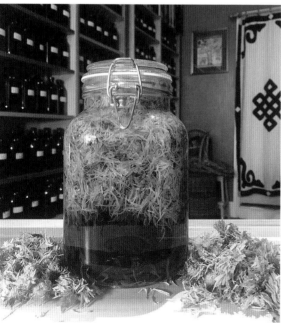

ties of Calendula flowers were gathered and sent to hospitals for their wound-healing and anti-infective properties.

Magical

Many sources refer to Calendula's ability to help us see more clearly. Scattered under the bed, they give rise to prophetic dreams. It is said that if one has been robbed, Calendula will send a dream that will reveal the identity of the thief. Carrying Calendula flowers in one's pocket while attending court was considered to help bring favourable justice. If a girl touched the petals with her bare feet, she would understand the language of birds. Garlands of Marigolds were traditionally strung on door posts to stop evil from entering the house.

Suggestions for the home apothecary

Calendula footbath for athlete's foot

Make a strong infusion of Calendula, and soak the feet in it daily for 20 minutes while it is still warm. I once suggested this to a nurse who had been plagued with persistent athlete's foot for several years despite trying many allopathic treatments. A couple of weeks later she said to me that in ten days Calendula had done what conventional medicine had failed to do in the past three years.

Calendula tincture as a lymphatic support

Loosely fill a jar with dried whole Calendula flowers, and fill to the top with 25% ABV alcohol. Leave to macerate for 4 weeks in a cool, dark place before straining, pressing, and bottling. If there is lymphatic congestion, avoid mucus-forming foods (especially dairy), and take 5 ml in hot water daily. Please note, if making this with fresh flowers, you will need a higher ABV alcohol percentage (probably 50%), otherwise it may not keep at room temperature.

Pulsatilla 🌿 *Anemone pulsatilla*

'Pulsatilla relaxes tension in sensitive nerve-rich areas.'

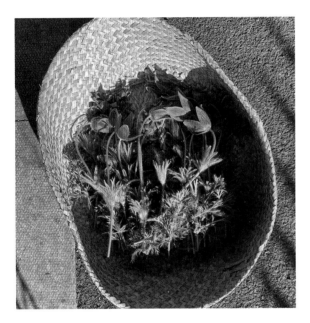

Pulsatilla is known as 'Pasqueflower' because it flowers around Easter-time and was traditionally used to colour Easter eggs. It is a relaxing nervine especially indicated for tension in the reproductive system or other sensitive areas, such as the ears. It is specific to those conditions where mental worry or repetitive thought patterns are playing an aggravating role in the manifestation of the symptoms. Consider Pulsatilla for very sensitive folks prone to nervous depression.

Medicinal parts

  ▷ Aerial parts

Aerial parts are gathered when the plant is flowering. I was taught that Pulsatilla should be dried before being prepared as a medicine, as the fresh plant contains caustic compounds that can cause burning and blistering of the skin and mucous membranes. This applies to both topical and internal prescribing.

Physiological actions

Summary

  ▷ Nervine
  ▷ Antispasmodic
  ▷ Antimicrobial

Physiological virtues

Pulsatilla is a nervine herb with particular application to pain in the reproductive tract, such as ovarian pain or pain in the testes. It can be very helpful for neuralgia in other areas too, such as shooting pains in the face and head, earache or toothache. It can be applied as an infused oil for earache.

It is antispasmodic. Maud Grieve describes administering Pulsatilla tincture at a dose of 2–3 drops in a spoonful of water to allay the spasmodic cough of asthma, whooping cough, and bronchitis. She also considers it helpful for catarrhal conditions of the eyes.

Pulsatilla is also antimicrobial and is excellent to resolve boils. I prescribe it internally within an individually formulated blend or infuse it in oil with Echinacea flowers for topical application in these circumstances.

Energetics

Pulsatilla is bitter, hot, and astringent, cooling and heating. Energetically, it is the best herb to consider where there is tension linked in some way to the reproductive process, stress over trying to conceive, regret over deciding not to have children, stress arising from difficulties in mothering or being mothered. All sorts of situations call for a little Pulsatilla, and it is especially good for sensitive people who are prone to tearfulness and who take on other people's troubles as well as their own.

In Tibetan medicine

Pulsatilla is known as *Chee mong* [དྲེ་མོང་]. It stops tissue deterioration and generates digestive heat while drawing out serous fluid.

In my dispensary

In my clinic I work with Pulsatilla mostly in tincture form, adding it to individual tincture blends as required. The following is a case where Pulsatilla was well indicated.

'Janice' was a single mum in her 30s who worked very hard to juggle a full-time job with being a fun and engaged mum to her 8-year-old daughter. She had a persistent and painful pilonidal cyst and wanted to try a natural approach rather than immediately opting for the surgery that was being offered. Her circulation and elimination needed support, so I prescribed a tailor-made herbal mix to support her. I decided to include Pulsatilla because it was indicated twice: once for the cyst and once for the tension around being a great mum while managing to work full-time. Janice also had a topical lotion based on Myrrh and Calendula. This approach resulted in complete healing of the cyst within a period of five months and no surgery being necessary. Of course, I cannot say categorically how much influence the Pulsatilla had in the prescription, but my feeling is that it played a valuable role within the formula.

Historical applications

According to Greek legend, Pulsatilla sprang from the tears of Venus. Dioscorides mentions it as a herb to consider for ophthalmia, and this advice is also echoed by Culpeper and Gerard.

Gerard wrote that '*All the kinds of Anemones are sharp, biting the tongue, and of a binding facultie.*'

Magical

Tradition has it that if you gather the blossoms in the spring, wrap them in a red cloth, and wear or carry them, they will prevent disease.

Suggestion for the home apothecary

Pulsatilla ear oil

Dry your Pulsatilla thoroughly, cut it into small pieces, and place it into a clean, dry jar. Cover with mild olive oil. Leave for 4 weeks, then strain and bottle. Apply 3 drops into the ear.

Please note: Fresh plant material is not suitable.

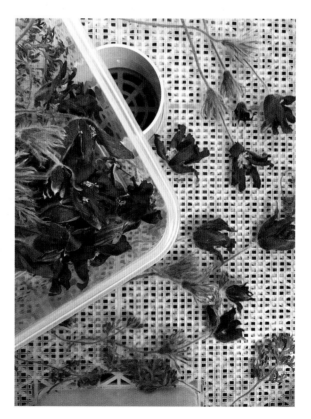

Raspberry 🍂 *Rubus idaeus*

'Raspberry is much more than just a uterine toner and strengthener.'

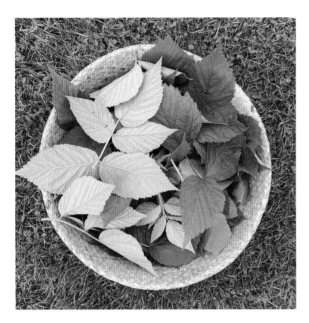

Raspberry's Latin name means 'The Bramble of Mount Ida', where it was abundant; Gerard calls it Hindberry, a derivation of the Saxon name 'Hindbeer'. Raspberry leaf is generally known as a herb for women's issues. If you look at the leaf, you will see that the undersides of the leaves are very pale; this helps to distinguish the plant from its close relative, the Blackberry. On a moonlit night you will notice that Wild Raspberry seems to glow, compared to the surrounding vegetation. You could rationalize this and say that this is entirely due to the pale undersides to the leaves, but I cannot help having more fanciful notions to do with the Moon, Venus, and the Doctrine of Signatures. However, do not fall into the trap of categorizing this as a herb just for women and for pregnancy. It is an excellent all-round anti-inflammatory and astringent and is a specific for prostate inflammation.

Medicinal parts

Western herbal medicine

- ▷ Leaves
- ▷ Fruit

Tibetan medicine

- ▷ Inner bark

Physiological actions

Summary

- ▷ Astringent
- ▷ Anti-inflammatory
- ▷ Antispasmodic
- ▷ Uterine tonic
- ▷ Galactagogue
- ▷ Diuretic
- ▷ Prostate tonic
- ▷ Vulnerary

Physiological virtues

Raspberry leaf is widely known as a herb to take during pregnancy in order to tone and relax the uterus. It is rich in iron, astringent, and gently antispasmodic. Taking the infusion (one cup a day) during the final trimester helps to strengthen the efficiency of contractions during labour and reduce haemorrhage. Raspberry leaf's iron content makes it a valuable tonic, and its antispasmodic properties reduce the tendency to spasm as well as lessening general tension. Some sources specifically advise avoiding Raspberry leaf in early pregnancy, as it could stimulate the uterus. Raspberry leaf is a gentle galactagogue, so if you continue to drink the tea after the birth, it will help to encourage milk production and reduce the severity of after-pains.

Raspberry leaf's astringency is also very useful to help reduce excessive menstrual bleeding. This is probably the reason I most prescribe Raspberry leaf in my clinic. I combine it with other herbs depending on the individual circumstances of the case, and it plays its part very well. It is not just for women, though. It is a gentle cleansing diuretic, and in France it is considered an excellent tonic for the prostate gland.

Raspberry leaf is a really good, easily accessible first aid herb. For the digestive system, its astringency can help to ease diarrhoea or soothe inflammation, while the fruit is a gentle laxative. Another valuable first aid application is for sore throats. I am a big fan of prescribing Raspberry leaf to reduce pain and inflammation in the throat. Just sipping the tea, gargling with it, or taking the tincture will bring almost instant relief, even in tonsillitis. This property has saved the day more than once for patients who are professional singers and, closer to home, when my children were in the village pantomime and needed to sing their hearts out several nights in a row. You can also make a vinegar with the fresh fruit for the same purpose.

Topically applied, the cooled infusion can be helpful for wounds, varicose ulcers, and sores. Also consider it for sitz baths, applied intravaginally, or in a steam for excessive discharge. It makes a good soothing eye wash, too.

Energetics

Raspberry is astringent. As a strengthener of tissues, Raspberry leaf is one of the herbs associated with promoting healthy boundaries. See the magical section for how this translates into a protective role.

In Tibetan medicine

Raspberry is known as *Gadra* [ག་ཟྲ]; the inner bark is called *Kandakari* [ཀནྡ་ཀ་རི]. It has a sweet-to-astringent taste, with a sweet post-digestive taste and a heavy, cool, and oily potency. It restores the body to a healthy state and is good for treating *rLung* fever, cold, unripe infectious fever, cough, and lung diseases. It is one of the ingredients in *Manu Zhi Thang*.

In my dispensary

As well as prescribing Raspberry leaf for sore throats, I most often include it in tincture blends for women experiencing menorrhagia. I also like to prescribe it in infusions blended with Marshmallow leaf and Peppermint to ease the discomfort of diverticulitis. In these cases, it is essential that dietary changes are implemented, so that the root cause of the problem is addressed, but Raspberry leaf is a valuable anti-inflammatory to support the patient while changes are being made.

Historical applications

Gerard felt that Raspberry fruit was of '*temperate heat*' and more easily digested than Strawberries. He wrote: '*The fruit is good to be given to those that have weake and queasie stomackes.*'

In 1735, the Irish herbalist John K'Eogh wrote that '*an application of the flowers bruised with honey is beneficial for inflammations of the eyes, burning fever and boils. The fruit is good for the heart and diseases of the mouth*'.

Raspberry leaf's effectiveness at promoting relaxation of the uterus and allowing a smoother birth experience has become accepted to some extent within allopathic circles. In the 1940s Dr Violet Russell wrote that '*Somewhat shamefacedly and surreptitiously I have encouraged any expectant mothers, who felt so inclined, to drink this infusion. . . . In a good many cases in my own experience*

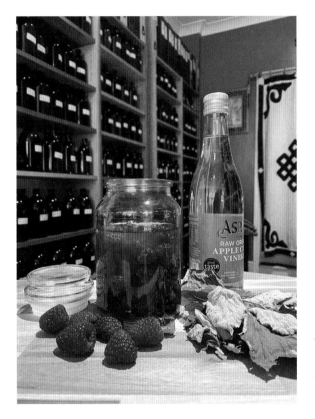

the subsequent labour has been easy and free from muscular spasm. . . . More labours are held up by muscular tension than are delayed by muscular weakness.'

Magical

Raspberry is associated with protection. Branches of Raspberry were hung above the doors for general protection or to prevent a recently departed spirit from re-entering the house.

Suggestion for the home apothecary

Raspberry vinegar

This is a great recipe for sore throats and coughs. Steep 250 g fruit in 500 ml of vinegar for 2 weeks, then strain. Add a couple of teaspoons to a cup of hot water, and sip when needed. You can add infused Poplar bud or Elecampane honey to this, if you like. Alternatively, blend it with other less pleasant-tasting cough blends, or dilute with 2 parts water and take as a gargle.

Red Clover 🍃 *Trifolium pratense*

'Red Clover is an alterative with lymphatic, antispasmodic, and antitussive virtues.'

Red Clover is primarily an alterative. I know that many people think of it as a herb to choose for its oestrogenic properties, especially to help reduce menopausal symptoms, but if I am honest, this has never sat comfortably with me. It feels as though we are turning to herbs in a rather allopathic way when we do this. I have helped a great many women feel well again after being plagued by distressing menopausal symptoms, and I am pretty sure that the vast majority of mixes that I have prescribed in these cases did not contain Red Clover. I know that many women swear by Red Clover, and I do not want to dismiss their experience, but I do wonder whether a large part of its action is through its ability to help clean the blood and support the lymphatic system rather than just to manipulate levels of oestrogen, or the appearance of oestrogen, in the body.

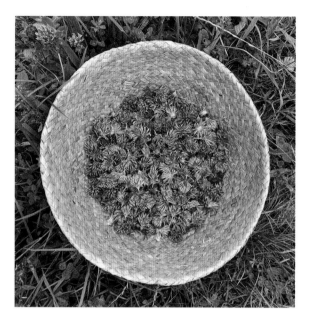

Medicinal parts
 ▷ Flowers
 ▷ First leaflets

Physiological actions

Summary
 ▷ Alterative
 ▷ Lymphatic tonic
 ▷ Antispasmodic
 ▷ Oestrogenic

Physiological virtues

Red Clover was first introduced to the British Isles in the mid-seventeenth century as a soil-improving crop. Later on, it was discovered to have oestrogenic properties when sheep grazing on pure Clover swards were much less fertile than expected. Nowadays, it is a very popular over-the-counter menopause-supporting herb and is widely considered to be helpful in supporting healthy bone density due to its phytoestrogens.

Traditionally, though, it is a blood cleaner and a lymphatic tonic. It has antispasmodic properties that are helpful for those suffering from bronchial ailments or spasmodic coughs such as whooping cough (pertussis).

As an alterative, it is very helpful in all sorts of skin conditions including acne, eczema, and psoriasis. It is an excellent lymphatic tonic and can be helpful in resolving benign cysts of the breasts or premenstrual breast tenderness. There is a long tradition of applying fomentations, poultices, and pastes made with Red Clover in order to shrink cancerous growths.

A Red Clover compress can be helpful in cases of arthritic pain and gout. It makes a good eye wash for conjunctivitis. Add 5–10 drops of the tincture to an eye bath full of cooled boiled water.

Energetics
Red Clover is bitter, sweet, and astringent.

In my dispensary
In my clinic I see Red Clover mostly as a lymphatic system support and an expectorant that calms coughs. This wonderful cleansing herb also plays a very useful role in clearing skin conditions.

Historical applications
Gerard described this herb as a '*three-leaved grasse*' or meadow trefoil.

In their *King's American Dispensatory* (1905), Lloyd and Felter described it as '*an excellent*

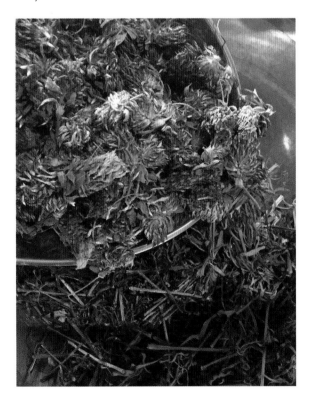

internal agent for those individuals disposed to tibial and other forms of ulcers', which can no doubt be attributed to Red Clover's alterative and lymphatic actions. They also wrote that it is one of the few herbs that favourably influence pertussis. A strong infusion of the plant is said to suspend a spasmodic cough for 2–3 days. This was edited in later editions to say that it is not always effective but that it does, however, help other spasmodic coughs, including those associated with measles and bronchitis.

Magical
Red Clover is associated with protection, success, money, love, and fidelity. It was employed in exorcisms due to its three-lobed-leaf shape, which was considered to represent the Holy Trinity. This is why the three-leaved Clover is worn as a protective amulet, and the infusion is sprinkled around the house to remove negative spirits.

Red Clover has the reputation of helping financial dealings to go well. The way to benefit from this is to add Red Clover to your bath. This brings to mind the term being 'in clover', which implies being wealthy and having abundance in all areas of one's life. It is also worth knowing that, worn over the right breast, it brings success in all undertakings. A four-leafed Clover is a well-known good luck charm.

Suggestion for the home apothecary
Herbal tea for skin cleansing and premenstrual breast tenderness

Take a small handful of the blossom and infuse covered in hot water for 10 minutes before drinking. You could also add some Cleavers or a Calendula flower head for added lymphatic support. If you dry the herbs, you will have access to them year-round.

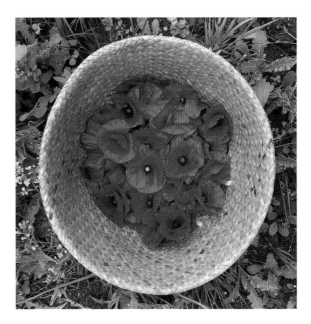
'Poppies help us to embrace the present moment.'

Beautiful, ephemeral Red Poppies are associated with mid-summer. They grow on disturbed ground and create huge swathes of red across the landscape when conditions and the seed bank allow. They are forever associated with death, loss, and remembrance, as well as with hopes for peace. For me, Poppies symbolize impermanence. The fleeting nature of their flowers and their very brief season reminds us that we need to live in the moment and make the most of what life offers us. Poppy can help us to let go of hopes for the future and regrets about the past and let us drift into a peaceful sleep, waking refreshed in the morning with a new perspective on life. In the language of flowers, Red Poppy represents remembrance and moral integrity.

Medicinal parts

- Flowers
- Petals

The seeds are a culinary ingredient: use whole or crushed for oil.

Physiological actions

Summary

- Sedative
- Hypnotic
- Antitussive
- Anodyne

Physiological virtues

Red Poppy has long been prescribed as a mild sedative, sleep aid, and gentle cough remedy. It is much gentler than its cousin, the Opium Poppy. It does not ask us to let go of this world completely when we are under its gentle influence. It just helps us to relax enough to sleep more deeply. Red Poppies do smell of Opium when fresh, but the narcotic odour disappears when they are dried.

Officially, the flowers are described as being anodyne, emollient, emmenagogue, expectorant, hypnotic, slightly narcotic, and sedative. Red Poppy can help to calm over-activity in children, and its relaxing influence can also be helpful for nervous digestive disorders. It was traditionally prescribed in the treatment of jaundice.

The petals (or whole flowers) should be harvested on a dry day as the flowers open. They can be dried for later use in infusions or as a decorative ingredient in pot pourri. Alternatively, you can infuse them fresh if your need is immediate. The main medicinal constituent of the fresh flowers is the red colouring matter, which consists of slightly sedative rhoeadic and papaveric acids. This red colour is darkened when in contact with alkalis. The seed pods contain latex, which is narcotic and slightly sedative. It can be taken in very small quantities, and under expert supervision, to help induce restful sleep. The leaves and seeds are tonic, said to be useful in the treatment of low fevers.

Energetics
Red Poppies are bitter. They remind us of impermanence and to appreciate the present moment.

In Tibetan medicine
Although Blue Poppies (*Meconopsis* genus) are perhaps the most famous herb in the Tibetan pharmacopoeia, the genus Papaver is also prescribed medicinally. *Papaver rhoeas* is known as *Tsun pa metok* [བཙུན་པ་མེ་ཏོག] or *Gyamen* [རྒྱ་མེན]. It is considered to have a sweet-to-astringent taste and a sweet post-digestive taste. Its potency is cooling. It is beneficial for disturbed blood and

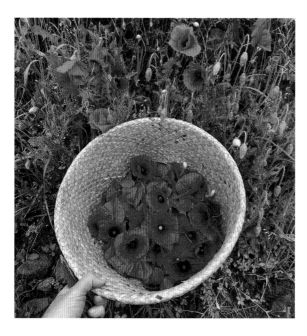

all types of pain in the body, especially back pain.

Another Poppy species in the Tibetan pharmacopoeia is *Papaver nudicaule* (Iceland Poppy); its Tibetan name is *Metok Sair Chen,* which means 'Large gold flower'. It has a bitter taste, with a cool, light, rough, and slow-acting potency. The leaves, stems, flowers, and fruit are the medicinal parts gathered. It is considered to heal wounds and to restore blood vessels after they have been damaged.

Historical applications
The *Bald's Leechbook* suggests that applying Poppy ointment to the temples will relieve sleeplessness.

Gerard was sceptical about Red Poppy: '*Most men being led rather by false experiments than reason, commend the floures against the Pleurisie, giving it to drinke as soon as the pain comes, either the distilled water, or syrup made by often infusing the leaves. And yet many times it happens, that the paine ceaseth by that meanes, though hardly sometimes.*'

Parkinson said: '*The wild or red Poppy that groweth in the corne, while it is young, is a Sallet herbe in Italy, in many places, and in the territory of Trent especially, as Matthiolus saith, as also to prevent the falling sicknesse which Theophrastus also saith in his 9. Booke and 13. Chapter, was common in his time.*'

He also said that '*the Syrupe made of the flowers is with good effect, given to those that have Plurisie*', and the dried flowers '*boyled in water and drunke*' were prescribed for headaches and chest pains. He described it as being more cooling than any other Poppy and recommended it for '*hot agues, frensies and other inflammations, either inward or outward*'.

Magical
Poppy seed heads were gilded and worn as talismans in order to draw wealth to the wearer.

If you wish to know the answer to a question, write it in blue ink on a piece of white paper and insert it into a Poppy seed head. Place this beneath your pillow, and the answer to your question will appear in a dream. Eating the seeds is said to promote fertility and attract love and money.

Suggestion for the home apothecary

Fresh Poppy tincture

Pack a jar with flowers picked on a dry day. Pour over 50% ABV alcohol (this is 100% proof if you are using vodka and you work with the 'proof' system in your country), ensuring they are properly submerged. Leave in a cool, dark place for 4 weeks, then strain and bottle.

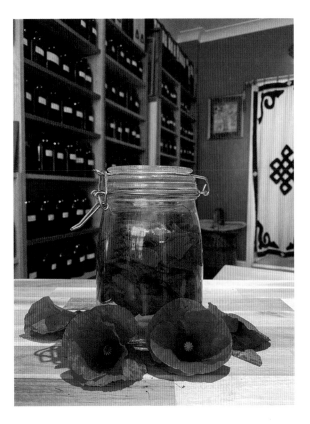

Rose 🖤 *Rosa* spp.

'Rose opens the heart.'

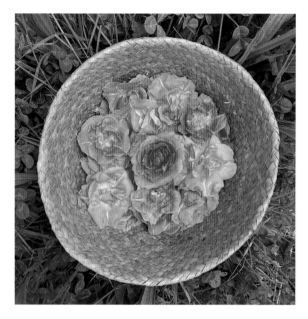

Rose is most is most often thought of as being associated with beauty products, yet it is not just a herb for superficial purposes, it can go deep. When I think of Rose, I see it as a relaxing and supportive herb with a special affinity to the heart. It is a valuable herbal medicine in its own right, a medicine that helps us release long-held trauma or grief.

The Rose species, *Rosa* spp., includes, among others, *Rosa canina*, *Rosa rugosa*, and *Rosa gallica*.

Medicinal parts
- Flowers
- Petals
- Hips

Physiological actions
Summary
- Nervine
- Relaxant
- Astringent
- Anti-inflammatory
- Bitter
- Antidepressant
- Aphrodisiac
- Antibacterial
- Antiseptic
- Antiviral
- Vulnerary

Physiological virtues

In considering the action of the flowers, Culpeper says that Rose strengthens the heart and '*stomach*'. The phrase '*Rose strengthens the heart*' is very succinct, but here we are talking about many different levels of action. On the deepest level, Rose is a medicine that helps us to release trauma or grief that we have not been able to digest fully. When our very being has been rocked by intense experiences of trauma or loss, it can feel as though the intensity of what we have experienced is trapped in our physical body, especially in our heart area. It feels as though, even though we may be mentally able to understand that it is time to let go of the trauma, our body simply cannot release it. The trauma is held tight and woven into the fabric of our being. Sometimes it pops up unasked, as in cases of the flashbacks of PTSD or rushes of anxiety in anxiety disorders, but when this happens, it can feel too painful and too difficult to deal with the underlying trigger. If we have experienced deep grief or trauma, we cannot just deal with it on an intellectual level. We need to actually release it from our body. This is where Rose comes in.

I think of Rose as holding our hand while we begin to face the things that we have shut away inside, pushing them down while we get on with our life. Rose is absolutely wonderful for 'broken hearts', loss, grief, bereavement, trauma – from violent situations, conflict, serious accidents, or, sadly perhaps most commonly encountered among patients, sexual abuse.

Sometimes we can mentally process our grief or trauma and feel that we have reached a state of real acceptance, yet still the physical effects linger on. We may develop unexplained cardiovascular symptoms – often hypertension that seems to be considered 'an accepted part of aging'. In these cases, Rose can help to gently encourage the body to 'catch up' with the mind.

It might surprise you to think that we can be greatly affected by the experiences we hold in our bodies. Yet we can all relate to the ill effects of chronically stiff shoulders or a habitually tight neck. It should not be such a crazy idea that the smooth functioning of our body and circulation is intricately influenced by patterns of tension that we hold.

The influence of tension held within our bodies may not show up as dramatic or life-threatening conditions and is therefore easily disregarded as being a causative factor for health conditions that arise after several years of consistent imbalance. Yet, I have to say that again and again I have seen how the body functions better and in a more balanced way when the patients reach a new level of 'ease' with themselves and with the experiences that have brought them to this point in their lives.

Rose provides physical support to our bodies as well as emotional support. The petals are astringent and cooling, and their cooling nature can be helpful to enliven the liver if it has become a bit stagnant. This particular virtue of Rose means that it can be a good antidepressant and can assist in regulating menstrual periods that have become disrupted. It is also an aphrodisiac. Its astringency tones the digestive tract, reducing inflammation, easing diarrhoea, and encouraging the appetite if this has been lost or diminished. It is a kidney tonic and a blood tonic as well as being gently sedative and relaxing.

As a topical treatment, Rose is antibacterial, antiviral, and antiseptic and is a good toner and wound healer. *Rosa canina*, the Dog Rose, is so named because in mediaeval times it had the reputation of being able to cure the bite of a mad dog.

Rose leaves are medicinal and can be applied as a poultice to wounds. The young leaves make a good infusion as a mild laxative. Older leaves and long steeping times will bring out more astringency and are likely to have the opposite effect.

The hips are also a valuable medicine, high in Vitamin C. In fact, they contain more than twenty times more Vitamin C than Oranges, which have been shipped long distances before they reach our fruit bowls. They are popular as a supplement taken to ease the inflammation of arthritis and are traditionally made into syrups and vinegars to support a healthy immune system during the winter. Take care to remove the tiny irritant hairs in the centre of each hip if you are processing them for food or ingested medicine.

Energetics

Rose is sweet, bitter, and astringent. Rose petals are a gentle heart opener, encouraging the body to release deeply distressing experiences that could not be 'digested' at the time they occurred and so have been shut away in the heart area. Shutting distress and trauma away in the body may be the only way that we are able to carry on with life's responsibilities following intense and distressing events. Once it has been shut away, it can be very daunting to contemplate facing what has been buried. Rose can help with this process, slowly, gently, and beautifully. Its action on the heart allows it to begin to loosen its grip on hidden experiences, and its action in supporting our livers and digestion helps us to better digest the emotions as they arise.

Bach associates Rose with resignation and apathy, a situation that results in an unwillingness to change. I would agree that Rose encourages us to let go of what is holding us back, but I would not call it apathy: I would describe it as self-defence.

In Tibetan medicine

In Tibetan, Rose is called *Sé wi metok* [སེ་བའི་མེ་ཏོག]. Its taste is sweet and bitter, and it has a sweet-to-sour post-digestive taste. Its potency is heavy, cool, and smooth. It is said to cure *Tripa* and to fight *rLung* diseases. It is beneficial for headaches and dizziness caused by *Tripa* and *rLung* flare-ups. It is also prescribed for certain channel and respiratory ailments. Rose hips are considered to help clear up eye disorders and increase bodily strength.

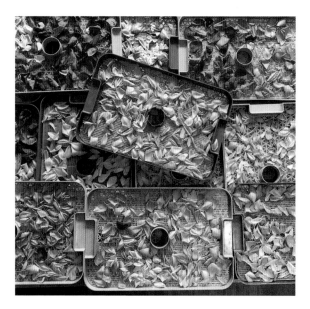

In my dispensary

I often reach for Rose tincture to add to prescription blends in my dispensary. I usually choose Rose tincture for those who need its special emotional support after experiencing grief, heartbreak, or trauma. I also sometimes prescribe it for patients who need to get back in touch with their softer and more feminine side, regardless of their biological gender.

I especially like to prescribe capsules made of equal parts of Rose petals and Hawthorn blossom. These assist with opening up the heart area and releasing chronic tension that has been held there for a long time. If the trauma is deeply buried and very significant, be careful to start gently. I feel that the capsules – usually two a day, but in very sensitive cases only one – are best saved for once a certain amount of time, perhaps a few years, has passed since the triggering incident. As the capsules gently start to relax the tension in the heart area, patients may experience more vivid dreams than usual and find that the events surrounding the incident begin to offer themselves up into the conscious mind for consideration. When this happens – although it does not always work like this – patients usually find that they are able to view the experience in a more constructive and detached way. They report that they feel differently about things, somehow understanding the role the trauma has played in shaping their attitudes but knowing that it does not define them. When a traumatic incident happened very recently, we need to try to work through the shock that has engulfed us. If we need herbal support to cope with day-to-day functioning, we will probably need nervine herbs, which are a bit stronger in action than Rose. Having said that, the occasional cup of Rose petal tea can help to bring some relief to that gnawing physical ache that is felt in the heart area after a bereavement or trauma. I feel that at this point I should say that holistic herbal medicine is never intended to 'heal' bereavement – that is not possible or desirable. Bereavement is a natural process that we have to go through in our own way. However, herbal medicine, and Rose in particular, can really support the process and make it a little easier to bear.

The following case is an example of where Rose can help us to better process an 'older bereavement' that we may have thought had been fully digested. 'Cassie' was 40 years old; she suffered with a long-standing tendency to slow-healing boils around her jaw line, and she was experiencing some digestive bloating. She mentioned that she had experienced two very traumatic close bereavements ten years previously but felt that she had processed the grief and was getting on with her life. Her skin issue called for Calendula, with its specificity for states of lymphatic congestion in areas 'where the sun doesn't shine' and for its gentle digestive support, so I created a tailor-made blend with Calendula as the lead herb, alongside Cleavers and a few others. I also included some double-infused Rose tincture, partly because it is such a good gentle digestive support, but also because I felt that perhaps she had not been fully able to digest her grief. People with poor digestion have a much tougher time processing grief. As well as giving the tincture, I also asked her to take a break from eating both dairy and gluten.

She was a very motivated and determined patient, embracing the dietary changes that I had suggested. After four weeks she reported that her skin and digestion were already much improved. She told me that she was 'feeling really great' and that she realized that she had forgotten that it was possible to feel spontaneously happy. When I heard that feedback, I immediately knew that her experience had been greatly influenced by the Rose in her prescription.

Another patient in a similar situation as regards an 'older bereavement' had Rose in her blend; a couple of months later she told me that she had caught herself spontaneously humming a happy tune – something she had not done for many years.

Historical applications

The medicinal Rose, *Rosa gallica*, comes originally from Iran, where it has been cultivated for at least 3,000 years. The Greek poet, Sappho, who lived in the sixth century BC, famously described the Rose as '*The Queen of Flowers*'. The Arabian physician, Avicenna, distilled Roses to extract the oil and to create fragrant Rose water.

The Romans were very fond of Roses, and it was customary to scatter Rose petals around their homes. It is recorded that Emperor Nero ordered that the fountains of Rome should run with Rose water.

In the Middle Ages, the hips of Dog Rose (*Rosa canina*) were a popular sweetmeat and a popular folk remedy for chest problems. The galls found on the Dog Rose were considered to be a specific herbal remedy for kidney stones, and Rose petals were an esteemed remedy for depression.

Of the flowers, Gerard wrote: '*The conserve of Roses, as well that which is crude and raw, as that which is made by ebullition or boiling, taken in the morning fasting, and last at night, strengtheneth the heart, and taketh away the shaking and trembling thereof, and in a word is the most familiar thing to be used for the purposes aforesaid, and is thus made: Take Roses at your pleasure, put them to boyle in faire water, having regard to the quantity; for if you have many Roses you may take more water; if fewer, the lesse water will serve: the which you shall boyle at least three or foure hours, even as you would boile a piece of meate, until in the eating they be very tender, at which time the Roses will lose their colour, that you would thinke your labour lost, and the thing spoiled. But*

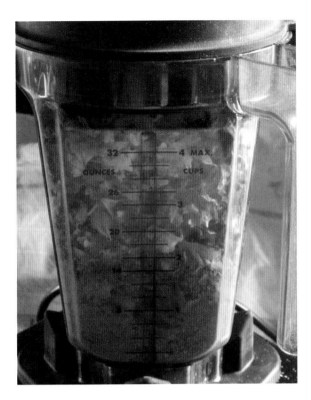

proceed, for though the Roses have lost their colour, the water hath gotten the tincture thereof; then shall you add one pound of Roses, foure pound of fine sugar in pure powder, and so according to the rest of the Roses. Thus shall you let them boyle gently after the sugar is put therto, continually stirring it with a wooden Spatula untill it be cold, whereof one pound weight is worth six pound of the crude or raw conserve, as well for the vertues and goodnesse in taste, as also for the beautifull colour.'

Magical

Rose is typically associated with love. Making beads from Rose hips is said to attract love, and drinking a cup of Rose petal tea before bed can encourage prophetic dreams. There is an old tradition that says that women choosing between three potential suitors can choose the 'right' one by taking three green Rose leaves and assigning one to each man: then the one that stays green the longest is the right one. I am sure this will work for all of those finding themselves choosing between three potential lovers, not just cis women.

Suggestion for the home apothecary

Rose petal honey

Powder carefully dried Rose petals in a Vitamix or a dedicated coffee grinder that is used only for herbal medicines. Sieve the resulting powder so that it is even. Stir the powder into runny honey, aiming for a proportion of around 1 part by volume of Rose powder to 3 parts by volume of honey, but you can vary the proportions according to your own preference. Stir well and leave in the jar to cure. Over the next few weeks, the honey will become much firmer in texture and will be filled with the fragrance of the dried Rose petals. Stir 1 tsp into hot water or add to your herbal tea when you are feeling in need of a concentrated boost of Rose.

'Rosemary enlivens the circulation without heating the system.'

I should not admit to having favourites, but Rosemary (*Salvia rosmarinus*, formerly *Rosmarinus officinalis*) is one of my all-time favourite garden plants. I love that the word '*rosmarinus*' means 'dew of the sea', the name alluding to its preferred habitat of Mediterranean shores.

I am sure that we would all agree that Rosemary's scent is absolutely divine. John Evelyn said that the flowers '*are credibly reported to give their scent above thirty leagues off at sea*'. According to the sixteenth-century Richard Banckes' *Herball*, written in 1552, '*Smell of it oft, and it shall keep thee youngly.*'

Medicinal parts

▷ Leaves
▷ Flowers

Physiological actions

Summary

▷ Circulatory stimulant
▷ Cardiotonic
▷ Antidepressant
▷ Digestive
▷ Hepatic
▷ Cholagogue
▷ Sedative
▷ Analgesic
▷ Expectorant
▷ Anticatarrhal
▷ Diaphoretic
▷ Diuretic
▷ Immune tonic
▷ Antiseptic
▷ Antiviral
▷ Antifungal
▷ Anti-inflammatory

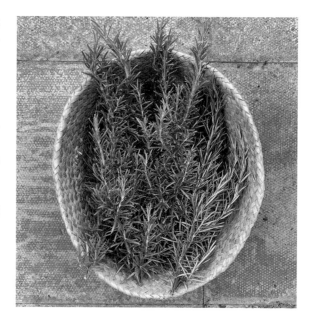

Physiological virtues

As well as traditionally being associated with youthfulness and improved memory, this gorgeous herb has a wealth of helpful properties when taken internally. I prescribe it frequently in my practice, usually as a tincture blended with other herbs in a tailor-made prescription for patients.

It is a very helpful circulatory support, being less heating that many of the traditional herbal circulatory herbs such as Ginger and Chilli. It strengthens the heart and acts as a hypotensive, encouraging peripheral circulation and reducing capillary fragility. It improves the circulation to the head and brain, which is probably why it is considered so good to help the memory, and why it is traditionally prescribed to help to treat hair loss. It is worth considering Rosemary in prescriptions for patients with poor circulation who have developed vertigo or tinnitus. Rosemary also stimulates the circulation throughout the body, making it a very good choice for Raynaud's disease and for varicose veins.

It supports the digestion, relieving flatulence and promoting healthy functioning of the liver and gallbladder. This action may explain some of its action as a gentle antidepressant, but Rosemary also relieves tension and lifts the spirits. It is a mild pain killer and sedative, being a herb to consider for anxious tension headaches, and it also helps to relieve migraine. It can be good to relieve period pain, especially in cases when period blood is dark and clotted.

Rosemary has significant antiviral properties, containing oleanic acid, which has displayed antiviral activity against influenza viruses, along with herpes viruses and HIV, in test tube studies. It has the added quality of supporting the respiratory system, clearing the sinuses, encouraging expectoration, and resolving phlegm. By increasing peripheral circulation, it can support fever management through its diaphoretic action. It is also a diuretic, encouraging increased elimination through the kidneys.

Rosemary is a great choice to restore normal energy levels if a viral infection has left you feeling washed out and exhausted. It is very rich in antioxidants and can be a good and accessible way to support the immune system in general.

It is fabulous as a topical treatment, being antiseptic, antifungal, and anti-inflammatory. It stimulates the circulation without bringing too much heat to the area. Long before I was a herbalist, I was a shepherdess and a cheesemaker, and Rosemary was my main first aid choice for the flock and the humans that cared for them. It was my go-to herb to treat sore feet, cuts and scrapes, sprains, and inflamed udders. Mixed with boiling water and brown bread, it makes a very good antiseptic drawing poultice for infected cuts or stubborn splinters.

Nowadays I infuse Rosemary in olive oil with Nettle seeds as a potent topical anti-inflammatory for arthritis in smaller joints, such as fingers and toes. This is a Roman formula that I found many years ago while investigating old herbals. Rosemary is also included in my scalp lotion for encouraging healthy hair regrowth.

Please note that if you suffer from seizures, you will need to avoid Rosemary. Also avoid medicinal doses during pregnancy.

Energetics

Rosemary is bitter, warm, and astringent. It enlivens us and improves our mental processes. It helps us to have a more outgoing perspective instead of withdrawing into ourselves, if that feels as though it has been waning.

In Tibetan medicine

Rosemary is good for *Péken* states that involve sluggishness, depression, poor circulation, and oedema.

In my dispensary

I prescribe Rosemary a great deal in my herbal practice, both in internal and in topical medicines. I harvest it and make infused oils for topical treatments with the fresh herb. I dry it for tincture making and for infusions if a patient does not have access to their own fresh herb. It is one of the herbs that I always include in my daily pot of 'garden tea', not just because it tastes so good but because it has so many health benefits. If you are keen to introduce Rosemary into your health regime, it is best to mix a little of it with many other herbs, rather than taking it daily on its own over a long period.

The following case is typical of a case Rosemary was well indicated. 'Ruth' was 71 years old. She had had poor circulation as a child, and it had worsened throughout her life. She now suffered with Raynaud's syndrome and had painful varicose veins in her lower legs, which had been treated when she was in her 40s, but this had left her with venostasis and a tendency to varicose eczema. She also had tinnitus and worsening eyesight. Despite all of this, Ruth was active and positive in her outlook. She walked every day and had a healthy diet. She came to see me because she hoped that herbal medicine could reverse the worsening of her symptoms.

I prescribed a personalized tincture blend with Rosemary and Hawthorn as the lead herbs, supported by Cramp bark, Ginger, and Ginkgo. She also had a topical treatment in the form of a Horse Chestnut and Witch Hazel ointment to apply daily to her lower legs. Four weeks later she reported a very noticeable difference. Her fingers were no longer going white when she drove her car, and her varicose eczema was lessening. The appearance of the varicose veins was reducing too. On top of that she felt better in herself, and her energy levels had increased. She continued to improve over the next four months, at which point she was signed off, very happy with her health outcome.

Historical applications

Gerard was very keen on Rosemary. He wrote: 'The Arabians and other Physitions succeeding, do write, that Rosemary comforteth the braine, the memorie, the inward senses, and restoreth speech unto them that are possessed with the dumbe palsie, especially the conserve made of the floures and sugar, or any other way confected with sugar, being taken every day fasting . . . the floures made up into plates with Sugar after the manner of Sugar Roset and eaten, comfort the heart, and make it merry, quicken the spirits, and make them more lively. . . . The distilled water of the floures of Rosemary being drunke at morning and

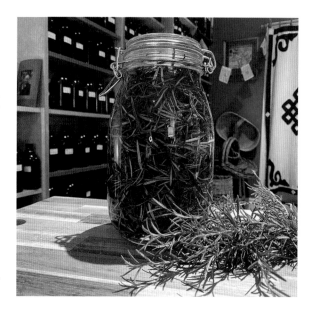

evening first and last, taketh away the stench of the mouth and breath, and maketh it very sweet, if there be added thereto, to steep or infuse for certaine daies, a few Cloves, Mace, Cinnamon, and a little Annise seed.'

Parkinson said that by the 'warming and comforting heate thereof it helpeth all cold diseases, both of the head, stomack, liver and belly: the decoction thereof in wine helpeth the cold distillations of the braine into the eyes, . . . and all other cold diseases of the head and braines, as the giddiness or swimming therein, drowsinesse or dulnesse of the mind and senses like a stupidnesse, the dumbe palsie, or loss of speech, the lethargie and falling sicknesse, to be both drunke, and the temples bathed therewith. . . . It helpeth also a weake memory by heating and drying up the cold moistures of the braines, and quickening the senses.'

He also described Rosemary as a liver tonic: 'It helpeth also those that are liver-grown, by opening the obstructions thereof, by warming the coldnesse extenuating the grossness, and afterwards binding and strengthening the weakness thereof.' He recommended smoking dried Rosemary leaves for coughs and adding the leaves to baths and ointments to '*helpe cold benumbed joynts, sinews or members*'.

Culpeper wrote that it '*helps all cold diseases of the head...drives melancholy vapours from the heart, refreshes the vital spirits, comforts the heart . . . opens the obstructions of the liver, treats yellow jaundice . . . helps to treat dim vision and clear the sight*'.

Magical

One of the magical names of Rosemary is 'Elf Leaf'. It is associated with protection, purification, mental powers, and youthfulness. Burning it as an incense purifies the home and drives away negativity. When placed beneath the pillow, it will protect the sleeper from nightmares, and hanging some in the porch or on doorposts will keep thieves away. Wearing Rosemary is said to help the memory and preserves youthfulness. Wrap some powdered leaves in a linen cloth and bind it to the right arm in order to banish depression and make the emotions light and merry.

Suggestion for the home apothecary

Rosemary salt

Finely chop fresh Rosemary and mix it into some coarse mineral salt at a ratio of 1 part by volume fresh Rosemary to 2 parts by volume mineral salt. Spread the mixture only about 1 cm deep onto a wide flat dish. Cover with

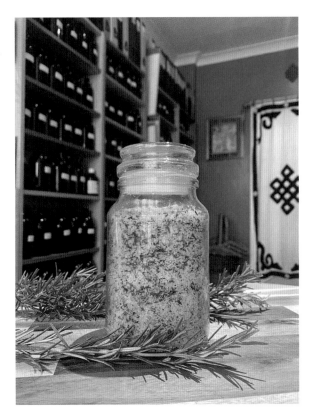

a clean cloth, and leave it in an airy place to cure. Stir the salt daily for the next two weeks, then store it in an airtight jar. Fill a salt grinder with this salt and add it to your food when you feel like it. I especially love it on poached eggs, boiled new potatoes, or roasted nuts, but it is delicious on pretty much every savoury dish.

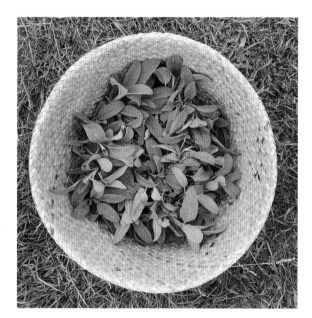

'Why should a man die while Sage grows in his garden?'

The saying quoted above was popular in the Middle Ages and is a translation from the Latin: '*Cur moriator homo cui Salvia crescit in horto?*' The fact that Sage's generic name, 'Salvia', means 'I save', or 'I heal' says it all. Sage is a fabulous and adaptable healing herb, worthy of a place in every apothecary garden. Not surprisingly, there are many sayings lauding its healing attributes – for example, an old English proverb that goes: '*He that would live for an aye, must eat Sage in May*'. This refers to the tradition of eating Sage daily during the month of May as a way of promoting good health through the rest of the year. Another saying, this time from France, focuses on Sage's action in treating tremors and palsy: 'Sage helps the nerves and by its powerful might Palsy is cured and fever put to flight.'

Sage supports all bodily systems and is a traditional tonic for longevity. These days, though, it is most often considered as a go-to 'menopause herb', or as a culinary herb, with the odd leaf being picked here and there for the pot. Sage has so much more to offer us than that.

Medicinal parts
> Leaves
> Flowers

Some people prefer purple Sage as a medicine, but I work with the green version very happily.

Physiological actions

Summary
- Cholagogue
- Tonic
- Nervine
- Antispasmodic
- Antisudorific
- Blood sugar balancer/hypoglycaemic
- Astringent
- Antiinflammatory
- Anticatarrhal
- Antiseptic
- Antibacterial
- Oestrogenic
- Anti-galactagogue

Physiological virtues

Overall, Sage is a very good tonic herb: consider it for nervous exhaustion, post-viral fatigue, and general debility. It supports the nervous system, calming it when there is nervous excitability causing tremors or palsy associated with disorders of the brain and nerves. In these cases, it should be taken in small doses, little and often. Sage been shown to inhibit an enzyme that breaks down acetylcholine, making it potentially valuable in supporting patients with Alzheimer's disease. As well as its nervous system support, it reduces excessive salivation – a virtue that is of particular interest when supporting patients with Parkinson's disease. Sage is antispasmodic, and a cup of Sage tea can also be a good remedy for a simple nervous headache.

Sage acts as a stimulant to the digestive system: hence its association with the culinary preparation of fatty foods. It stimulates the liver and improves the efficiency of digestion where there is debility. It can relieve the discomfort associated with biliousness, improve the appetite, and relieve colic. It reduces blood sugar, so it is worth considering where there is insulin resistance.

It is also a remedy for the respiratory system, relaxing the airways and clearing catarrh. A hot infusion is an excellent treatment for upper respiratory tract infections. It is antiseptic and antibacterial, with specificity against *Staphylococcus aureus*, making it really good for throat infections. Its astringency is helpful to resolve mild haemorrhage from the lungs, and the leaves were traditionally smoked in a pipe to relieve asthma.

Sage's virtues do not end there. It supports the circulatory system, improving the peripheral circulation, and it can be helpful for angina. Its astringency makes it a popular gargle for problems located in the mouth and throat, such as sore throats, bleeding gums, excessive salivation, and tonsillitis. Its antiseptic properties mean that the strong cooled tea makes an excellent wound wash, especially for slow-healing, dirty wounds. The fresh leaves, rubbed onto the teeth, will whiten them as well as strengthening the gums, and as a hair wash it darkens the hair. Bruised in vinegar and heated, the leaves are a helpful first aid fomentation in the treatment for sprains: apply this in a folded muslin cloth, as hot as can be tolerated.

Sage is oestrogenic in nature and acts as an emmenagogue, helping to bring the menstrual cycle into a better rhythm if it is irregular or scanty. It has a drying tendency, which has led to it being a popular and oft-recommended herbal choice for menopausal women experiencing excessive sweating, especially as its oestrogenic properties can act to reduce menopausal symptoms. I do not work with Sage in this way though, preferring to get to the underlying cause of any imbalance that is causing the distressing symptoms to arise. At this point I would just like to point out that menopause is not a disease state, any more than puberty is. These are healthy and natural phases of the body as it adapts to different phases of life. Despite Western society's persistent negative health messages around menopause, our transitions can truly be symptom-free and joyous if our body is in healthful balance. If distressing symptoms arise, they are usually due to an existing imbalance that has not been known or has been ignored for too long, made worse by the negative 'baggage' around the idea of this natural life transition. Menopause simply flags it up. The good news is that a holistic approach can be very effective indeed and bring lasting, safe relief even when the treatment with herbs ceases. Let us stop blaming menopause as the culprit and see it as a messenger, reminding us to take better care of ourselves.

Sage should not be taken in medicinal doses during pregnancy, although small amounts taken in culinary dishes are not harmful. It does reduce lactation, so do not take it while breastfeeding. Cold Sage tea drunk every few hours will dry up breast milk, if this is needed. Sage contains thujone, which is potentially toxic, so it is advisable to view Sage as a short-term support rather than a herb to take daily for many years. Avoid in epilepsy.

Energetics

Sage is bitter, warming, and astringent.

In Tibetan medicine

In Tibetan medicine, the Sage that is prescribed is *Salvia nubicola,* or *Jibtsi karpo* [འཇིབ་རྩི་དཀར་པོ།]. *Jibtsi karpo* has a sweet-to-bitter taste, with a sweet post-digestive taste and a cooling potency. It is mostly prescribed for mouth and throat diseases, including toothache. It is also good for treating hot disorder of the stomach and liver.

In my dispensary

As well as prescribing Sage in tailor-made prescriptions, as appropriate, I especially like to make a mouthwash, generally combined with Spearmint and Myrrh, as a gargle.

'Ellie' had suffered a bereavement in the last couple of years and found that her gums had been in bad shape since then. They were bleeding and receding, and her dentist had told her that she was at risk of losing some teeth. As well as an internal mix to support her poor peripheral circulation, I prescribed a mouthwash based on Sage, Myrrh, and Spearmint tinctures. She was to mix 5 ml of mouthwash with 20 ml of water daily and swill it thoroughly for as long as she could manage before spitting it out. Within four weeks her gums were no longer hurting or bleeding.

Historical applications

Dioscorides recommended Sage as a diuretic as well as to stimulate menstruation and help to '*expel the dead child*'. It was considered to be a valuable wound-healing herb and a treatment for '*foule ulcers or sores*'. He also wrote – as reported by Parkinson – that '*the decoction of the leaves and branches made with wine, doth taketh away the itching of the cods, if they be bathed therewith.*' The word '*cods*' refers to the scrotum.

Sage's warming and drying qualities were described by Agrippa being used to treat women whose wombs were too moist and slippery and so preventing conception. They were advised to take '*a quantity of the juyce of Sage with a little salt, for foure days before they company with their Husbands, it will helpe them to conceive, and also for those that after they have conceived, are subject often to miscarry upon any small occasion, for it causeth the birth to be better retained, and to become more lively.*'

Parkinson described Sage as being prescribed for consumption. It was made into pills, as follows: '*Take of Spikenard (Nardostachys grandiflora) and Ginger of each two drammes, of the seed of Sage a little toasted at the fire eight drammes, of Long Pepper twelve drammes, all these being brought into a fine powder, let there bee so much juyce of Sage put thereto, as may make it into a masse, formable for pills, taking a dramme of them every morning fasting, and so likewise at night, drinking a little pure water after them.*'

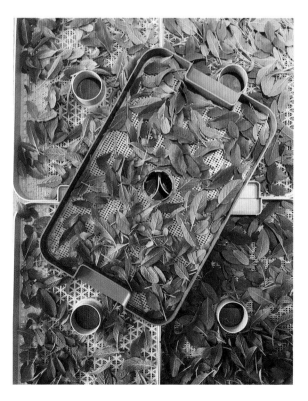

'*Matthiolus saith, that it is very profitable for all manner of paines of the head, comming of cold, and rheumaticke humours, as also for all paines of the joynts, whether used inwardly or outwardly, and therefore it helpeth such that have the falling sicknesse, the lethargie or drowsie evill, such as are dull and heavie of spirit, and those that have the palsie, and is much use in all defluxions or distillations of thin rheume from the head, and for diseases of the chest or brest.*'

Parkinson also recommended Sage for hoarseness: '*the juyce of Sage taken in warme water, helpeth an hoarseness and the cough*' and a gargle was made up using '*Sage, Rosemary, Honisuckles, and Plantaine boyled in water or wine, with some Honi and Allome put thereto*'. This was used to treat sore mouths and throats, or '*the secret parts of man or woman as need requireth*'.

It was favoured for treating palsy, too. Parkinson wrote that '*the leaves sodden in wine and laid upon any place affected with the Palsie, helpeth much, if the decoction be drunke also.*'

Sage taken with Wormwood was prescribed for dysentery (*the bloody fluxe*), and it has long been prescribed to moderate women's periods. Pliny wrote: '*it procureth women's courses, and stayeth them coming downe too fast*'.

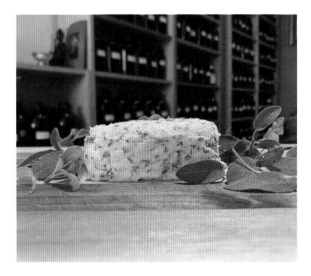

Gerard wrote: '*Sage is singularly good for the head and brain, it quickeneth the senses and the memory, strengthening the sinews, restoreth health to those that have the palsy, and taketh away shakey trembling of the members.*'

A conserve made from Sage flowers was said to improve the memory, and eating Sage daily during the month of May was a tradition that promoted good health through the rest of the year. In Sussex, England, there was a traditional cure for the ague that involved eating Sage leaves on nine consecutive mornings, while fasting.

Magical

Sage is associated with immortality, longevity, wisdom, and protection. A small horn filled with Sage can be worn as a protective amulet – something that is especially considered to protect against the evil eye. Sage is also a wishing herb. Write your wish on a Sage leaf and sleep with it beneath your pillow for three nights. If you dream of the thing that you are wishing for, it will come true; but if you do not, bury the Sage leaf and accept that it was not to be. It is considered better luck to get a friend to plant Sage in your garden for you than doing it yourself. Also it is best grown in a bed with other herbs.

Suggestion for the home apothecary

Sage butter

Finely chop fresh Sage leaves and mash them into some butter. Once it is evenly mixed into the butter, form it into a convenient pat in a piece of greaseproof paper. Refrigerate. Spread the butter onto a daily sandwich during the month of May. You could also mix the chopped Sage into Coconut oil as a plant-based alternative, if preferred.

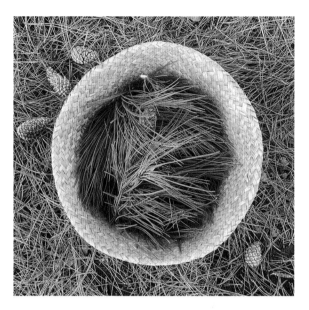
'Scots Pine helps us to breathe more easily and to let go of troubling emotions.'

There are many species of Pine throughout the world. Most of them are medicinal. Here in the United Kingdom, Scots Pine is our beautiful native pine. It grows tall and majestic, with warm pinkish/reddish bark, and it exudes a sense of regal calm. As it is so tall, it can be quite hard to gather the shoots, but occasionally you come across a recently fallen branch. If you do, make the most of it.

Pine has very many medicinal attributes, one of them being that it helps us to breathe more easily. It can also help us to let go of troubling, negative emotions that are often held as tension and congestion in the lungs. Pine is a medicine for the soul as well as the body.

Medicinal parts

▷ Shoots
▷ Needles
▷ Pollen
▷ Cones (sometimes)

Physiological actions

Summary

▷ Expectorant
▷ Antitussive
▷ Antiseptic
▷ Diuretic

Physiological virtues

The leaves and young shoots are antiseptic, diuretic, and expectorant. You can take Pine internally to help with kidney, bladder, and respiratory complaints, and you can add it to bath water to treat fatigue, nervous exhaustion, sleeplessness, and skin irritations.

It is a popular herb in inhalants, easing respiratory congestion. Extracts from the buds, harvested in spring, are an antitussive and are antimicrobial, with a particular affinity to the respiratory system. Pine can also increase the production of gastric juices, which is helpful in tackling the build-up of mucus and phlegm in the system generally. A decoction of 3–4 buds per cup can be made up, and a spoonful of the liquid taken three or four times daily. The seeds can be eaten to help with bronchial and muscular complaints.

Oil, distilled from the needles of Scots Pine, is a common ingredient of cough and cold remedies, especially as inhalants. It is also popular in liniments for muscular aches and pains, rheumatism, and arthritis. It is said that the root tar promotes hair growth.

Energetics

Pine is warming and aromatic. It can help us to let go of troubling, negative emotions, which are often held as tension and congestion in the lungs.

Since it is so prominent in the landscape, Pine was often planted in high places or at the junction of ancient trackways to serve as a way marker. In the Celtic Tree Ogham (a Celtic system of divination based on trees), Pine is known as *Ailm*. It stands for seeing clearly and developing foresight. It is most powerful as winter moves into spring. This is helpful, as the power of foresight helps us to set our intentions wisely for the year ahead.

Bach associates Pine with self-reproach and guilt, especially indicated when someone apologizes for being ill and, in some way, feels that they deserve it.

In Tibetan medicine

In Tibetan medicine, Pine is known as *Dreun shing* [སྦྲོན་ཤིང་]. It has a taste that is considered sweet, with a post-digestive taste that is also sweet. Its potency is hot and dry. The texts describe it as remedying *Pekén/rLung* conditions, and it is specifically recommended to treat the build-up of serous fluid in the limbs and joints. It is also prescribed for dropsy, cold ailments, and suppurating wounds.

In my dispensary

In my clinic I predominantly work with Pine as a tincture, choosing it in blends for patients who need respiratory support. It really calls out to be included when people are holding on to troubling emotions and are not comfortable with vocalizing their feelings. Sometimes, when taking a patient's pulse, I notice that the lung pulse feels quite different from the rest of the organ pulses, yet the patient has not complained of any respiratory symptoms or past medical issues concerning the lungs. In these cases, there is either a physiological change that is as yet asymptomatic, or there is a tendency to hold on to troubling emotions. When I explain this and ask for the patient's feelings on this, they very often tell me immediately that they have been holding on to and suppressing a difficult emotion. I always say that they do not need to tell me what it is, unless they particularly want to, but I suggest that adding Pine to their blend will help to start the process of letting the emotion go. Pine does, after all, help us to see more clearly and expansively, helping us to move forward in our lives.

Historical applications

Gerard, in his *Herball* of 1597, says: '*The whole Cone or apple being boiled with fresh Horehound, saith Galen, and afterwards boiled again with a little honey till the decoction doth come to the thickness of honey, maketh an excellent medicine for the cleansing of the chest and lungs.*'

Magical

Pine is associated with the element of air and, when burnt as incense, clears negativity from a space. It is also associated with strength, fertility, and vigour. The cones develop as a spiral that turns to the right, so a Pine cone gathered in mid-summer (with its seeds still inside) is considered to be a potent magical object. Eating one pine nut from it daily is said to make one immune to gunshots.

The cones are carried to increase fertility, and Pine needles are burnt to drive away evil and cleanse the house. You can add them to the bath water as a cleansing ritual. In Japan pine branches were placed over the door of the house to ensure continual joy within (because it is an evergreen).

In the Welsh Celtic tradition, the upper shamanic realms (known as 'Gwynfyd') can be accessed by visualizing oneself climbing a large Pine tree, guided and held by its clear and steady presence. The Pine reaches above the normal forest canopy – the everyday world – and offers us a clear view and a higher perspective. It clears confusion and stuck energy: an action that reveals hidden truths. Pine can help us to move forward in spiritual growth by acknowledging the things that we have buried.

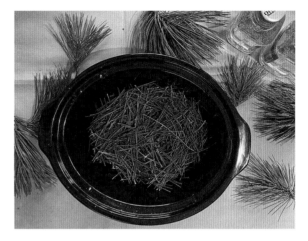

Suggestion for the home apothecary

Pine-infused oil

On a dry day, harvest Pine needles, cut them into small pieces with scissors, and place them into a slow cooker. Pour over mild olive oil to cover the needles completely, stirring the oil with a spoon or a chopstick to get rid of any air bubbles. Set the slow cooker to the 'warm' setting for one hour, then switch off and allow it to infuse passively until the next day. Repeat the following day and again for another two days, then leave lidded, to infuse passively for a couple of weeks. Keep checking to make sure that the plant material is covered by the oil. Alternatively, you can infuse the oil in a jar passively for 4 weeks. When your oil is ready, strain it through a colander lined with muslin cloth, and then bottle it. If you like, you can reinfuse the oil with further Pine needles to get a stronger extraction.

Pine is often chosen as an invigorating massage oil and is especially valued as a chest rub for colds and bronchitis, and also as a breast massage oil for painful lumps and tumours. You can also make your oil into an ointment to soothe headaches.

Shepherd's Purse 🌿 *Capsella bursa-pastoris*

'Shepherd's Purse reduces heavy periods and flooding. It helps us to hold something of ourselves back.'

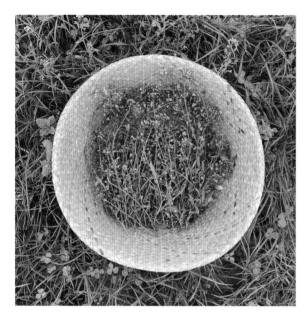

Shepherd's Purse is a ubiquitous wild plant around where I live, standing out with its little heart-shaped seed pods. They look similar to the shape of a sheep's scrotum – something that was, in times gone by, used by shepherds to store their coins. In Tibetan it is, perhaps more palatably, known as 'shoulder blade'. The Irish name for this herb is 'Clappedepouch', named after lepers who begged at crossroads with a bell (clapper) and a long pole with a cup at the end of it to receive alms from passers-by.

As I write this, Shepherd's Purse has chosen to spring up on the pavement right outside my clinic. While I will not be harvesting it from there, it does make me smile each time I arrive at work. Shepherd's Purse is a potentially life-saving herb deserving of much respect.

Medicinal parts

- ▷ Leaves
- ▷ Stems
- ▷ Flowers
- ▷ Seed pods

This is a plant that is best prepared from fresh material, so make a tincture or vinegar with fresh plants.

Physiological actions

Summary

- ▷ Astringent
- ▷ Haemostatic
- ▷ Vulnerary
- ▷ Diuretic

Physiological virtues

Shepherd's Purse is astringent, haemostatic, and vulnerary. It is a specific for reducing heavy menstrual bleeding (menorrhagia) and menopausal flooding and was traditionally prescribed for post-partum haemorrhage. It must have saved many lives in the past. It contains flavonoid glycosides, amino acids, oxalic acid, glucosinolates, volatile oils, fumaric acid, and minerals.

It is a urinary antiseptic and diuretic, helpful where there is haematuria. It is hot in nature and stimulates the circulation as well as supporting the integrity of the venous system. This makes it helpful, for example, in the case of haemorrhoids and varicose veins. Herbalist Julie Bruton-Seal reports clinical and first-hand experience of Shepherd's Purse helping to rectify prolapses of both the uterus and the urinary bladder. This is a herb to be avoided by patients with kidney stones due to its oxalic acid content, and one should be cautious in prescribing for those who are pregnant or breastfeeding.

Energetics

Shepherd's Purse has a sweet and hot taste. Energetically, it helps us to generate the momentum and motivation to establish boundaries. It is well indicated for those who give of themselves too much and deplete their vital energy because of it. When people have been giving out too much to others, they become exhausted and depleted and are no longer able to generate the momentum to make positive changes, particularly the setting of healthy boundaries. It is not selfish to take care of ourselves. We need to do this if we are to have the strength to care for others. In fact, people who need Shepherd's Purse often understand that they need to hold back something of themselves, but they are so exhausted by over-giving that they feel powerless to make the necessary changes. Shepherd's Purse can provide the extra support needed to make this change.

In Tibetan medicine

Shepherd's Purse is known as *Sog Ka* [སོག་ཀ།], which means 'shoulder blade'. Its taste is sweet, hot, and astringent, with a sweet post-digestive taste. Its potency is heavy, stable, and oily.

In Tibetan medicine it is primarily considered to be an antiemetic. It also supports the kidneys, treating kidney diseases in general, and it removes retained urine. It is prescribed mostly to reduce oedema, but it also treats consumptive lung disease. It is good for infiltration of hot disorders in the channels (nerves) as well as hot disorders associated with poisoning.

In my dispensary

I tend to prescribe Shepherd's Purse when there is menorrhagia, usually giving it as a simple or with an equal part of Cramp Bark if there is period pain. The mix is taken only during the period. This is to manage symptoms while the underlying root cause is responding to treatment. Most patients no longer need their 'period mix' after a couple of months of holistic treatment.

'Samantha' was in her early 40s and cared for her elderly mother alongside a demanding full-time job. She had fibroids and suffered from extremely heavy and debilitating periods. She was chronically anaemic and was tired all the time. She wished to pursue a natural approach before opting for surgery. She had tried to boost her iron levels through dietary changes and by taking ferrous sulphate supplements, but she had been unable to make headway with this strategy, and her periods had remained consistently very heavy. We started by going very thoroughly through her diet and lifestyle. Although Samantha had a pretty healthy diet, she was not eating as much iron-rich food as she could have done. Her digestion was rather sluggish, and I suspected that she was not absorbing the nutrients from her diet efficiently. She had a longstanding tendency to constipation, which, I believed, could be contributing to oestrogen dominance, which, in turn, contributed to a better terrain for the development of fibroids. My priority was to support a healthy bowel function while boosting her iron intake and absorption. I hoped that with more balanced oestrogen levels and improved haemoglobin status, her periods would naturally become lighter. I thought that this would allow us to make further headway with her long-standing low iron levels. I could see that she needed to find the motivation to look after herself better, and she needed to create better boundaries with her mother. I knew that Shepherd's Purse would be a key herb for her.

I prescribed a daily digestive formula containing sour and bitter herbs to improve her digestion in general, to help normalize her bowel habit and to support her liver function. I also prescribed some iron-boosting herbal capsules based on Spirulina and Nettle and, since she was a meat-eater, I advised her to eat red meat at least three times a week, if possible. I also prescribed a 'period mix' tincture based on fresh Shepherd's Purse with Cramp Bark. She was to take this mix at a dose of 2.5 ml in hot water up to a maximum of four times a day during the heaviest days of her period. I cautioned her to take it only as needed, since over-prescribing could potentially slow down her bowels, and we did not want that.

She was a very conscientious patient and followed my advice religiously. The first time

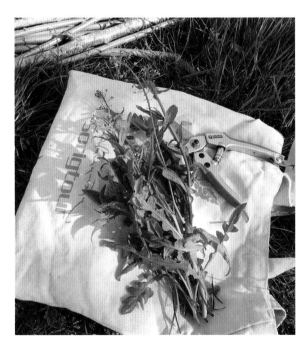

she tried the 'period mix', she noticed that her period immediately became considerably lighter, and she did not feel quite as exhausted after it had finished. Over the next few months her periods continued to become lighter and less prolonged, and her iron levels began to pick up. As her energy levels improved, she developed the strength and the motivation to take up more outside interests and establish healthier boundaries with her mother.

Historical applications

Gerard says the following of Shepherd's Purse: '*Shepeards purse is called in Latine, Pastoris bursa: in French, "Bourse de Pasteur ou Curé": in English, Shepeards purse or scrip: of some, Shepheards pouch, and poor man's Parmacetie: and in the North part of England, Toy-wort, Pick-purse, and Case-weed. . . . Shepheard's purse staieth bleeding in any part of the body, whether the juice or the decoction thereof be drunk, or whether it be used pultesse wise, or in bath, or any other way else.*'

Culpeper says that it helps to stop bleeding, either from external or internal wounds. He also wrote that '*If bound to the wrists or soles of the feet, it helps the jaundice. The herb made into poultices, helps inflammation and St Anthony's fire. The juice dropped into the ears, heals the pains, noise and matterings thereof. A good ointment may be made of it for all wounds, especially wounds in the head.*'

Maud Grieve wrote that during the First World War, a liquid extract of Shepherd's Purse was applied to wounds sustained by soldiers on the battlefield. The more commonly chosen haemostyptics, ergot and Goldenseal, became unavailable, and Shepherd's Purse stepped up to the plate.

Dr Ellingwood records that '*This agent has been noted for its influence in haematuria . . . soothing irritation of the renal or vesical organs. In cases of uncomplicated chronic menorrhagia it has accom-*

plished permanent cures, especially if the discharge be persistent. The agent is also useful where uric acid or insoluble phosphates or carbonates produce irritation of the urinary tract. Externally, the bruised herb has been applied to bruised and strained parts and to rheumatic joints.'

Suggestion for the home apothecary

Shepherd's Purse tincture

Pick the aerial parts of Shepherd's Purse on a dry day, cut them up, and fill a jar loosely with this. Pour over at least 50% ABV vodka, making sure that the plant material is covered. Leave it in a dark place for 4 weeks, shaking it occasionally to make sure no bits of herb are sticking out of the liquid. Strain and press (or squeeze) and pour into a clean bottle. Take 2.5 ml diluted in a third of a mug of hot water up to four times a day during the period if experiencing excessively heavy bleeding. Be sure to address the underlying causes of menorrhagia and not to rely on this as a long-term strategy.

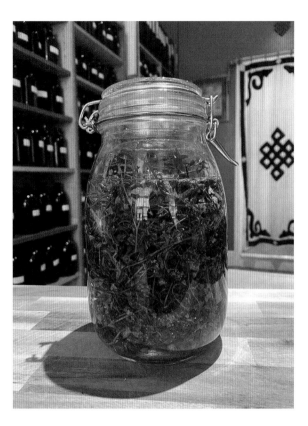

Skullcap 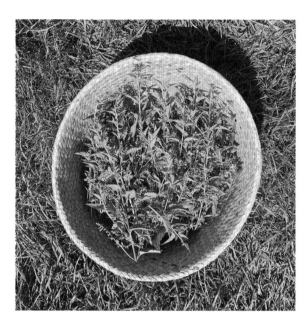 *Scutellaria lateriflora*

'Skullcap is a very deep tonic to the nervous system.'

Skullcap is a native of North America, and it was traditionally prescribed by indigenous peoples to stimulate menstruation and to support the passing of the placenta. Later, the Physiomedicalists thought of Skullcap primarily as a nervine but recognized that it had a much deeper action on the nervous system than most other herbal nervines. They prescribed it for epilepsy, convulsions, spasms, and serious mental illnesses such as schizophrenia. It was also found to be effective to counteract the effects of rabies, hence one of its folk names is still 'mad dogweed'.

If you are learning the Latin binomials of the herbs that you work with – and I thoroughly recommend that you do – please take care with its specific name, which refers to the fact that the flowers are held on the side of the stem, not all around it. Many sources erroneously refer to its specific name as being to do with the position of the leaves rather than the flowers. If you realize that the leaves are held all around the stem and the flowers are not, you should find it easy to remember that the correct specific name is '*lateriflora*'.

Medicinal parts

▷ Aerial parts

Physiological actions

Summary

▷ Nervine
▷ Sedative
▷ Antispasmodic
▷ Bitter

Physiological virtues

Skullcap is a sedative, a nervine tonic, and antispasmodic and a mild bitter. It helps to support and nourish the nervous system while alleviating the symptoms of stress and anxiety. This means that it can treat the root cause while also acting symptomatically. It is a very good choice for nervous exhaustion. It has a significantly antispasmodic action, so is worth considering when there is a lot of tension in the body. Choose it in blends for anxiety, panic attacks, insomnia, tension headaches, and period pain as well as premenstrual syndrome.

Skullcap is a gentle bitter so can play a helpful role in stimulating a digestive system that has been weakened by a long period of stress. This is one of the few herbs that I always tincture from fresh.

Energetics

Skullcap is bitter, astringent, and cooling.

In Tibetan medicine

According to Tibetan medicine, nervous system imbalances such as anxiety, panic attacks, and insomnia are linked to *rLung*, and this, in turn, can be heightened by the intake of too high a proportion of bitter foods and medicines. Skullcap is a mild bitter but can still be helpful for those with *rLung* imbalances, especially if prescribed alongside appropriate dietary changes and other sweeter and more nourishing herbs. Examples of these herbs are Wild Oat, Ashwagandha, and Caraway seed.

In my dispensary

I absolutely love Skullcap and often reach for it when prescribing. Some of that is perhaps a reflection on the number of patients who come for help because they are suffering with stress, tension, and anxiety. Skullcap is a deep tonic to the nervous system, especially helpful for those who have been suffering with nervous system disorders for many years.

This case shows the action of Skullcap in supporting the nervous system as well as gently encouraging better digestion: 'Jane' was 52 years old and had been suffering with severe anxiety for over sixteen years. She had been taking various antidepressants during this time and was currently taking 60 mg daily of Fluoxetine. She also had digestive issues, suffering with frequent bloating and alternating constipation and diarrhoea. We started by getting her to reduce her caffeine intake from four cups down to a maximum of one per day and to increase her water consumption. I asked her to remove gluten from her diet and reduce her intake of simple carbohydrates in general. I also suggested that she introduced bone broth in order to provide a nourishing and grounding influence. I chose Skullcap as her main nervine support because it would also gently support her digestion. I teamed it with Agrimony, Wild Oat, Valerian, and Ashwagandha.

Within four weeks she reported 'feeling so much calmer' and after another four weeks she felt better still, reporting that she had already started the process of gradually reducing her antidepressant medication with the full support of her GP.

The following case illustrates how Skullcap can help shift things quite quickly when there is anxiety combined with weak digestion. This is especially the case when dietary changes are combined with a tailor-made supportive tincture blend. 'Eddie' was 30 years old and was feeling very run down and tired, scoring his average energy level as only 5 out of 10. He was having a pretty stressful time both with his work and with his relationship with his partner, which was proving to be turbulent. Also, his digestion had always been a problem. He had suffered with bloating and rumbling for many years and regularly had constipation alternating with diarrhoea. He was especially worried because he was experiencing significant left upper abdominal pain. During the consultation he told me that he often had bad colds, his ears felt blocked, and he was prone to sinusitis.

He was not eating breakfast because, he said, he never felt hungry in the morning, and he was then eating badly later in the day, because he was so hungry. I explained that he would need to start to eat at least a small, healthy breakfast to start to break this cycle of low energy and unstable blood sugar. I also suggested that he should drink less coffee and hydrate better. Finally, I suspected that, due to his weak digestion, he was not tolerating dairy very well; so I asked him to stop it completely for the time being. I prescribed a tincture blend containing Skullcap, Agrimony, Chamomile, Vervain, Blessed Thistle, and Caraway. He was to take 5 ml in hot water twice a day.

Two weeks later he came for his first follow-up and said that he felt 'so much better' and that I was 'so right about dairy'. He described a 'drastic difference' in his digestion. The bloating and rumbling was much diminished, and his episodes of constipation had gone completely, along with his upper left abdominal pain. The rest of the time he had fewer daily stools, and these were better formed than they had been. He was eating breakfast and making better food

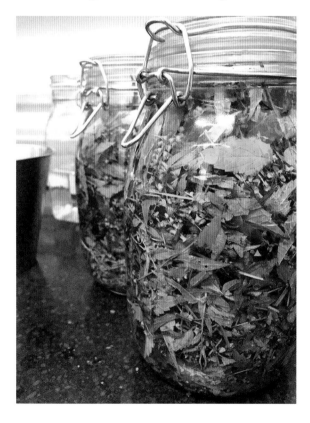

choices during the day, and his energy levels were already picking up. Although his life was still stressful, he was feeling less anxious and was sleeping better. He continued with his lifestyle changes for a few more months before he was signed off from herbal treatment. He said that he was feeling as though he were a different person, compared to how he had felt when he first came to my clinic.

Historical applications
Skullcap's reputation as a cure for rabies started in the late eighteenth century, when a Dr Van Derveer apparently prescribed it to prevent '*400 persons and 1,000 cattle from becoming hydrophobus after being bitten by mad dogs*'.

Magical
Skullcap is associated with love, fidelity, and peace. It is said that if a wife wears it, her husband will be protected against the charms of other women. Perhaps the truth of the matter is that the wife will be less worried and suspicious, leading to more harmony in the home.

Suggestion for the home apothecary
Skullcap tincture

Roughly chop fresh Skullcap, and loosely fill a jar with it. Cover completely with alcohol that is at least 50% ABV, and leave in a dark place for 4 weeks. Drain, press, and bottle. Take 5 ml daily in hot water if you feel your nervous system needs deep support. You can also combine it in a dropper bottle with other calming herbal tinctures, such as Rose, Motherwort, Lemon Balm, and Passionflower. Take a few drops on the tongue when you feel especially anxious.

Slippery Elm   🌰   *Ulmus fulva / U. rubra*

'Slippery Elm nourishes and calms tissues. While supporting us, it also invites us to look at the ways that we may perpetuate an exploitative attitude to our health and our herbs.'

Wild populations of Slippery Elm are at great risk of over-exploitation due to the fact that there is a worldwide insatiable demand for its bark, and cultivated stands are not able to keep up with the enormous human desire to 'use' this herb. Slippery Elm is a truly amazing medicine, supporting us in many ways with its soothing, demulcent bark, but it may be too tempting to rely on its support when we do not really need to.

Slippery Elm eases away the intense rawness and pain of inflamed mucous membranes, such as those associated with gastritis, IBS, dry coughs, or sore throats. When prescribed in the right circumstances, it can be absolutely life-changing, especially as a temporary support while lifestyle and dietary causal factors are adjusted. Sadly, it is all too easy to reach for this herb over a long time frame rather than making changes to address underlying causes of the symptoms.

Slippery Elm is such a supportive herb that taking it can allow us to continue to eat and drink the 'wrong things for us' or to have a lifestyle that is causing us to deplete our health. We may be able to 'get away with it' because we take Slippery Elm, but in doing so we are not really respecting our body, our health, or the precious herb that we are taking. If we think about it rationally, I am sure that the majority of us would rather make some sensible adjustments to the way that we live than to contribute to the over-exploitation of a scarce species and inflict continued stress on our body.

These days, a great many herbalists avoid prescribing Slippery Elm, choosing alternatives

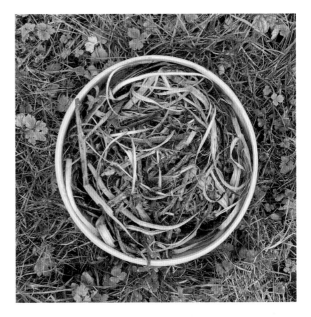

such as Marshmallow root, which is much more plentiful and a wonderfully effective choice. I fully appreciate and support this stance.

Medicinal part
- Inner bark

Physiological actions

Summary
- Demulcent
- Anti-inflammatory
- Nutritive
- Expectorant

Physiological virtues

I do still work with Slippery Elm medicinally, but I am extremely conscious of how I prescribe it. I have a small population of Slippery

Elm trees that I grew from seed ten years ago and manage by pollarding. This produces bark that helps to supply the needs of my patients, especially as I always blend it with other herbs and only see it as a temporary support rather than a long-term treatment strategy. I have lost count of the number of times that I have persuaded patients that they no longer need Slippery Elm, whether self-prescribed or pre-scribed by me.

Slippery Elm is demulcent, nutritive, and emollient. It can be prepared as an infusion, cap-sules, a gruel, pessaries, suppositories, lozenges, a poultice, and paste. It soothes, lubricates, and protects any tissue with which it comes into contact. In the digestive tract it is especially indicated in cases of acid reflux, gastritis, IBS, ulcerative colitis, and enteritis. It not only acts as a moistening demulcent, but it also neutral-izes excess acidity. It is especially good when there is alternating constipation and diarrhoea associated with IBS. The beauty of this is that there is no need to keep swapping treatment between astringents and aperients. It is helpful, whichever is being manifested.

Slippery Elm is a moistening expectorant that is excellent in cases of bronchitis, consump-tion, and bleeding from the lungs. It soothes the lungs, promoting a feeling of relaxation and expansion and helping to breathe more easily. Its high calcium content is said to be especially helpful in cases of tuberculosis. Taken as a decoction or as a lozenge, it calms the inflammation and discomfort of sore throats, tonsillitis, and inflammations of the oral mucosa such as found in *lichen planus*.

Slippery Elm can, in theory, also be a help-ful option for cystitis or irritable bladder, but I would prefer Marshmallow or Plantain leaf for these indications.

Slippery Elm is nutritive, providing easily digestible nutrition when nothing else will be tolerated. It can be prepared as a gruel, the nutri-tious value of which is equivalent to oatmeal. Slippery Elm gruel is well worth considering in cases of severe malnutrition and stomach can-cers. To make it, take 1 tsp of powder and mix well with an equal amount of honey or maple syrup. Slowly add 570 ml/1 pint of boiling water or non-dairy milk, mixing all the while to form a smooth gruel. It can be flavoured with a little Cinnamon or Nutmeg.

Here in the United Kingdom it is not possible to source the whole bark, only the powder. This is because shards of bark were historically used to procure abortion. Apparently, a sliver was inserted into the cervix, encouraging it to open as the bark absorbed moisture and softened the tissue around it. Because of this, selling the bark is not allowed. If you do have access to home-grown bark, it can be prepared as an infusion or decoction. Take 1 tsp of inner bark and pour on a cupful of boiling water. Steep for one hour or overnight. It can also be simmered and reduced to make a thick syrup. This can be taken in small amounts throughout the day.

Whichever internal prescription of Slippery Elm is chosen, I must emphasize again that it should be viewed as only a temporary health support, not as a long-term prop.

Topical applications can be prescribed to treat skin conditions and to draw out foreign bodies and poisons. A drawing poultice is made by mixing 2 parts Slippery Elm powder with 2 parts Cornmeal and 1 part each of Bloodroot, Hypericum-infused oil, Chickweed, and Bur-dock. Mix well and add warm water until a thick paste is formed. Apply this to boils, abscesses, wounds, swollen cervical glands, and enlarged prostate glands. If applying to a hairy skin sur-face, coat the face of the poultice with olive oil. Use clean white cotton and change the poultice if there are any signs of drainage.

As a pessary, it can be helpful to treat growths

or inflammation of the womb as well as cases of prolapse. In his book *Back to Eden*, Jethro Kloss describes mixing Slippery Elm powder with pure water to create a thick paste. This is shaped into roughly 2.5-cm × 2.5-cm pieces. Three of these are inserted and held in place with a sponge. The pessaries are left in place for three days; then the sponge is removed and the patient given a thorough douche to remove all traces of the Slippery Elm. It could also be given as a rectal suppository that is renewed following each bowel movement.

Energetics
Elm is sweet. It helps us to see the 'bigger picture' and to live up to our responsibilities. Edward Bach describes the energetic qualities of Elm as helping people who feel overwhelmed.

In Tibetan medicine
Although *Ulmus fulva* is not included within the Tibetan pharmacopoeia, it is sweet and nutritive, so we can infer that it will help to reduce both *rLung* and *Tripa*. Its action to reduce the heat and inflammation of *Tripa* would perhaps seem to be the more obvious of the two, but Slippery Elm is also excellent to counteract excessive *rLung*. It exerts a stabilizing and earthing influence. It is interesting to discover, via Matthew Wood, that Herbalist William LeSassier felt that Slippery Elm had a relaxing influence on the nervous system. He said that it helped to clear emotional imbalances. This clinical observation would be seen in patients who had been suffering with excess *rLung* that had now been calmed.

Ulmus androssowii is a species of Elm the bark of which is included in the Tibetan pharmacopoeia. It is known as *Yo bog* [ཡོ་འབོག]. Its taste is astringent and slightly hot with a post-digestive taste that is bitter. Its potency is cool and rough. It is considered to be helpful for osteoarthri-

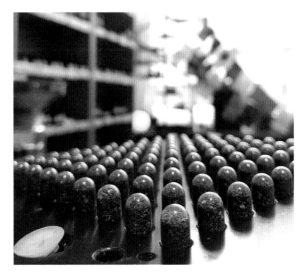

tis, fever, and inflamed wounds. It is added to incense blends as it helps to stick them together and acts like glue.

In my dispensary
I was taught the benefits of Slippery Elm by my tutor and mentor, Edith Barlow. She used to prescribe it, blended with Marshmallow root and other herbs, to help heal an inflamed gut and as an ingredient in a respiratory capsule blend. As a result of her teaching, I most often prescribe it in capsules made with equal parts of Marshmallow root and Meadowsweet. These are very effective in the early stages of the treatment of acid reflux, IBS, diverticulitis, stomach ulcers, and ulcerative colitis. In very severe cases, the capsules can be taken before and after each meal. Once the inflammation has calmed, the number and frequency with which it is taken is gradually reduced. The dosage of capsules may start at 9 per day in the most severe cases, reducing down to 1–2 a day once the lifestyle and dietary changes have been implemented and the positive effects of this are beginning to be felt. In case you are wondering about the size of the capsules, I should tell you that I always

work with size '0' capsules in my dispensary. I find that many patients prefer that size and tell me that they find larger ones (size '00') much more daunting to swallow.

Some people feel that taking Slippery Elm immediately before eating could reduce the absorption of nutrients. However, as a short-term treatment measure I would say that, even if this is the case, the benefits far outweigh the 'costs'. In very severe cases of digestive-tract inflammation, absorption is already likely to be significantly compromised. Time and time again I have seen how a short course of Slippery Elm blend capsules heals long-standing inflammation, leading to more 'ease' and less 'disease' as well as to much better absorption going forward.

I also prescribe Slippery Elm, alongside many other expectorants and demulcents, in a respiratory-system-supporting capsule blend. The proportion of Slippery Elm is quite low in this blend, around 5%, but it feels a very important part of the mix nonetheless.

When prescribing Slippery Elm in blends, I make sure that patients understand its preciousness. I explain that it is a temporary support

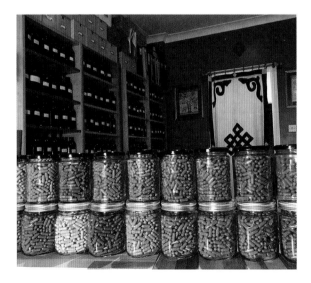

while they get themselves back on track. In my practice I never prescribe Slippery Elm as a simple.

Here are a couple of cases to illustrate some of the points I have raised about this herb.

I had a patient in his 20s who, after suffering from an infection of Covid-19, experienced a very severe flare-up of pre-existing IBS symptoms. This caused him to develop persistent diarrhoea. When I first saw him, the situation had been going on for a couple of months. He looked thin and drawn and was losing weight at an alarming rate. He was spending many hours on the toilet each day, which prevented him from not only from eating normally but also from getting on with the rest of his life and his university studies. Not surprisingly, he was feeling weak and disheartened. His allopathic health-care team were not sure what was going on but continued to investigate various angles, ranging from parasites and coeliac disease, to mast cell activation disorder – so far with no conclusive results. We agreed to start by removing potentially challenging foods from his diet, especially caffeine, carbonated drinks, dairy, and gluten, and to increase wholesome, easily digestible foods. He was to take nine Slippery Elm blend capsules each day, two before and one after each meal. He was also to take two capsules of Cat's Claw (*Uncaria tomentosa*) each day, one after breakfast and one after supper. Within three weeks the improvement was remarkable. He looked better, and his diarrhoea was already much less troubling. After a further twelve weeks he began to have normal bowel movements again. He was gradually reducing his intake of Slippery Elm and Cat's Claw, maintaining his improvement through continued adherence to his new dietary regime.

Another, much older, patient had been suffering with acid reflux for many years and was feeling irritable and fed up. She ate late most evenings and enjoyed a glass of wine with her supper. She admitted that she never drank any water at all; between meals she liked to eat plenty of butter, cheese, and crackers. My priority was to encourage her to hydrate properly and change her eating habits for the better. This meant avoiding eating too late and having a break from the dairy products and the wine. I also recommended that she slept propped up with extra pillows to help fix the inflammation and incompetence of her oesophageal valve. Meanwhile, we were going to soothe the inflammation with Slippery Elm blend capsules and strengthen her digestion with gentle bitters, so that food was not hanging around for so long in her stomach.

She responded very well to the regime of capsules, and within a short space of time she was not experiencing any reflux and felt much better. She was, however, very resistant to making any dietary changes. After a couple of months of treatment, it came to light that she was continuing to indulge in all of the contraindicated foods at the same rate as when I had first met her. She was able to do this without flare-ups, provided she continued to take her relatively high doses of Slippery Elm. I explained about the conservation status of Slippery Elm and said that I could not in all conscience continue to supply her long-term at that rate if she was not prepared to at least try to follow my dietary advice. I reminded her that my intention was for her to have a temporary break from contraindicated foods so that she could reach a point where her oesophageal valve was healed and her digestive power was restored. She flatly refused to do this and demanded that I continue to supply her with heroic doses of Slippery Elm in order that she could continue with her preferred lifestyle. I sided with the Slippery Elm, and the patient and I parted company.

I find that this is a common problem with Slippery Elm. It produces such good results that patients can be lulled into thinking of it as an allopathic solution rather than a long-term holistic cure. For some patients the cost of the medicines proves to be no obstacle, and they do not see beyond their own desire to continue with their preferred damaging lifestyle habits. They love the fact that Slippery Elm gives them the ability to carry on as they have always done without too much discomfort, but this is simply not sustainable. It is not sustainable for their health and not sustainable for the planet. I do not believe that it is healthy to use any herb to prop up an unsustainable lifestyle in the long term, let alone a scarce or endangered species.

Historical applications

Slippery Elm is a medicine taught to us by the indigenous people of America. They have been living in harmony with it and respectfully harvesting what was needed for medicinal support for centuries.

Wych Elm (*Ulmus glabra*) inner bark was officinal in the British pharmacopoeia in 1864 and 1867. Like Slippery Elm, it is very mucilaginous and contains a significant amount of starch. It also contains some tannins, which give it astringent and anti-inflammatory virtues. A decoction of the bark was prescribed as a demulcent, and a medicinal tea was made from the flowers. Although Dutch Elm Disease has now devastated our native hedgerow Elms, they still regrow from suckers and tend to reach a height of 10–12 metres before being targeted by the beetles that spread the fungal disease. There are Elm suckers in every hedgerow here, and these could be a plentiful source of potentially valuable medicine. I am just beginning to explore our native Elm inner bark as a substitute for Slippery Elm, but I cannot report any clinical experience yet.

Magical

Slippery Elm is said to have the power to halt gossip. Burn it and throw a knotted yellow cord or thread into a fire with it. English Elm was once known as 'Elven' due to its popularity among elves. It protects against lightning strikes and attracts love when carried.

Suggestion for the home apothecary

Digestive system healing capsules

These capsules can be a helpful temporary support for patients with inflammatory gut symptoms, from acid reflux or stomach ulcers to diverticulitis and IBS. Blend equal parts of the powders of Slippery Elm, Marshmallow root, and Meadowsweet, and put them into size '0' capsules. You can also add Liquorice to this blend, although I prefer not to. You may think that decoctions would be easier, but in my experience capsules make it much easier for patients to comply with the strict dosage regime in the early stages of treatment. As a short-term measure, the patient should take 1–9 per day, depending on the severity of the inflammatory symptoms. It is absolutely essential that the patient makes the necessary dietary and lifestyle changes, no matter how daunting this may seem at first. In the majority of cases dairy, gluten, and caffeine need to

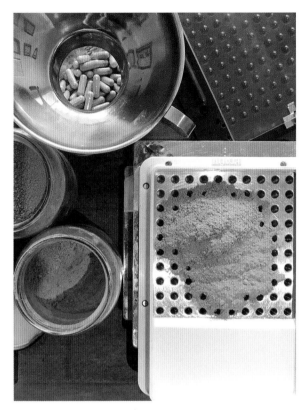

be removed while the healing process is taking place. When symptoms are very severe, 2 capsules should be taken before and 1 after each meal. It can be helpful for the patient to take a couple of Cat's Claw capsules per day alongside the healing capsules.

Small-flowered Willowherb 🌼 *Epilobium parviflorum*

'Small-Flowered Willowherb is a specific for supporting prostate health.'

I work solely with *Epilobium parviflorum*, because I was taught that it is a specific for supporting the prostate. Its cousin, Rose Bay Willowherb (*Epilobium angustifolium*), is well known as a substitute for tea and is prescribed as an astringent and a respiratory antispasmodic.

Medicinal parts
▷ Aerial parts

Physiological actions
Summary
▷ Diuretic
▷ Anti-inflammatory
▷ Antimicrobial

Physiological virtues

Small-flowered Willowherb can be very helpful in benign prostatic hyperplasia and also in some cases of prostate cancer. Research has indicated that it activates aptosis in human hormone-dependent prostate cancer cells. It is also a good general support for the urinary system. All of the Epilobium species also have anti-inflammatory, antioxidant, and antimicrobial virtues.

It is best harvested before the seed heads form if you want to avoid explosions of fluffy seeds in your processing area.

Energetics
Small-flowered Willowherb is astringent and bitter.

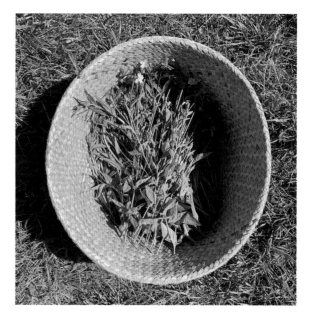

In Tibetan medicine
In Tibetan medicine this is called *Dukmo nyoong* [དུག་མོ་ཉུང་]. Its taste is bitter-to-sweet with a bitter post-digestive taste. It has a cool and rough potency. It is considered to be good to clear excess *Tripa* and is prescribed to stop diarrhoea due to fevers.

In my dispensary
I regularly prescribe Small-Flowered Willowherb, either as part of a tincture blend or in a capsule, to patients who suffer from benign prostatic hyperplasia. It is generally combined with other prostate-supporting herbs such as Nettle root, Saw Palmetto, and Pellitory-of-the-Wall.

Soapwort 🍂 *Saponaria officinalis*

'A saponin-containing expectorant and a cure for visceral obstructions and itching.'

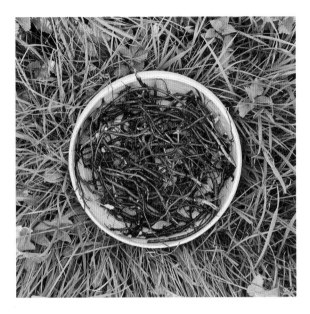

Soapwort is a beautiful, if rather enthusiastic, addition to the herb garden. The roots are harvested as a helpful expectorant due to their saponins. This also means that you can make natural shampoos or washing liquid from this plant. One of its country names is 'Latherwort'.

Medicinal parts
- Roots

Physiological actions

Summary
- Expectorant
- Emetic
- Antipruritic

Physiological virtues

Soapwort is, as its name suggests, rich in saponins. It is primarily an expectorant, thinning the mucus and making it easier to be expelled. When ingested in therapeutic doses, either as a tincture or a decoction of the finely chopped roots, it acts as a mild irritant to the stomach, encouraging expectoration due to a process known as reflex expectoration. When prescribed with skill, this herb is highly effective to support patients with bronchitis, asthma, and coughs in general. Ingesting large quantities of Soapwort is not recommended though, as it will result in emesis. In the past it was prescribed for jaundice and other visceral obstructions. It was considered a good cure for old venereal complaints 'where mercury had failed' and was recommended for any rheumatism or cutaneous issues that had arisen in consequence of syphilis infection.

A strong decoction applied topically is excellent to soothe itching. If you have Soapwort in your garden, try crushing a leaf and applying it to an itchy bug bite. You will immediately see what I mean.

Energetics

Soapwort is bitter. It is a good treatment to calm itching. On an energetic level, if we are experiencing significant itching, we may find it helpful to ask ourselves, 'What are we itching to do in our life?'

In my dispensary

I tend to work with Soapwort as an expectorant in tincture or capsule form. I blend it with other herbs, as indicated by the individual case. This means that Soapwort is kept at a low dose within each prescription. It is also an excellent herb to prescribe topically for patients experiencing significant itching (see below).

Historical applications

Culpeper wrote that it was: '*opening and attenuating and somewhat sudorific . . . it cures virulent gonorrhoeas by giving the inspissated* [i.e. reduced] *. . . juice of it to the amount of half an ounce daily.*'

Soapwort was used for cleaning cloth before the commercial production of soap began in the 1800s. It is gentle but effective. It is said that an infusion of Soapwort was used to gently clean the Bayeux tapestry during its restoration. If you are keen on using Soapwort as a cleaning agent, please bear in mind that even though the soapy compounds are totally natural, they can still be damaging to ponds and aquatic environments, just as ordinary soaps are.

Suggestion for the home apothecary

Decoction to soothe itching

Take a small handful of Soapwort roots and simmer them gently in 1 litre of water for 20 minutes. Strain and cool, then apply topically to the affected area. Any leftover decoction

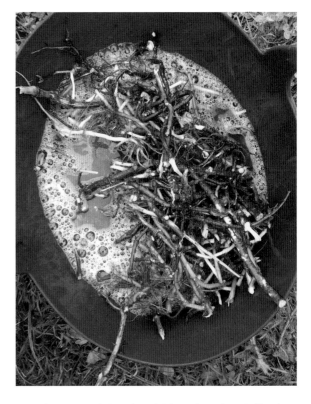

can be stored in the fridge for the following day. Alternatively, add the entire amount of the decoction to the bath water and soak in it. The image shows fresh roots being washed.

Solomon's Seal 🌿 *Polygonatum multiflorum/P. biflorum*

'Moistens, balances, and restores tissues which need to move and flex.'

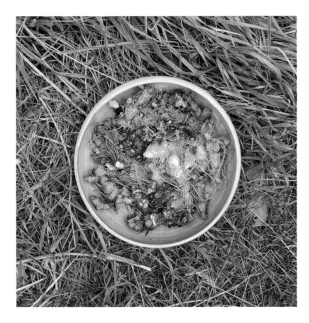

Solomon's Seal is also known as Lady's Seal or Dropberry. In the Lake District of England it was known as 'Vagabond's Friend' – a reference to its ability to quickly fix black eyes, bruises, and broken bones. It is one of those plants whose signature is quite clear. The word 'Polygonatum' means 'many knees', and its white fleshy rhizomes are jointed, with the appearance of knees. Also, the way that the leaves are held on the stalks is reminiscent of the way that muscles are attached to bones. The interior of the roots, when cut, bears a mark reminiscent of the Star of David, which was the seal of King Solomon – hence its common name.

I grow it in a shady area of my garden and love to see the flowers in the spring. I do not have an abundance of it, so I tend to work with it only in very specific situations – namely those relating to joints – rather than exploring its

wider medicinal actions in the respiratory and urinary systems, for example. If I had more of this beautiful herb available to me, I am sure that I would be turning to it much more often.

Medicinal parts

- ▷ Roots
- ▷ Rhizomes

The berries are poisonous.

Physiological actions

Summary

- ▷ Musculo-skeletal tonic
- ▷ Bone and ligament knitter
- ▷ Astringent
- ▷ Demulcent
- ▷ Anti-inflammatory
- ▷ Cardiotonic
- ▷ Adrenal tonic

Physiological virtues

Solomon's Seal promotes protein synthesis and is a very good herb for joints, supporting ligaments, cartilage, synovial fluid, and bone health. It is moistening and astringent, as well as a tonic, at the same time. This gives it the ability to act as an amphoteric support. For example, it is really helpful when the joints are inflamed and sore through a loss of synovial fluid, but it can also support joints and ligaments that are too pliable and prone to dislocation. Small doses help to tighten and tone them. Solomon's Seal is therefore worth considering as a support for patients with Ehler's Danlos Syndrome or other inherited hypermobility. It can play a very helpful role in reducing dislocations and improving tolerance to exercise. In cases of hypermobility, appropriate careful exercise is the best treatment, with Solomon's Seal being best prescribed at a very low dose (less than 10 ml of tincture per week). Its ability to tighten loose ligaments also makes it a suitable choice in cases of prolapse. Where there is uterine prolapse, be sure that any constipation is alleviated at the same time. Using a squatting rather than a 'sitting' position for defaecation is essential for those hoping to resolve this.

Solomon's Seal is anti-inflammatory and has the ability to help broken bones and ligaments to knit together. Consider it for repetitive strain injury, tennis elbow, carpal tunnel syndrome, mild tears of the meniscus of the anterior cruciate ligament, or partial tears of the rotator cuff. It is also helpful for intervertebral disc injuries or sacroiliac joint pain. It is especially good for slow-healing bones after major operations such as hip replacements. In these cases, prescribe it in a blend internally and apply the infused oil daily to the area around the wound (avoiding the wound itself until it is completely healed).

Solomon's Seal contains low levels of cardiac glycosides. This seems to support the heart, encouraging increased circulation through the capillary beds, nourishing it, and helping it to beat more regularly. It works on the venous system as a cardio tonic and is useful for mild cases of congestive heart failure when dyspnea and dry cough are present. It relaxes the heart and the tendons in the chest and lungs. Herbalist Christopher Hedley taught that Solomon's Seal was a good herb for elders, being especially good for elderly patients with thin, dry chests. I remember him teaching that it can be burned as a smudge to bring people back from the point of death, but this is not something I have tried.

Solomon's Seal is demulcent and moistening, so it can play a role in treatment for inflamed lungs or gastrointestinal tract. It can be prescribed for irritable bowel syndrome, dry constipation, a dry cough, and dry difficult-to-shift mucus. Please remember that it is essential to check that hydration is adequate rather than relying solely on herbs to treat 'dry' conditions. Too many people prefer to take a medicine or to rub something on rather than address unhelpful dietary or lifestyle factors. We should always aim to treat the root cause of a problem.

Solomon's Seal is said to help decalcify areas of excessive bone growth: bone spurs or bunions, for example. Matthew Wood wrote that this action is through correcting tensions in hips and legs that can cause uneven bone growth. When these tensions are resolved, the bone spurs dissolve. As a long-standing traditional 'bone-knitting' herb, we can see that Solomon's Seal has the ability to encourage recalcification when needed. It is also likely that part of Solomon's Seal's mode of action is the invigoration of the circulation to the affected area. It is worth noting that it is also very helpful in cases of osteoporosis. Christopher Hedley liked to combine it with a little Black Cohosh (*Actaea racemosa/Cimicifuga racemosa*) and some Vitamin K2 'to force the calcium into the bone'.

It is also a herb worth considering for adrenal insufficiency and cortisol excess, but keep it at a low level within the blend.

Energetics

Solomon's Seal is sweet, bitter, moistening, cooling, and astringent. It is a herb that has the ability to moisten and relax tissues at the same time as astringing and toning them.

In Tibetan medicine

Polygonatum cirrhifolium or *P. macrophyllum* are known as *Ra nye* [ར་སྙེ།]. They have a sweet, bitter, and astringent taste, with a sweet post-digestive taste. Their potency is mild, being cool, oily, and heavy. '*Ra nye*', the 'goat' version, cures cold *rLung* disorders, helps to resolve disorders of serous fluid, and encourages the digestive heat, prolonging life and making one more robust in old age. *Polygonatum oppositifolium* is the 'sheep' version, not the 'goat' version. It is called *Lug nye* [ལུག་མཉེ་]. It is also sweet and bitter-to-astringent but has a warming potency. It restores bodily strength and treats pain in the kidneys and waist region, fluid retention in the joints, weak digestive heat, first-stage oedema, as well as *rLung* diseases and erectile dysfunction. The Solomon's Seals are chosen for *chudlen* (life-prolonging treatments) as well as for cold-natured diarrhoea and belly pain when the patient drinks cold things. They reduce inflammation in the small intestine.

In my dispensary

In my own practice I especially reach for Solomon's Seal when there are joint issues associated with dryness or there is a tendency to hypermobility. If I had more abundant supplies available, I am sure that I would prescribe more liberally and in more situations.

'Jilly' was 65 years old and came for help because she was suffering with quite severe scleroderma and felt tired and low. This is an autoimmune condition associated with inflammation and the production of excessive collagen in connective tissues, particularly skin and joints. She described the tendons and joints in her wrists as feeling constricted and 'squeaky', so I immediately knew that she needed Solomon's Seal in her blend. Her digestion and circulation also needed support, and I advised removing gluten and dairy from her diet. I also prescribed a tincture blend made up of digestive and circulation-supporting herbs that she was to take twice a day. I included Solomon's Seal at a rate of approximately 10% of the blend.

Jilly enthusiastically embraced the lifestyle and dietary changes that I suggested and took her herbal medicine consistently. The constric-

tion and 'squeakiness' in her wrists disappeared within a month, and over the next few months her energy levels gradually began to increase and her skin began to look and feel more supple. Although the Solomon's Seal made up only a relatively small proportion of the blend, I knew that it had a very large influence on her joint 'squeakiness', partly because this is typical for Solomon's Seal, but also because the response was so swift compared to the gradual improvement in other areas.

'Ellie' was in her early 60s and had always suffered with hypermobility. As a result of her joint instability, she found that her muscles were prone to being very tight, and her pelvis and sacroiliac area tended to be out of balance. She wanted to feel more stable and hoped that herbal medicine could help her. I prescribed a tincture blend to help relax her muscles and support her circulation, and I added Solomon's Seal. Within four weeks she reported that she felt 'much less floppy'.

Historical applications

Gerard referenced Dioscorides: '*Dioscorides writeth, That the roots are excellent good for to seale or close up greene wounds, being stamped and laid thereon; whereupon it was called "Sigillum Salomonis", of the singular virtue that it hath in sealing or healing up wounds, broken bones, and such like. Some have thought it took the name "sigillum" of the markes upon the roots: but the first reason seems to be more probable. . . . The root of Solomons seale stamped while it is fresh and greene, and applied, taketh away in one night, or two at most, any bruise, blacke or blew spots gotten by fals or womens wilfulnesse, in stumbling upon their hasty husbands fists, or such like.*'

'*Galen saith, that neither herbe nor root hereof is to be given inwardly: but not what experience hath found out, and of late daies, especially among the vulgar sort of people in Hampshire which Galen, Dioscorides, or any other that have written of plants so much as dreamed of; which is, That if any of what sex or age soever chance to have any bones broken, in what part of their bodies soever, their refuge is to stampe and apply outwardly in manner of a pultesse, as well unto themselves as their cattell.'*

'The root stamped and applied in manner of a pultesse, and laid upon members that have been out of joynt, and newly restored to their places, driveth away the paine, and knitteth the joynt very firmly, and aketh away the inflammation, if there chance be any. . . . The same stamped, and the juyce given to drinke with aleor white wine, as aforesaid, or the decoction thereof made in wine, helps any inward bruise, diperseth the congealed and clotted bloud in very short space.'

Parkinson described the qualities of Solomon's Seal as *'having partly a binding and partly a sharpe or biting quality, as also a loathesome bitternesse therein, hardly to be expressed, whereby it is of little use in inward medicines; which sharpenesse and loathsomenesse we hardly perceive in those that grow with us . . .'.*

Magical

During the late Middle Ages there was some debate about the most appropriate name for the plant. The great Solomon had been a conjurer, enchanter, and philosopher. His seal was a star of David, and this carried with it connotations of magic, mysticism, and the occult. Herbalist, Turner, who was a staunch Protestant and disapproved of the name 'Solomon's Seal', tried to encourage the use of the name 'Whyte Wurt' from the German name *Weiss Wurz*, but luckily – in the English language at least – the original name 'Solomon's Seal' has stuck and is much more memorable than White Wort.

Solomon's Seal is ruled by Saturn and is associated with the element of Water. It is said that if you place it in the four quarters of the house, it will provide protection for the inhabitants. Sprinkling an infusion of the roots is considered to clear away evil. It can be chosen as an ingredient in offertory incenses.

Suggestion for the home apothecary

Solomon's-Seal-infused oil

Take fresh, clean, surface-dry Solomon's Seal root, and slice it thinly. Place the slices into a clean, dry jar and cover completely with olive oil. Leave in a dark place for at least 4 weeks, then strain and bottle. Fresh Solomon's Seal root has a rather 'cheesy' aroma, so you may prefer to add some Lavender flowers to the blend to improve the fragrance. Apply daily to weak or injured joints. If the patient has a broken bone, apply above and below the cast. It may be more convenient to set the infused oil into an ointment. (See Plantain for instructions.)

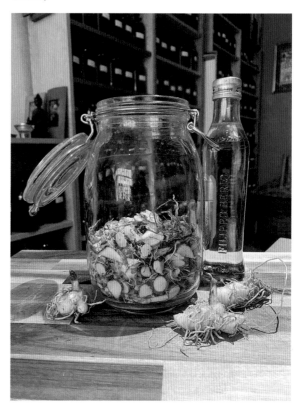

Spearmint 🌿 *Mentha spicata*

'Spearmint helps to counteract excessive androgens in women.'

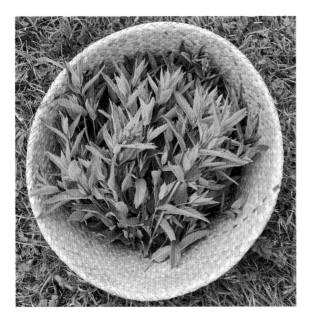

Spearmint shares many of the same medicinal virtues as Peppermint, but it has its own entry in this book because it has the very special and helpful property of counteracting excessive androgens. This makes it a great herb to consider for patients suffering from polycystic ovary syndrome (PCOS).

Medicinal parts

▷ Aerial parts

Physiological actions

Summary

▷ Antiandrogenic
▷ Blood sugar balancer
▷ Nervine
▷ (For other actions, see Peppermint)

Physiological virtues

Spearmint is a specific for counteracting excessive androgens in women with PCOS and thereby reducing the symptoms associated with such excess, including hirsutism. This can be through drinking the tea regularly, taking the tincture, or by applying topically. Spearmint is full of antioxidants, is anti-inflammatory, and can assist in balancing blood sugar – another reason why it can be helpful for those with PCOS.

It is a good herb to choose for hiccoughs, indigestion, and wind. It gently increases sweating and can help to reduce fevers, but it is more relaxing in action than its cousin, Peppermint. This makes it a good choice for soothing feverish children.

Like Peppermint, it should be avoided by those who suffer with acid reflux or hiatus hernia.

Energetics

Spearmint is warming, drying, and astringent.

In my dispensary

I work with Spearmint in tincture and tea blends, according to the individual needs of my patients, especially those with excess androgens. I also love it, mixed with Sage, Myrrh, and Calendula, as part of a mouthwash tincture blend. The patient dilutes ½ tsp of this in a quarter of a cup of water and swills thoroughly.

Historical applications

Spearmint has a long history of medicinal and culinary use. The ancient Greeks added it to bath water and chose it for oral hygiene. It was probably introduced into Northern Europe by the Romans, and by Chaucer's time – the 1300s – it was a garden plant. In those days people rubbed the leaves onto their teeth and gums as a cleanser.

In Greek mythology, the beautiful water nymph Minthe was pursued by Pluto, God of the Underworld. His wife, Persephone, in a rage, turned her into a plant that would be trodden underfoot. Unable to reverse the spell, Pluto caused mint to release a beautiful fragrance.

Although Spearmint seems 'cooling' due to its fever-reducing effects, Dioscorides described it as having '*a heating, binding and drying quality*'. He suggested that '*taking two or three branches in the juice of four pomegranates would alay the choler*'.

Suggestions for the home apothecary

Garden tea

Add Spearmint to your daily 'garden tea'. Garden tea is designed to vary with each day and should consist of as many different medicinal garden or foraged herbs as possible. The idea is that you are not having an intense dose of any one particular herb. This means there is much less chance of your system being inadvertently thrown off balance if you are not totally sure which herbs will be best for your circumstances.

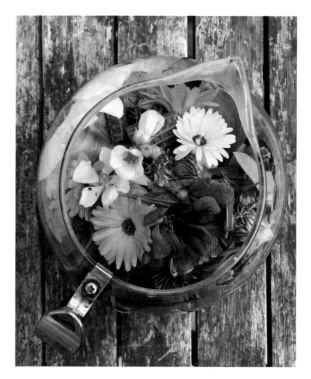

Try to include at least 8 different herbs, and aim to vary them each day.

If you need inspiration, you could consider the following: Spearmint, Peppermint, Rosemary, Sage, Lavender, Marshmallow, Lemon Balm, Rose petals, Red Clover, Plantain leaves, Echinacea flowers, Mallow flowers, Wild Strawberry, Raspberry leaf, Lemon Verbena, Hollyhock flower, Mugwort, Calendula, Honeysuckle, and many, many more.

St John's Wort 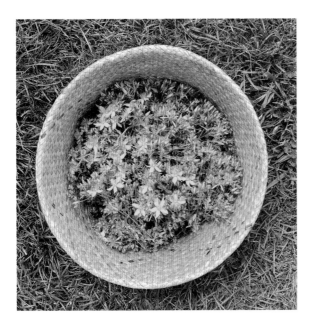 *Hypericum perforatum*

'St John's Wort is so much more than a natural antidepressant.'

The generic name '*Hypericum*' comes from the Greek and means 'over an apparition'. This is because it was believed to strongly repel evil spirits. In the Middle Ages it was prescribed as a psychotherapeutic remedy. This was a time when evil spirits were considered to be responsible for much health mischief. One of its folk names is 'Fuga Daemonum', which means 'Devil's flight'. Its specific name comes from the fact that, when held up to the light, the leaves appear to be full of tiny holes. These are oil glands producing the well-known and much loved bright red healing sap.

Many people like to make a gorgeous red infused oil with fresh flowers during the summer, and St John's Wort is a very well-known topical treatment. Yet it also has a myriad medicinal virtues when prescribed internally. Nowadays, it is most frequently prescribed as an antidepressant. This does not, in my view, properly respect its holistic potential. In fact, I most often prescribe St John's Wort as an expectorant.

Medicinal parts
- Flowers
- Tops

Physiological actions

Summary

- Expectorant
- Bitter
- Vulnerary
- Antiseptic
- Anti-inflammatory
- Antiviral
- Nervous system healer
- Antidepressant
- Antispasmodic
- Hypotensive

Physiological virtues

St John's Wort is first and foremost an expectorant herb, traditionally prescribed in cases of chronic consumption or chronic catarrhal states. It is a bitter, so, as well as encouraging the removal of catarrh through expectoration, it helps to enliven the digestive system. This reduces the formation of catarrh at the source.

Its antiseptic and astringent properties make it an excellent wound healer, whether taken internally, as in the case of peptic ulcers, or applied topically for cuts, eczema, scrapes, burns, and insect bites. It is pain-relieving, which makes topical applications especially soothing. It is also antiviral so is well indicated for shingles and cold sores. It can be applied either as an infusion or as an infused oil or ointment.

It is a gentle diuretic, helpful in cases of urinary retention, and it can also be good as part of a strategy to treat nocturnal urinary incontinence in children.

It has long been known as a herb for the nervous system. It is a specific for inflamed or damaged nerve endings – think of an injured coccyx or recurrent shingles, for example. It is also very helpful for any neuralgia or sciatica, even when the cause is not known.

It has antispasmodic properties and can help to relieve spasms in the gastrointestinal tract and the biliary system. It relaxes the peripheral circulatory system, so can be effective in reducing hypertension. Lastly, it helps to support patients with nervous exhaustion and depression. It may be helpful in the treatment of addictions.

Much research has been carried out on St John's Wort since the discovery that it acts as a natural serotonin reuptake inhibitor. It is perhaps more researched than any other herb; but the downside of this is that it now has a very long list of contraindications, based on non-holistic prescribing practices. One of the reasons that I rarely prescribe St John's Wort as an 'antidepressant' is that I prefer to prescribe herbs in short courses rather than creating long-term dependency. I would much rather treat the underlying root cause and encourage the patient to maintain their new healthful balance with dietary and lifestyle adjustments. If herbs are taken in very large doses – perhaps based on predicted levels of constituents required to produce a therapeutic effect – or are taken daily over a period of many years, the potential for contraindications is increased.

Like many other bitter herbs, St John's Wort can increase detoxification activity within the liver; it is therefore often considered contraindicated with allopathic medications. In this case, the activity of both the CYP3A4 and the CYP2C9 enzyme pathways is increased. The CYP3A4 enzyme pathway is involved in the metabolism of more than 50% of allopathic medications. While enhanced detoxification via the liver is usually considered to be a positive thing, it could be cause for concern when patients are taking a carefully calculated dose of allopathic drugs, such as HIV protease inhibitors, insulin sensitizers, antibiotics, chemotherapy agents, or the contraceptive pill. Additionally, like many herbs, St John's Wort could, theoretically, with large enough regular doses, cause blood thinning, and it is known to cause photosensitivity.

Energetics
St John's Wort is bitter, astringent, sweet, and cooling.

In Tibetan medicine
The species of Hypericum included in the Tibetan pharmacopoeia is *Hypericum bellum*. It is called *Ja shing dwang phyug* [ཇ་ཤིང་དྭང་ཕྱུག]. It has a bitter-to-astringent taste with coarse and light characteristics and a cooling potency. It treats hot disorders of the liver, fever accompanied with cold, oral inflammation, dysentery, itching, and skin disorders.

According to the wisdom of Tibetan medicine, taking St John's Wort over a long period will increase *rLung*. Since much anxiety, insomnia, and mental agitation is due to excess *rLung*, the Western practice of prescribing St John's Wort over a long period to support mental health is likely to worsen the underlying root cause. In these cases, symptoms would be very likely to return as soon as the St John's Wort was ceased, meaning that the treatment strategy had created dependence on the medicine. This tendency can be lessened to some extent if the patient increases the quantity of oily, rich, nutritious foods in their diet – by consuming, for example, bone broth, sesame oil, and Oats.

In my dispensary

I work with St John's Wort in the form of tincture, teas, capsules, and topical treatments. I especially love it for patients needing respiratory support or physical nerve healing. I very rarely prescribe it for its antidepressant activity.

'Mary' was in her early 70s and, after a period of stress, came down with a painful attack of shingles. She had animals to care for and could not afford to be incapacitated. She came to one of my drop-in sessions for help, and I gave her some St John's Wort-infused oil, telling her to apply it frequently to the affected area. She told me that the relief was almost instantaneous, calling it a 'miracle oil'.

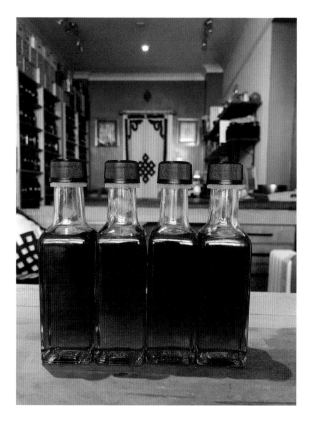

The shingles healed quickly, and she was not troubled with it again.

'Maisie' was in her late 70s and had recently developed severe adult-onset asthma. She had had a frightening episode of breathing difficulties and was admitted to hospital, and she wanted to avoid it happening again. She had been prescribed two inhalers but often still felt wheezy. She was nervous and wanted more support. When I went through her case, she told me that her digestion was sluggish, and for the past forty years she had suffered with regular episodes of shingles and post-herpetic neuralgia. She had also had a bad skiing accident in the past in which she had injured her coccyx, and it still gave her trouble. It was clear that St John's Wort was needed here on several levels.

I prescribed it in her personalized tincture blend as well as in the respiratory-system-supporting capsules that I gave her alongside. She also had some St John's Wort-infused oil to apply topically, as needed. I had a long chat with her about her lifestyle and diet, which resulted in her resolving to make some much-needed big changes, quitting smoking being one of them. She did well with her herbal support, her breathing improving greatly, her post-herpetic neuralgia being much less troubling and her digestive system was much better. She is still working on giving up smoking, but she is smoking much less than she had been.

Historical applications

Gerard wrote: '*Saint Johns wort hath brownish stalks beset with many small and narrow leaves which if you behold betwixt your eis and the light, do appeare as it were bored or thrust thorow in an infinite number of places with pinnes points . . . the leaves, floures, and seeds stamped, and put into a glasse with oile olive, and set in the hot sun for certain weeks together, and then strained from those herbs, and the like quantitie of new put in and sunned in like manner, doth make*

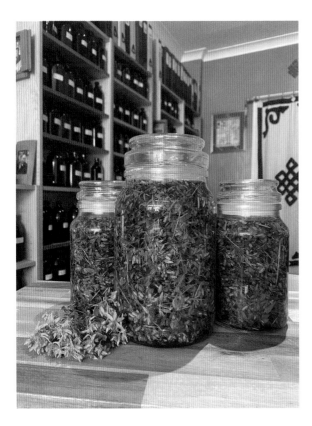

an oile of the colour of bloud which is most pretious remedie for deep wounds and those that are thorow the body, for the sinues that are prickt, or any wound made with a venomed weapon.' This last point refers to the infused oil being considered the best treatment for deep sword wounds.

Parkinson said that this herb: '*hath power to open obstructions, to dissolve tumours, to consolidate or soder the lips of wounds, and to strengthen the parts that are weake and feeble*'.

He described how to make a triple infusion of St John's Wort flowers in oil using the warmth of the sun – a formulation which appeals to me much more than his description of another compound oil made with St John's Wort flowers: Dittany of Crete, Gentian, Blessed Thistle, Tormentil, and earthworms '*washed and slit*'.

Magical

St John's Wort has a traditional association with scaring away devils or evil influences. If gathered at Midsummer and worn, it was considered to keep mental illness at bay and cure sadness. It was placed in the window to protect against thunderbolts, fire, and evil spirits. Soldiers would wear it to make them invincible. When placed against the mouth of accused witches, it was believed that this would force them to confess. It is perhaps surprising that it is also considered as attracting love.

Suggestion for the home apothecary

Infused oil

Loosely fill a jar with freshly harvested St John's Wort flowering tops and cover it with mild and light olive oil. Cover the jar with muslin cloth to allow moisture to escape and leave it on a sunny windowsill. If you do not have a sunny windowsill, you can warm the jar in a gentle water bath made in a slow cooker. Once the oil has turned a deep red, it is ready to drain and bottle. Be careful to leave the bottom watery layer behind when decanting the oil. Apply as needed to cuts, scrapes, burns, and areas with nerve pain – such as sciatica, shingles, or peripheral neuralgia. Do not take the infused oil internally.

Teasel 🌱 *Dipsacus fullonum*

'Teasel strengthens ligaments and helps us to better carry our loads in life.'

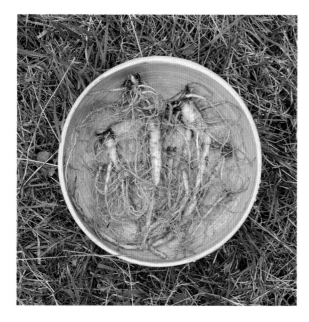

Teasel is specific for strengthening joints and ligaments while also acting as a tonic for liver and kidneys. It is a biennial, and it is the vibrant young roots of the first-year plant that are harvested. In its second year the plant grows tall and produces its iconic spiky flower heads, but at this stage the root system becomes woody and depleted. It has done its job.

Medicinal part
▷ Roots (first-year)

Physiological actions

Summary
▷ Anti-inflammatory
▷ Alterative
▷ Bitter
▷ Tonic

Physiological virtues

Teasel root has long been used in traditional Chinese medicine to 'tonify the liver and kidneys' and to ease painful joints. In general, it promotes healthy circulation and reduces inflammation.

Herbalist Matthew Wood describes Teasel root as 'invaluable' for joint injury and chronic muscle inflammation. It is especially valuable for patients with injuries to large joints, such as shoulders or hips. Consider Teasel in cases of fibromyalgia, chronic arthritis, and Lyme disease.

Japanese Teasel root is known as *Xu Duan*, which means 'restore what is broken'. As well as healing damaged tissues, it is prescribed for arthritis, to promote healthy blood circulation, as well as kidney cleansing.

Energetics

Teasel is bitter and slightly sweet. It is a strong and structural plant. It helps us to better carry the loads that we take on in life. When we experience joint pain or injury, it can often be associated with doing too much or carrying excess weight, either in terms of our own body weight or in terms of a physical burden. Teasel helps us to strengthen our joints and ligaments, making us more resilient. It also helps us to see that we need to be mindful of the loads that we take on.

In my dispensary

I usually prescribe Teasel in tincture form for patients who have joint injuries or whose ligaments need support. I especially think of it if I have a patient who is prone to taking on too

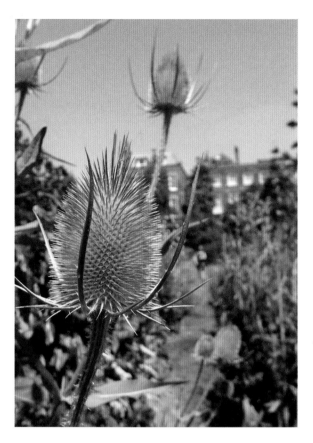

much and who has a longstanding injury to one of the large joints in their body.

Historical applications

The old name for Teasel is "Venus' Basin" due to the way that water collects in the hollow formed by the leaves joining the stem. The water there was considered as curative, especially for warts and as an eye wash. Romany lore teaches that Teasel water cures wrinkles and dark circles under the eyes.

Culpeper wrote that the roots of Teasel '*have a cleansing faculty*'; he also described how Dioscorides recommended an ointment made out of the roots for warts, wens, cankers, and fistulas.

Other old writers recommend Teasel roots for improving the appetite and as a remedy for jaundice.

Magical

A bouquet of dried Teasel kept in the house is considered to repel mischievous sprites that come in and hide your possessions.

Thyme 🍃 *Thymus vulgaris/T. serpyllum*

'Thyme helps us to breathe more freely.'

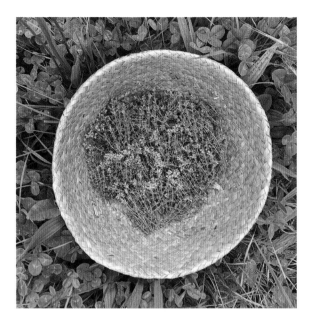

I grow Thyme in my garden and love it, but I have a very special affection for Wild Thyme (*Thymus serpyllum*). When I lived in Dorset, I had permission to gather Wild Thyme from a beautiful area of unspoiled chalk downland. I used to love climbing up the steep track through the trees and coming out onto this glorious herbal paradise. It always reminded me of the famous lines from Shakespeare's *A Midsummer Night's Dream*:

> *'I know a bank where the wild thyme blows,*
> *Where oxslips and the nodding violet grows,*
> *Quite overcanopied with luscious woodbine,*
> *With sweet musk-roses, and with Eglantine.'*
>
> [*A Midsummer Night's Dream*, II.1.249–252]

Wild Thyme has a serpent-like growth habit, hence its Latin name. It has medicinal properties that are very similar to those of garden Thyme, but it is gentler and more subtle. Wild Thyme is known as 'Mother of Thyme'.

Medicinal parts
▷ Aerial parts

Aerial parts are gathered while flowering.

Physiological actions

Summary

▷ Antiviral
▷ Antimicrobial
▷ Diaphoretic
▷ Expectorant
▷ Antispasmodic
▷ Sedative
▷ Antitussive
▷ Bitter
▷ Vermifuge
▷ Diuretic

Physiological virtues

Thyme is a heating diaphoretic, so it pushes the blood to the surface of the body and encourages sweating. It has a significant antimicrobial and antiviral action as well as helping to thin mucus and disinfect the mucous membranes. It encourages the expectoration of stubborn phlegm. As an antispasmodic, it eases coughs, too, so all in all it is an ideal herb to take as a tea if you have a cold. It is such a good respiratory herb that it is considered particularly helpful in severe influenza, whooping cough, chest infections, and bronchitis. If taken regularly, Thyme can reduce asthma.

It contains bitter principles that encourage the secretion of gastric fluids so can be helpful for dyspepsia and sluggish digestion. It is a vermifuge and can be a good herb to include in a herbal strategy to help rid children of threadworms. Thyme helps to eliminate uric acid from the body. Consider it in gout, arthritis, and rheumatism.

Thyme is a gentle diuretic and that action, combined with its antimicrobial action, makes it a useful first aid treatment for cystitis. This is worth remembering, because even if you are travelling away from home, it is very likely that you will be able to source it. Drink as a tea, and, if possible, combine it with a demulcent herb such as Marshmallow Leaf, Plantain, or Cornsilk.

Thyme is so readily available that it is worth knowing about all of its first aid actions. Applied topically, it is an excellent antiseptic wound wash, also for boils and dermatitis. As a compress, it can be excellent at shifting slow-healing skin disorders.

Its calming and antispasmodic action makes it a good first aid option to reduce period pains. It has an overall soothing and sedating action. If you have a child prone to nightmares, try giving them a foot bath of Thyme before bed.

Above all, Thyme helps us to breathe more freely. For patients struggling with respiratory issues, a chest or back poultice can bring quick relief from severe coughing. It can help to remove the panic associated with not being able to catch your breath.

Medicinal doses of Thyme should be avoided in pregnancy and hypertension.

Energetics
Thyme is pungent, slightly bitter, warming, and drying.

In Tibetan medicine
As a warming and drying herb, it is a good one to consider for patients suffering with increased *Pekén*. This is consistent with its Western herbal application to drive away phlegm and support digestion.

In my dispensary
In my practice, I prepare Thyme as a tincture, in teas, and also in capsules. I often reach for it in cases requiring respiratory support. The following case is quite a good example of where Thyme is well indicated.

'Adrian' was 48 years old and often had colds that would go to his chest. He had a permanently streaming nose and found it challenging to walk up hills without coughing and wheezing, especially in cold weather. He looked pale and said he was exhausted all the time. He had recently been diagnosed with adult onset asthma and had been prescribed a preventer and a reliever inhaler that had helped a bit, but he wanted to feel better.

I felt that Thyme would be a good support for him and prescribed it in a personalized tincture blend as well as in a respiratory-system-supporting capsule blend. I also asked him to cut out dairy and drink more water. I warned him that he was likely to experience increased expectoration once he started taking his herbal medicines. Four weeks later he reported that he had been coughing up 'gunk', but his energy level was better, and his appetite was improved. His lower conjunctiva, which had been very pale at the first consultation, looked a better colour. He said he had had a couple of breathless episodes at night, but on the whole his breathing felt much better. Another four weeks later he noticed that his tendency to breathlessness on exertion was less, and he did not need his reliever inhaler as often. His streaming nose seemed to have calmed down too. After another couple of months of treatment, he reported that his energy level was now quite good, and he was noticeably much less breathless. I noticed that he was no longer pale and had some colour in his cheeks. He told me that he was very happy because he had been able to walk up a local steep hill without needing to stop on the way up, as he had used to have to.

Historical applications

The Romans believed that burning Thyme would repel scorpions. Pliny considered Thyme to be an antidote for snake bites, '*poison of marine creatures*', and headaches.

John Pechey, in his '*Compleat Herbal of Physical Plants*' published in 1694, said of Thyme: '*Tis hot and dry. It forces the Courses, and Urine. Tis Cephalick, Uterine, and Stomackick. Tis good for spitting of Blood, and convulsions, and for Gripes. Outwardly applied, it cures Headaches, and Giddiness; and disposes to Sleep.*'

Parkinson recommended Thyme '*to purge flegme*'. It was prescribed in the form of a decoction with honey, salt, and vinegar.

Culpeper wrote: '*It is a noble strengthener of the lungs, as notable a one as grows; neither is there scarce a better remedy growing for that disease in children which they commonly call the chin-cough, than it is. It purges the body of phlegm, and is an excellent remedy for shortness of breath. It kills worms in the belly, and being a notable herb of Venus, provokes the terms, gives safe and speedy delivery to women in travail, and brings away the after-birth. It is so harmless you need not fear the use of it. An ointment made of it takes away hot swellings and warts, helps the sciatica and fullness of sight, and takes away pains and hardness of the spleen: it is excellent for those that are troubled with the gout; is also, to anoint the testicles that are swelled. It eases pains in the loins and hips. The herb taken any way inwardly, comforts the stomach much, and expels wind.*'

Of Wild Thyme, he wrote: '*It is excellent in nervous disorders. A strong infusion of it, drank in the manner of tea, is pleasant, and a very effectual remedy for headaches, giddiness, and other disorders of that kind; and it is a certain remedy for that troublesome complaint, the nightmare.*'

Carolus Linnaeus liked Thyme to ease hangovers and headaches.

Magical

The folklore of Thyme is fascinating. The souls of the dead were said to rest in the flowers, and sprigs of Thyme were added to a ritual drink to commune with the departed. In England it is not considered advisable to bring Wild Thyme into the house because of this association. For me, Thyme is associated with healing and the restoration of life. I guess it depends on your perspective.

In a magical context, Thyme is burned to attract good health and to purify a space. Highlands and Islands folk have a tradition of drinking Wild Thyme tea to prevent bad dreams and to impart strength and courage. Wearing Thyme on one's person is considered to help one develop and strengthen one's psychic powers, and it is said that women who wear a sprig of Thyme in their hair make themselves irresistible to potential lovers.

Suggestions for the home apothecary

Thyme tea

Drinking a cup of Thyme infusion daily is a great preventive measure. Simply use 1 tsp of dried herb per cup and pour on boiling water and leave, covered, to steep for at least 10 minutes so it is quite strong. If you do succumb to a respiratory infection, you can increase the dosage to 5 cups per day.

Thyme tea as bath

Thyme also works very well as a foot or hand bath. This is useful for those who struggle to consume the required amount internally. Make

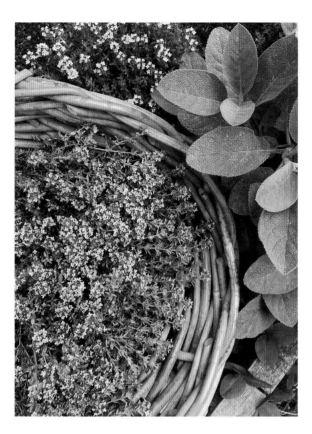

570 ml/1 pint of strong Thyme tea and add it to a bowl. Once cooled to a bearable temperature, soak the feet or hands in it for 30 minutes. You can combine a hand bath with a steam inhalation if you cover your bowl and your head with a cloth.

Thyme poultice or soak

You can also make a chest poultice with Thyme. Alternatively, you can soak cloths in the hot tea, wring them out and apply them to the chest area (taking care to avoid scalding). Replace the cloths frequently so that the treatment continues for 30 minutes each session. Keep the area warm with a hot water bottle while it is in place. You will need to cover the fomentation area with extra layers so the hot water bottle does not burn the patient.

Thyme syrup

If you make a strong jug of Thyme tea and add an equal amount of honey, you have made a simple syrup that may be more palatable for children.

Turmeric 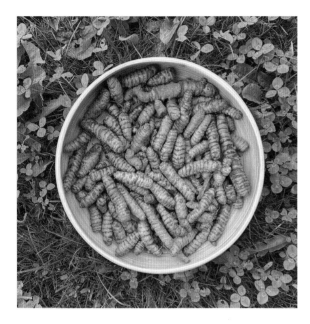 *Curcuma longa*

'Turmeric is a golden herbal treasure trove.'

The name 'Turmeric' is thought to come from the Latin '*terra merita*', which means 'meritorious earth'. Known as '*Haldi*' in Hindi and '*Jiang huang*' in Chinese, it is a very valuable medicine for a wide range of health conditions as well as being a delicious culinary ingredient. It is often described as a universal cure-all, but medicinal doses do not suit all constitutions.

Medicinal part
- Rhizomes

Physiological actions

Summary
- Anti-inflammatory
- Bitter
- Cholagogue
- Blood sugar balancer
- Antidepressant
- Cardiovascular tonic
- Antibacterial

Physiological virtues

Turmeric is a potent anti-inflammatory herb and can be a good choice in cases of inflammatory bowel disease or gastritis. It is an excellent digestive and liver support, helping to normalize blood sugar response. This makes it applicable in cases of insulin resistance and blood sugar swings. It also stimulates the secretion of bile, helping to improve the regularity of bowel function, and it acts as an overall tonic to the liver, being a traditional remedy for jaundice. Turmeric can alleviate depression and is a mood stabilizer, perhaps through its liver-supporting action.

Its anti-inflammatory action can help to reduce the pain of arthritis, and through this mechanism it may have a comparable effect on reducing joint pain to that of hydrocortisone. For the same reason it is also an excellent herb to consider for the treatment of eczema and psoriasis.

Turmeric promotes cardiovascular health as it inhibits blood clotting, reduces inflammation in the vessels, and helps to lower cholesterol levels. It seems that it may have a protective effect against Alzheimer's too. It is rich in antioxidants; in India is traditionally considered to slow the aging process. It is a very good support for cancer patients and those in recovery from cancer.

Turmeric stimulates the uterus and may reduce fertility. It may be worth avoiding taking large doses if you are trying to conceive.

It has become a hugely popular herb that is often touted as being suitable for every patient and in every health condition. However, be aware that it is rather heating and drying, and it does not suit everyone. Certain constitutions do not do too well taking Turmeric without balancing it with other cooling and moistening herbs, such as Marshmallow or Plantain.

The absorption of Turmeric is greatly enhanced when it is mixed with a little – for example, 1% – Black Pepper. It is also better to take it with fats, so mix the powder in with hot milk (or plant milk) or take your capsules with a balanced meal.

Topically, Turmeric can be applied to wounds to prevent infection and speed healing. Just mix it with a little coconut oil to make a paste. When applied to the skin and exposed to the sunlight, Turmeric is strongly antibacterial. This is due to the presence of curcumin, which is more strongly antioxidant than Vitamin E.

Energetics
Turmeric is hot, bitter, and astringent.

In Tibetan medicine
In Tibetan medicine, Turmeric is known as *Yung ba* [ཡུང་བ]. Its taste is slightly bitter and hot, with a bitter post-digestive taste. Its potency is oily, rough, and warm. The texts say that it reduces infection and inflammation, counteracts poisons, and stops tissue degeneration, such as in the case of necrosis. It is good to treat neurological disorders and haemorrhoids. It is said to 'defeat infectious diseases'. It is also helpful in cases of polyuria. When taken with whey, it is said to act as an anaphrodisiac.

In my dispensary
I often prescribe Turmeric capsules to patients suffering with inflammatory joint disease. I make these with the addition of 1% ground Black Pepper, to enhance absorption. Patients are advised to take the capsules with a meal

or some non-dairy milk, since absorption is enhanced when it is consumed with fats.

I infuse coconut oil with Turmeric and Ginger to make a topical anti-inflammatory preparation. Patients tell me that this blend is very effective for painful joints.

Historical applications
Turmeric was first mentioned as a Chinese medicinal herb in the Tang *Materia Medica*, written by Su Jing in 659 AD. It has an extremely long history of being considered a medicine and a food throughout Asia. It is, however, a relatively recent addition to the European *materia medica*. This is illustrated by Maud Grieve's entry for it, written in 1931: '*Turmeric is a mild aromatic stimulant seldom used in medicine except as a colouring.*'

Magical
Turmeric is a symbol of prosperity. It is also associated with purification. In Hawaiian magic it is mixed with salt water and sprinkled around the area that requires purification.

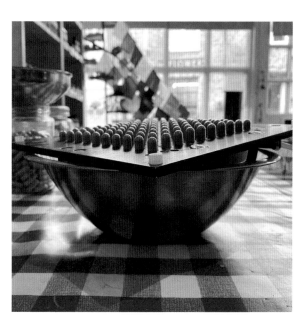

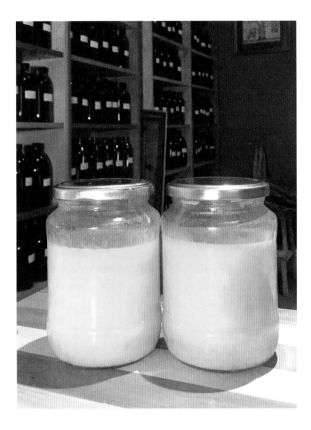

Suggestion for the home apothecary

Turmeric- and Ginger-infused Coconut oil for painful joints

Take equal parts of fresh Turmeric rhizome and fresh Ginger rhizome. Slice thinly and place in a slow cooker that has a 'warm' setting (the 'low' setting is too hot). Cover with Coconut oil and apply gentle warmth for just one hour per day for 3–4 days. Once it is ready and the oil is warm and melted, strain and pour into clean, dry jars. If you do not have a slow cooker or one with a 'warm' setting, you will need to use a water bath method. Place the herbs and the oil into a double boiler and warm gently for an hour before straining and pouring into jars. The oil should never be heated directly.

Massage into painful joints twice a day.

Valerian ❦ *Valeriana officinalis*

Valerian is a relaxing nervine, often prescribed for insomnia and anxiety. A cup of Valerian tea taken half an hour before bedtime is, in my view, far more effective and less damaging than a diazepam tablet. You will have to keep the cup away from your cat, though: cats love the smell of Valerian and become intoxicated by the fragrance. This is somewhat surprising, since many humans think that Valerian smells of sweaty socks; Dioscorides even named it '*Phu*' because of its odour. But even if you find the aroma unappealing – personally, I like it – it is worth getting over that, since it is an excellent herb.

Medicinal parts

▷ Aromatic roots
▷ Flowers (sometimes)

Physiological actions

Summary

▷ Nervine
▷ Sedative
▷ Antispasmodic
▷ Anodyne
▷ Stimulant (for some people)

Physiological virtues

Valerian contains a group of aromatic-oil-soluble compounds that are sedative in action.

The main virtues of this herb are that it is relaxing, pain-relieving, sleep inducing, and antispasmodic. This makes Valerian a hugely valuable and adaptable herb in the dispensary. Far from being a herb just for insomnia and anxiety, it can be constructively prescribed for a multitude of other conditions, including

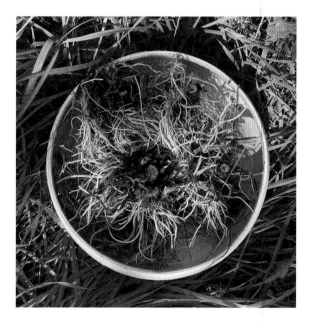

urinary-tract, respiratory, digestive, and circulatory issues, and for relaxing the muscles where tension or spasm is interfering with normal physiological function.

Consider Valerian when there is griping in the intestines or other stress-related issues in the gut. It is also a good choice for tension-related pains in the female reproductive system, for example dysmenorrhea.

Valerian relaxes the smooth muscles of the circulatory system, helping the blood to flow more freely when the vessels are narrowed by tension. This is why Valerian may be helpful in hypertension as well as in cases of impaired peripheral circulation such as Raynaud's syndrome. It also slows the heart and encourages it to beat more forcefully. Its ability to relax and encourage the circulatory system means that

Valerian, in a blend, can play a role in supporting the body's healing and immune response in a multitude of ways.

Valerian sedates the higher nerve centres. This virtue means that it has long been a choice to support those with tremors and spasms as well as historically being a specific for epilepsy. Its anodyne and relaxant properties mean that it can help many other patients to feel more comfortable during their healing process, especially those struggling after traumatic injury and shock. Its anodyne properties make it very helpful in cases of neuralgia, headaches, and joint pain.

Valerian can also be supportive for those going through withdrawal from addictions – benzodiazepines, for example. Remember, if supporting patients withdrawing from alcohol addiction, it is best to avoid tinctures.

Although it is a calming, sedative herb, Valerian does have a stimulating side to it. A small number of people are particularly sensitive to this aspect and find that Valerian causes them to feel agitated rather than relaxed. If you have tried Valerian and have found that it makes you feel 'hyped up', it is probably not going to be the herb for you. Even if Valerian produces the desired relaxing effect on your system, I do not recommend large doses of it as a simple over a long period of time.

Energetics
Valerian is bitter, hot, sweet, and astringent. Despite its bitterness, it has a hot nature. It is best avoided by people who are hot-tempered when they are in pain.

In Tibetan medicine
Valeriana officinalis is part of the Tibetan pharmacopoeia, although it is considered to be interchangeable with *Nardostachys chinensis* and *N. jatamansi*. Traditional Tibetan doctors work with herbs that are local to their area. This medicine is known as *Pang peu* [སྤང་སྤོས།] – a name that is fascinatingly similar to Dioscorides' name for this plant.

In Tibetan medicine the medicinal parts are considered to be the roots, leaves, and flowers. Its taste is bitter, and it has a bitter post-digestive taste, with a cool, rough, and light potency. It cures old fevers and 'poison fevers'.

In my dispensary
I reach for Valerian to support patients in a wide range of conditions. The dried flowers form part of my urinary-system-supporting tea, and I often include the root tincture in a blend for those who have tension in the respiratory tract. I also make a topical wound-healing tincture blend based on Myrrh, with a little Valerian, Calendula, and Capsicum. The Valerian is included

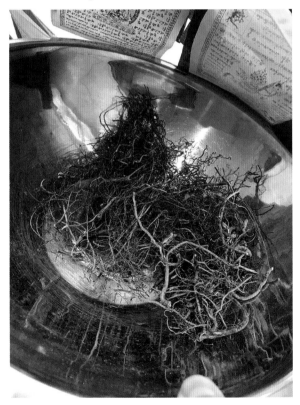

at a relatively low level (only 6%), but it acts as an anodyne and helps to relax the blood vessels in the area to be healed.

Historical applications

Culpeper wrote: '*The root boiled with liquorice, raisons and aniseed is good for those troubled with cough. Also, it is of special value against the plague, the decoction thereof being drunk and the root smelled. The green herb being bruised and applied to the head taketh away the pain and pricking thereof.*'

Gerard wrote of Valerian as being '*excellent for those burdened and for such as be troubled with croup and other like convulsions, and also for those that are bruised with falls*'.

Maud Grieve wrote that Valerian is effective in reversing failing eyesight when this is caused by the optic nerve '*lacking in energy*'.

Magical

Valerian root can be made into protective sachets. These are hung in the home to guard against lightning. If a couple is quarrelling, the introduction of some Valerian into the house will calm things down.

It is said that the Pied Piper of Hamelin owed his rat-attracting powers to the fact that he secreted Valerian roots about his person. It turns out that the scent of Valerian root is hugely attractive to rats as well as to cats.

Vervain 🌿 *Verbena officinalis*

'Vervain is specific for those who are perfectionists and carry the weight of the world on their shoulders.'

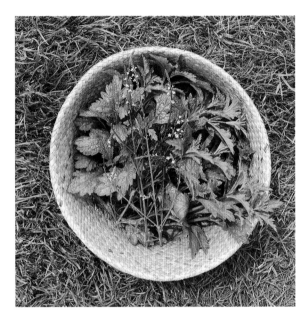

Vervain is especially suitable for people who feel that they have to do everything themselves if they want it done 'properly'. I always think of it for people who 'make lists' and 'carry the weight of the world on their shoulders'. Another way of viewing this is that they carry most of their tension in their neck and shoulders.

The name 'Vervain' is derived from the Celtic *ferfaen* from *fer,* which means 'to drive away', and *faen,* which means 'a stone'. This is said to be linked to its past association with curing people afflicted by bladder stones, a condition that was life-threatening before modern aseptic surgical techniques. Although I completely accept that etymology, I find that the name still feels very relevant today, as it brings to mind the strongly relaxing properties of this herb. Vervain encourages softness and relaxation when people have long-standing tension held in their bodies, especially in their shoulders. You could say that it drives away their hardness.

Vervain has a very rich and long-standing tradition of ritual and magic. One of Vervain's old names is '*Herba Sacra*'. The Latin name, 'Verbena', is from the general term used to describe plants that were offered on an altar. Romans called it '*Hiera Botane*', which means sacred plant. It was also known as 'Juno's Tears' by the Romans and as 'Tears of Isis' by the ancient Egyptians.

Medicinal parts
▷ Aerial parts

Physiological actions

Summary
▷ Nervine
▷ Bitter
▷ Antispasmodic
▷ Hepatic
▷ Blood sugar balancer/hypoglycaemic
▷ Emmenagogue
▷ Galactagogue
▷ Diuretic
▷ Astringent
▷ Diaphoretic

Physiological virtues

Vervain is primarily a nervine. It is very relaxing and is considered specific for long-standing nervous tension. It can be a good choice for insomnia associated with vivid dreams and feelings of paranoia. As well as relieving tension, it is a tonic to the nervous system. This is especially helpful when a patient has been chronically stressed for a long time.

It is strongly bitter and so acts as a good digestive support. The bitterness encourages bile secretion when this is deficient, but actually very many herbs can be chosen for this particular action, so I recommend choosing Vervain when it is also indicated in other ways. I feel that for best results it is always important to match the character of the herb to the character of the patient.

Vervain encourages better hormone balance to be achieved in the body, doing this through helping the liver to process spent hormones more efficiently. This supports overall hormone balance rather than pushing up the levels of any one particular hormone. This means that Vervain can be helpful in menstrual irregularities, period pain, and menopausal symptoms, as well as for premenstrual tension and headaches associated with the menstrual cycle. Its action in supporting the female reproductive system is so well established that Culpeper described Vervain as a women's herb.

Vervain's liver-supporting action means that it can also play a role in balancing blood sugar and counteracting depression caused by liverishness.

While it is contraindicated during pregnancy, it can be helpful during labour to stimulate contractions. It also helps to encourage milk flow after the birth.

Vervain is also traditionally a diaphoretic herb. It is regularly prescribed in China to manage fever in influenza and malaria. It is well worth considering for fevers when the patient is experiencing nervous-system symptoms as well. It is also a diuretic, increasing the flow of urine and flushing out gravel and stones as its traditional Celtic name, '*Fer Faen*', implied. Its ability to encourage excretion via the kidneys means that it is worth considering in cases of gout and

rheumatism if the character of the patient suggests that Vervain is a good match.

Vervain can also be applied topically. This is good to remember if, due to its intense bitterness, a patient is unable to tolerate much of it taken internally. A poultice can relieve headache, earache, neuralgia, and rheumatism. When applied, the skin becomes reddened, giving rise to the idea that Vervain draws the blood to the outside. Vervain as a poultice or fomentation is also a traditional application to relieve the discomfort of haemorrhoids. At the other end of the body, it can be good as a compress for eye inflammation. The infusion also makes a good mouthwash for mouth ulcers and bleeding gums.

Energetics

Vervain is bitter and astringent. I was taught that it is an especially good herb for people who hold their tension in their shoulders and find it hard to delegate tasks because 'if you want something doing well, do it yourself'. These folk may feel a huge level of pressure because they believe that everything would collapse without them. They are likely to make lists, too. Vervain soon counteracts the tension and rigidity, allowing people to accept help and be more relaxed about change.

Bach also wrote that Vervain flower essence is helpful for people with strongly fixed principles and ideas.

In my dispensary

The case of 'Danni' is a good example of where Vervain can be suitable. Danni was in her early 30s. Ever since she was a teenager, she had suffered with regular bouts of severe depression. She had taken various antidepressants for many years but had recently completed a process of gradual supervised withdrawal from them and was now completely free of allopathic medication. Although she was proud of herself for coming off her antidepressants, she was very anxious and worried that her mood was beginning to deteriorate. She was determined to avoid going back onto allopathic medication if she could possibly help it, since she was planning to have a baby in the following year or so.

Danni's energy level was at rock bottom. She did not sleep well, not only suffering with hot sweats but also getting up frequently to pee and then not getting back to sleep afterwards. She only got out of bed in the morning because she had to for her work. Unfortunately, her working environment was quite cold, and she often felt cold and sluggish during the day because of it.

Danni tried to eat a healthy diet, but it was quite high in carbohydrates and low in protein. She tended to drink large quantities of water (570 ml/1 pint) at each mealtime, and towards the end of the day she often turned to sweet snacks and caffeine in order to prop up her flagging energy. This pattern was clearly causing her digestive system to suffer. She told me that she had a very 'rumbly tummy' and often felt nauseous when she woke up.

Danni needed digestive support alongside nervines, and Vervain was an obvious choice as a main herb when she said that she was a perfectionist who held a lot of tension in her neck and shoulders. She wanted to throw everything at the problem, because she felt that she was at real risk of sinking back into full-scale depression. I advised a diet that was lower in carbohydrates and more 'nourishing' and for her to try to avoid drinking large quantities of water close to mealtimes. I also strongly suggested that she should take steps to be warmer during the day while she was at work. I wanted to create a herbal prescription that would calm and support her nervous system while toning her liver and digestion and stabilizing her blood sugar levels. She also needed temporary help with keeping warm, as she was cold so much the time, and I wanted her to feel more comfortable and 'at home' in her body.

Her personalized tincture blend contained, alongside Vervain, other herbs, including Wild Oats, Agrimony, Wild Lettuce, Chilli, Ginger, and Ashwagandha. She also had a blend of double-extracted medicinal mushrooms and two capsules per day each of Turmeric and a nervine herbal blend. After four weeks her sleep had improved, and her hot sweats had lessened. Her nausea had pretty much gone, but her mood was still volatile, and she felt a bit tearful. Another four weeks later she reported that she felt much more grounded and stable, and her anxiety was much, much better. Over time she continued to feel better and more relaxed. Her neck was less tense, and her energy levels were much improved. She realized that her work situation was not helping her to feel well and balanced, so she decided to make some major changes. She admitted that she would have liked to have done this sooner, but had not been able to face it before. Now she felt

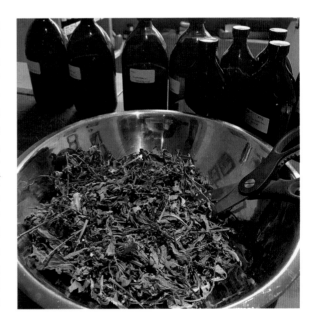

confident that the decision was the right thing for her. She told me that she had never believed that she could feel like this without allopathic medication and that it was wonderful.

Historical applications

Vervain was recommended for toothache by Hildegard of Bingen. She wrote: '*Whoever suffers from toxic blood, or through discharges from the brain to the teeth, should take equal parts of vermouth and Vervain and cook them in a clean container with pure natural wine. Strain the wine and drink it after adding some sugar. The cooked herbs, still warm, should be placed on the jaw, where the toothache is, and tied with a cloth before going to sleep. This the person should do until healed. The wine tempered with the above-mentioned herbs, then drunk, cleans the little vessels extending from the cerebral membrane to the gums from the inside. The herbs placed on the jaw placate the toothache from the outside, because the warmth of the vermouth with the warmth of the Vervain and that of the wine calms down the toothache.*'

Gerard was very scathing about the ritual and magic associated with Vervain, describing it as '*tending to witchcraft and sorcery*'. He did, however, subscribe to the idea that in order to treat intermittent fevers, you had to take a dose linked to the length of the fever's cycle. He wrote that Vervain '*is reported to be of singular use against the Tertian and Quartaine Fevers but you must observe mother Bombies rules, to take just so many knots or sprigs, and no more, lest it fall out so that it do you no good, if you catch no harm by it*'.

Parkinson said that it is '*hot and dry, bitter and binding, and is an opener of obstructions, clenseth and healeth: for it helpeth the Yellow Jaundies, the Dropsie and the Goute, as also the defects of the Reines and Lungs, and generally all the inward paines and torments of the body.*' It was '*applyed with some oyle of Roses and Vinegar unto the Forehead and temples, it helpeth to ease the inveterate paines and ache of the head, and is good also for those that are fallen into a frensy.*'

Magical

Vervain has also long been associated with magic and ritual. The Druids believed that Vervain opens the eyes and brings wisdom and inspiration. Vervain is traditionally gathered at Midsummer or at the rising of the Dog Star, when neither the sun nor the moon is out. If you carry any part of the plant, it is considered protective. It can be placed around the home to protect against lightning and storms, and an infusion can be sprinkled around to drive away evil influences. It is said that if Vervain is buried in the garden, wealth will flow to the household, and plants will thrive.

Magicians have long used it in love potions and divination. One of its names is '*Herba veneris*', due to its alleged aphrodisiac properties. Strangely, there is also a tradition that drinking the juice encourages chastity. For this, juice is obtained from plants harvested before sunrise on the first day of the New Moon. When drunk, it is said that all sexual desire will be banished for seven years.

Vervain's powers to generally protect and heal extend to topical applications. It is believed that if you smear Vervain juice on the body, it will cure all diseases and protect the patient against future sickness. As a bonus it is thought that it will allow the person to see into the future and have all of their wishes fulfilled.

Vervain has been associated with various forms of divination. For example, if someone is lying ill in bed, Vervain can help to indicate whether they will recover. Press some Vervain against them without them realizing and ask them how they are feeling. If they are hopeful, they will recover. If they are gloomy, they will not.

Wild Cherry 🍒 *Prunus avium / P. serotina*

'Wild Cherry is sedative and relieves coughs of all kinds.'

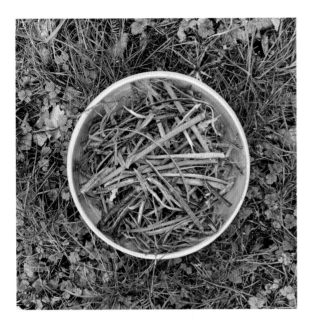

Wild Cherry is astringent, antitussive, and sedative. It is suitable for all sorts of coughs and is especially helpful as part of a respiratory-system-supporting blend.

Medicinal parts

▷ Bark
▷ Stem
▷ Fruit

Physiological actions

Summary

▷ Expectorant
▷ Antitussive
▷ Astringent
▷ Sedative
▷ Diuretic

Physiological virtues

Wild Cherry bark is astringent, diuretic, tonic, sedative, and antitussive. It is a very helpful herb in cases of catarrh and coughs, especially chronic dry coughs. Consider it to relieve coughs of all kinds, including bronchitis, nervous cough, whooping cough, and tuberculosis.

The stems are traditionally prescribed for cystitis, nephritis, urinary retention, and gout. Its sedative and astringent properties mean that it can also be a very good herb to treat indigestion and IBS, particularly when these are worsened by stress or anxiety.

Wild Cherry contains cyanogenic glycosides, which are metabolized to glucose and hydrocyanic acid, also known as prussic acid. It is mostly excreted via the lungs where it stimulates respiration to start with and then sedates the nerves that trigger the cough reflex. Although prussic acid is technically poisonous, the low medicinal doses prescribed are perfectly safe. Do not take large quantities of Wild Cherry bark as a simple over a long period, though. If treating chronic conditions such as asthma, combine Wild Cherry with other pectoral herbs, so that its dose is not too high within the formula. I usually stick to below 10% of a blend and find it very effective at that rate.

Energetics
Wild Cherry is sweet, sour, bitter.

In Tibetan medicine
In Tibetan *Prunus* spp. is known as *Kham bu* [ཁམ་བུ].

The texts say the oil from the seeds helps hair to grow and dries lymphatic fluid.

In my dispensary

I prescribe the bark as tincture within personalized blends, and I include it in my respiratory capsule formula. The following story illustrates how excellent it is as a foraged first aid for a cough.

Once I had travelled to Oxford to attend a conference on Tibetan medicine. I was very much looking forward to catching up with friends and participating in the conference. When I left home, I had been feeling well, but during the two-hour journey I realized that I was coming down with a feverish cold and a very tickly cough. I did not have any herbal medicine with me, but on arrival at my hotel I went out to gather some herbs to help me get through the next couple of days. I found Yarrow, Elderflower, Plantain, and some Cherry twigs from which I stripped the bark. Thanks to this tea, which I sipped throughout the following two days, I managed to concentrate on the conference and sit quietly without coughing. The Cherry bark played a very welcome role in relieving my cough.

Historical applications

Gerard wrote about the French custom of hanging Cherries in houses in order to ward off fever.

In the Cherokee tradition, Wild Cherry bark is a herbal support for women during labour. Other indigenous people in America took it for coughs and colds, as well as for its astringency to treat haemorrhoids and diarrhoea.

Culpeper said that '*The gum of the cherry tree dissolved in wine is good for cold, cough, hoarseness of the throat; mendeth the colour in the face, sharpeneth the eye sight, provoketh appetite and helpeth to break and expel the stone; the black cherries, bruised with the stones, and dissolved, the water thereof is much used to break the stone, and to expel gravel and wind.*'

Magical

Cherry is associated with new life and rebirth.

Suggestion for the home apothecary

Dried Cherry bark for respiratory-system-supporting teas and decoctions

Harvest coppice stems or prune some small branches in the spring. Scrape the bark from the stems using a sharp knife and lay the bark slivers out on a tray to dry in an airy place away from direct light. Once the bark is thoroughly dry and brittle, store it in an airtight jar in a dark place. Add a small piece of bark (about 0.25–1.25 cm long) to your respiratory-system-supporting tea infusion if you have a cough and cold. You could combine it with some or all of the following: Mullein, Red Clover, Cowslip, Thyme, Horehound, St John's Wort, Elecampane root, Coltsfoot, Daisy, Peppermint, Yarrow, and Lemon Balm. If the cough and throat feel dry and sore, add demulcents like Marshmallow, Plantain, Irish Moss, or Slippery Elm bark. If you have an unusual persistent cough not related to a viral infection please see a doctor.

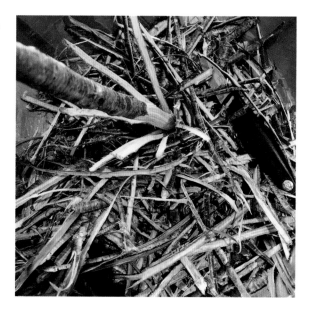

Wild Lettuce ❦ *Lactuca virosa*

'Wild Lettuce calms repetitive churning thoughts.'

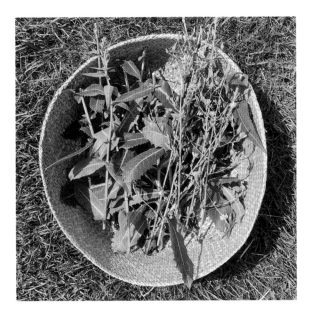

The name 'Lactuca' refers to the milky sap that is contained within the plant. It is sedative, relaxing, and pain-relieving. Wild Lettuce is especially helpful for people who lie awake at night with churning thoughts. A distinguishing factor is that the thoughts run along well-worn mental paths. The same worries, anxieties, and dissatisfactions constantly plague a patient's rest, yet they do not have the flexibility or motivation to make changes and resolve the situation – or, at least, to accept it.

Medicinal parts
  ▷ Aerial parts

Aerial parts should be processed while fresh.

Physiological actions

Summary
  ▷ Sedative
  ▷ Antispasmodic
  ▷ Anodyne
  ▷ Bitter
  ▷ Diuretic
  ▷ Diaphoretic
  ▷ Hormone balancer/antiandrogenic

Physiological virtues

Wild Lettuce is sedative, relaxing, and pain-relieving. The sap, known as 'lactucarium', contains small amounts of opiates and a trace of hyoscyamine as well as bitters, resins, and sesquiterpene lactones. In action it is like a very mild opium, and, unlike its more powerful Opium Poppy (*Papaver somniferum*) herbal colleague, it does not so readily upset the digestive system and is not addictive. It is quite safe and can be a helpful herb to calm over-excited children.

Wild Lettuce is bitter and can be helpful in supporting digestion and encouraging a more regular bowel habit.

Being a mild diuretic, it has a history of being prescribed for dropsy. It is also diaphoretic. It should be noted that it is a respiratory sedative, so large doses are to be avoided by those with chronic breathing difficulties. It does, however, effectively reduce chronic coughing. When prescribed appropriately, it can be helpful as long-term support for emphysema. It is not appropriate for severe acute coughs, though.

Wild Lettuce has always been prescribed to influence the reproductive system, in particular as a herb to reduce libido and to increase lactation. This understanding of Wild Lettuce's virtues has been developed further by Matthew Wood, in his book *The Earthwise Herbal* (2008, 2009). He shares fascinating insight into Wild Lettuce as a means of balancing hormones and encouraging the liver to break down androgens more effectively. This means that it can be very helpful in conditions such as acne and PCOS.

Topically, Wild Lettuce can be good as a pain-relieving application. Dr Christopher describes a formula that consists of equal parts Wild Lettuce and Valerian extracts and is applied to the site of pain. As it is a respiratory sedative, avoid prescribing large doses for patients who have chronic breathing difficulties.

Energetics
Wild Lettuce is bitter and acrid. It helps to soften and release old patterns of thinking.

In Tibetan medicine
Wild Lettuce is significantly bitter but has a warming acridity that can help to moderate its energetic influence when prescribed to those with a cold constitution.

In my dispensary
I like to prescribe Wild Lettuce for patients who have a tendency to insomnia with churning thoughts, especially when this is accompanied by weak digestion. These patients often also have multiple food intolerances and anxiety. I find Wild Lettuce a very good support when blended with California Poppy and other nervines, as indicated by the individual circumstances of the case. Establishing a better sleep pattern is an essential part of the healing process, so a temporary prescription of an evening sleep mix can be a very good herbal strategy. It will not be needed long-term if the root causes are addressed.

'Laura' was 58 years old and had been stressed and anxious for quite a few years. She was exhausted and struggling to get through each day. She never slept well, and during the first consultation she told me that she was having quite a restricted diet, because she suffered with bloating and discomfort after eating certain foods. She admitted that she was addicted to coffee and green tea and drank several cups of each every day, but she did not feel that she had the strength or the will to make any changes because 'she needed the caffeine to continue to function'.

First, I explained that she would have to cut down on caffeine and drink more water. I suggested that she reduced gradually over a couple of weeks to minimize the potential discomfort (headaches) that can be associated with caffeine withdrawal. I prescribed a personalized blend of calming, grounding, and digestion-supporting herbs to help her while she started the much-needed lifestyle changes. I also gave her a sleep mix tincture based on Wild Lettuce, California Poppy, Lemon Balm, and Passionflower. She was to take 5 ml in hot water about 30 minutes before bed. After four weeks she reported that she was beginning to sleep better and had managed to cut down to one caffeinated coffee and one green tea per day. She noticed that she was feeling more lively and less anxious. After a further four weeks she reported much better energy levels, and she was happy that she could think clearly and focus better. She had previously thought that her foggy-headedness was 'due to menopause or her age'. Her sleep and digestion had also continued to improve. She continued to have the support of the Wild Lettuce blend for a further four weeks, and then we began to reduce the dose, and until she no longer needed it. She still keeps a small bottle in her cupboard in case she cannot sleep, but she does not need to take it if she sticks to her recommended diet and lifestyle.

Historical applications
The Roman Emperor Augustus was saved from a critical illness by taking Wild Lettuce. In gratitude, he built an altar to it and erected a statue in its honour.

Gerard wrote: '*Lettuce cools the heat of the stomach, called the heart-burning: and helpeth it when it is troubled with choler: it quencheth thirst, and causeth sleep.*'

Lyte described Lettuce as being cold and dry in the third degree. He said that it '*reconcileth sleep, and swageth pains: also it is good against the stinging of scorpions . . . the juice . . . dropped into the eies, cleareth the sight, and taketh away the clouds and dimness of the same.*'

Culpeper wrote that '*the juice . . . mixed or boiled with oil of roses, applied to the forehead and temples procureth sleep, and easeth the head-ache proceeding of an hot cause. . . . It helpeth digestion, quencheth thirst, increaseth milk in nurses, easeth griping pains in the stomach or bowels, that come of choler. . . . It abateth bodily lust, represseth venerous dreams, being outwardly applied to the cods with a little camphor.*' It was strictly forbidden for anyone who had '*an imperfection in the lungs.*'

Magical

Wild Lettuce is associated with the Moon, Water, and the Feminine. It is magically associated with chastity, protection, love, divination, and sleep. It is said that rubbing Wild Lettuce juice onto the forehead will help with falling asleep. It is also associated with resisting temptations of the flesh and safeguarding chastity.

Suggestion for the home apothecary

Wild Lettuce tincture

If you make tinctures, Wild Lettuce is best extracted from fresh leaves before flowering. For that reason, it is a herb that you really need to wild craft or grow yourself, since bought-in stock is dried.

To make the tincture, take perfect fresh Wild Lettuce leaves picked on a dry day so that they are surface dry. Cut them up to release the medicinal latex, and loosely fill a clean, dry jar with them. Pour over 50% ABV alcohol, ensuring that the plant material is properly covered. If some leaves are on the surface, shake or invert the jar daily to keep them moist. Leave the tincture to macerate in the dark for 4 weeks, then drain, press, and bottle. Take 5 ml in hot water before bed as a temporary support for occasional sleeplessness. It will blend well with Lavender and Lemon Balm tincture, and this will improve the taste if you find it too bitter on its own.

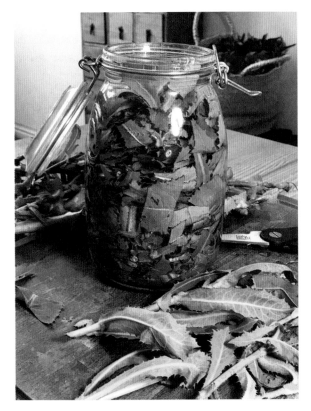

Wild Oat 🌿 *Avena fatua / A. sativa*

'Wild Oats are a sweet and nourishing nervine.'

Wild Oats are a fabulous support for a frazzled nervous system and are a particular favourite in my dispensary. I especially like the fact that they are energetically 'sweet' as opposed to having a 'bitter' quality, like many of our popular Western nervine herbs. They are grounding and stabilizing, providing nourishment and a calming influence.

Medicinal parts
▷ Stems
▷ Seeds

These should be harvested, both when green, as the grains are at the 'milky stage', and when the stems and seeds are more mature, for the 'Oat straw' stage.

Physiological actions

Summary
▷ Nervine
▷ Antispasmodic
▷ Tonic
▷ Demulcent

Physiological virtues

Wild Oats are a nourishing tonic to the nervous system as well as being antispasmodic. They are very different in character from the bitter sedating nervines, such as Vervain, Hops, Wild Lettuce, and Skullcap, which are popular within Western herbal medicine. In Tibetan medicine it is not considered helpful to introduce too much of a 'bitter' influence into the prescriptions of patients suffering from nervous states. Sweet and nourishing herbs are preferable, as they counteract *rLung* more effectively.

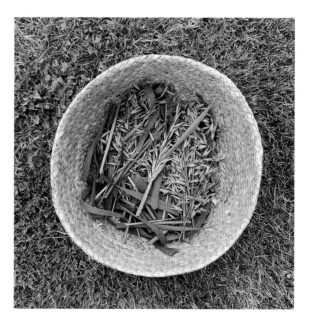

Wild Oats are excellent for recovery after a long and debilitating period of stress. They promote a feeling of balance, helping to lift our spirits, not through numbing our emotions, but through enabling us to see the bigger picture. They help us to see a way forward when previously there was none. Consider Wild Oats when patients have been ill for a long time and have forgotten what it feels like to be resilient and stable. Also choose them when the nervous system needs physical support, in degenerative illness such as multiple sclerosis, tremors, convulsions, acute inflammation in shingles, neuralgia, addiction, or when there has been a traumatic injury.

Wild Oats can also help in more immediate and raw situations: shock, grief, and anxiety attacks, for example. They support and hold us, giving us a sense of stability when we find it hard to see that within our own fractured body and mind. They help us to relax and accept, rather than mustering all our energy to hold a state of tension so that we can block out the unpleasantness of the situation. They say to us: 'Come on, you can face the situation.' In these cases, diet and lifestyle must also be given an overhaul, to change the emphasis from 'cleansing' to 'nourishing' and to remove the destabilizing effects of blood sugar spikes or stimulants.

Overall, Wild Oats are a deeply nourishing tonic helping us to feel more connected to our bodies and boosting our libido. They encourage healthy sweating. As they are so nourishing and mineral-rich, they are ideal for patients who are depleted and need building up after a long illness. Think of them in cases of chronic fatigue, especially where patients have been following a rigorous 'detoxing' or juicing regime for an extended period. They are also a good choice to include in prescriptions aimed at strengthening bones and maintaining bone density. If we were horses, they would give us glossy coats.

Oats are demulcent, soothing away trauma and inflammation, both internally and when applied topically. As a wash or in a bath, they are soothing and emollient – excellent to relieve itchy skin conditions. Fill a muslin bag with Oats or Oat straw and hang it under the hot tap while you are filling your bath.

Oat grains contain avenin, but not gluten. Some people who are sensitive to gluten are also sensitive to avenin, so if that is the case, they need to avoid Oat seeds. The main problem is that Oats are prepared in mills that also grind wheat grain, so there is usually significant contamination with wheat gluten. It is possible to buy Oats that have been processed in a dedicated gluten-free premises, in which case they will not contain gluten, but they will still contain avenin.

Energetics

Wild Oats are sweet, warm, and moist. According to Edward Bach, the flower essence of Wild Oat is indicated for when there is uncertainty as to the correct path in life and for people who waste their gifts through a lack of clear direction. These tendencies are very typically associated with raised *rLung*.

In Tibetan medicine

Oats are called *Seda* [སེ་དྭ་] in Tibetan. This medicine is sweet in taste, with a sweet post-digestive taste and a neutral and heavy potency. The sweet, nourishing, and heavy qualities of Wild Oats are mentioned in the *Gyudzhi* as being specific to counteract *rLung*.

In my dispensary

I often reach for Wild Oats as tincture or tea in order to help calm and ground patients who are suffering with *rLung* conditions. These may manifest as insomnia with racing thoughts, anxiety, panic attacks, palpitations, mood swings, or sudden lack of energy associated with blood sugar changes and rapidly shifting symptoms that cause the patient a great deal of worry and distress and are then forgotten about as other more intense symptoms take their place. When making tinctures or tea blends, I mix the milky Oat stage and the Oat straw stage together.

This case is typical of the gentle, nourishing, and focusing influence that Wild Oat brings to patients who need it: 'Lydia' was 58 years old and had been prone to feeling stressed and anxious for many years. She had been on antidepressants in the past but was now keen to try a natural and holistic route. She never slept well, and when we went through her diet, it was clear that she was having quite a bit of caffeine, mainly in the form of several cups of green tea each day. She also told me that she never sat still and was always busy. She was running her own business, but she knew that this was no longer what she really wanted to do. She would have liked to make some life changes, but she did not know where to start and felt that there was no time to think about it.

First, we agreed that she should cut down on caffeine and drink more water. I emphasized that no herbal treatment would be properly effective if she continued having so much caffeine. I prescribed a personalized tincture blend of calming herbs with Wild Oat as the main herb, with Skullcap, Vervain, and Cramp Bark and a few others to ground, relax, and calm her. After four weeks she reported that she was already feeling less anxious. Four weeks after that, she was sleeping much better, with her anxiety and tension being nearly a thing of the past. I was especially happy to hear that she was finding it more comfortable to spend quiet time alone, relaxing, instead of filling every moment with tasks that needed to be done. For the first time in a long while she was happy with her own company and was able to start thinking about new potential directions and ventures.

Historical applications
Gerard wrote disparagingly that '*Oatmeal is good to make a fair and well-coloured maid look like a cake of tallow.*'

Culpeper was more positive, writing that '*a poultice made of meal of oats and some oil of bay helpeth the itch and leprosy*'.

Magical
Wild Oats are associated with attracting prosperity and wealth. As our bodies are supported and nourished, so our external environment reflects a more abundant energy.

Suggestion for the home apothecary

Wild Oat blend tea

Mix equal parts dried Wild Oats, dried Agrimony, dried Skullcap, and dried Catmint. Store in an airtight jar, in a dark place. Have a cup of this herbal blend before bed. You can also have it during the day, if you are feeling especially anxious.

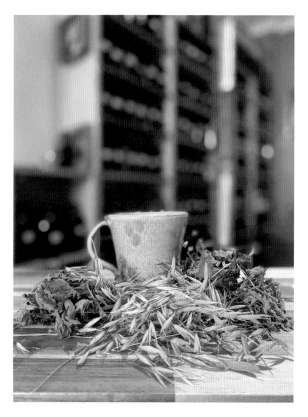

Willow 🌿 *Salix alba / S. nigra / S. fragilis / S. caprea, and others*

'Willow promotes flexibility, both physically and emotionally.'

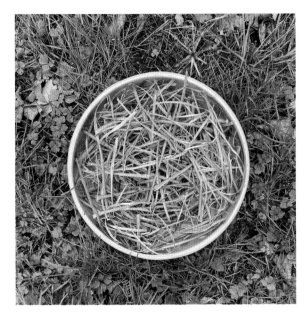

Willow is found in damp places, lining rivers and water meadows. It survives and thrives in boggy ground where other trees would not. In our bodies, it removes inflammatory sogginess and relieves pain and fever. It is often thought of as the original source of salicylic acid, which is a forerunner of aspirin. Salicylic acid was, in fact, first extracted from Meadowsweet, but it was later found that Willow was a more efficient source in the production of aspirin. Later, in 1899, aspirin began to be synthetically synthesized, so herbs were bypassed and left once again in the hands of those who love and respect them. Willow grows vigorously from a stick stuck into the ground. You could say that it grasps life. We could learn a lot from the resilience and determination of Willow.

Medicinal parts

▷ Bark
▷ Leaves
▷ Catkins

Physiological actions

Summary

▷ Anti-inflammatory
▷ Analgesic
▷ Febrifuge
▷ Astringent
▷ Bitter
▷ Vermifuge
▷ Diuretic
▷ Anaphrodisiac

Physiological virtues

Willow is high in salicylic acid, a compound that inhibits the production of prostaglandins. It reduces inflammation, relieves pain, and lowers fevers. In my – probably biased – view, it has an advantage over aspirin, as it does not thin the blood and is not irritating to the stomach lining. It can be taken safely over a long period to relieve pain and inflammation in joints, being particularly suited to easing the discomfort of arthritis and gout, for example. It is a herb to consider in order to reduce a patient's long-term dependency on aspirin or other anti-inflammatories. Its febrifuge properties can be helpful to relieve menopausal hot flushes when these are intense, and it can be a good first aid herb for a headache. Combined with antispasmodic Cramp Bark, it helps to reduce the pain of polymyalgia rheumatica, and fibromyalgia.

As well as the bark, the leaves were a well-established fever-reducing and pain-relieving tea in past times, leaves being better suited to passive infusion than bark.

Willow bark contains significant tannins which give it astringent properties and make it helpful for diarrhoea, especially when it is chronic. In these cases, if a sustainable cure is to be achieved, it is absolutely essential to take a good hard look at diet and lifestyle rather than just leaving herbs to do all the work. Willow is also a good bitter tonic, supporting the digestive system when this has become sluggish or tired through long-term illness or pain. Its vermifuge properties can be helpful here too if parasites seem to have got the upper hand in the gut.

Willow reduces libido if the intensity of this feels out of balance. It can be helpful for those experiencing premature ejaculation for example. Herbalist, Henriette Kress, makes a tincture from fresh Willow catkins as an anaphrodisiac when needed. Willow is also a diuretic so consider it for urinary inflammation and infections.

Topically, the bark is a popular ingredient in acne treatments since it is astringent, antiseptic and anti-inflammatory. A cooled infusion of the leaves was recommended for dandruff.

Even though, as herbalists we do not consider Willow to be as blood-thinning as aspirin, one should still exercise caution if there is a blood-thinning disorder or if the patient is on anticoagulants. It should be avoided in pregnancy and only prescribed very lightly in children with influenza or varicella as there is a theoretical risk of Reye's syndrome. It almost goes without saying that it is not suitable for those who are sensitive to salicylates.

Energetics
Willow is bitter and astringent, and cooling. Bach associates Willow with remedying resentment, self-pity, and bitterness. When we connect with Willow, it helps us to rejoice in others' good fortune instead of resenting it. On an emotional and energetic level, it helps us to cultivate flexibility and to reduce our egocentric tendencies.

In Tibetan medicine
Salix spp. is known as *Gya chang* [རྒྱ་ལྕང་]. Salix alba is known as *Keyag* [སྐྱེ་ཡག]. It has a taste that is bitter-to-astringent and a post-digestive taste that is bitter. Its potency is cool and rough. It is beneficial in poisoning, fluid retention in the joints, and neurological disorders due to both hot and cold conditions. It is also prescribed for gynaecological disorders and third-stage oedema. It is also generally appropriate to counteract heat and is considered especially suitable for gout and arthritis.

In my dispensary
I make a general pain-relieving blend with Willow bark for over-the-counter first aid prescribing.

Historical applications
Willow has a very long history of being considered a medicine. Sumerian clay tablets, produced in around 3200 BC, record it as a remedy for inflamed joints; much later, in around 400 BC, Hippocrates recommended it as a way of relieving pain and fever. Many members of indigenous American tribes have also long worked with the various Willow species that they had access to. Throughout the world and for thousands of years, Willow has been a valuable help and support to us as human beings.

Culpeper wrote that '*The leaves . . . stay the heat of lust in man or woman and quite extinguishes it, if it be long used; the seed also has the same effect.*' Regarding the bark, he advised that it be burnt, and the ashes '*mixed with vinegar,* [to] *take away warts, corns and superfluous flesh.*'

Lyte described the astringency and analgesic properties of Willow, which he called 'Withy': '*The leaves and barke of Withy, do stay the spetting of blood, the vomiting of blood, and all other flure of blood, with the inordinate course of womens flowers, to be boiled in wine and drunken. The leaves and rinds of the Withy boiled in wine, do appease the paine of the sinews, and do restore again their strength, if they be nourished with the fomentation or natural heat thereof. The greene leaves pound very small, and laid about the privie members, do take away the desire to lechery or Venus. The ashes of the barke of Willow mingled with vinegar, causeth warts to fall off, taketh away the hard skin or brawne that is in the hands or feet which is gotten by labour, and the cornes in a mans toes or fingers, if it be laid thereon.*'

Magical

Willow is associated with love, protection from evil, the moon, femininity, intuition, divination, and healing. The leaves can be carried to attract love, and willow wood is often chosen for wands especially when working with moon magic. The custom of 'knocking in wood' when speaking about something which might tempt fate, comes from the old custom of knocking on a Willow tree to avert evil. Willow's connection with water, intuition, and the emotions guides our awareness to cycles, rhythms, and the ebb and flow of life and our experience of it.

Willow is a tree that can help us with our wishes if we ask nicely. Make a connection with a friendly Willow and explain the reason for your wish. Choose a pliable shoot and tie a loose knot in it while focusing single-mindedly on your wish. Once your wish is fulfilled – or you have understood why it is not appropriate for you and can now let it go – return and untie the knot. Thank the Willow, and leave a gift.

Suggestion for the home apothecary

Willow bark blend

You will need:
- » *6 parts dried Willow bark*
- » *2 parts dried Valerian roots*
- » *1 part dried Valerian flowers (If you don't have Valerian flowers, just leave them out.)*
- » *0.5 parts dried Lavender flowers*

Put the herbs into a Kilner or Mason jar and pour on alcohol which is 40–50% ABV (alcohol by volume). If you work in 'proof' this is 80%–100% proof. Make sure all of the herbal material is properly covered by the liquid.

Choose a jar which allows you to loosely fill it with herbs to the top. Size does not matter. You could make only a small jam jar full or a

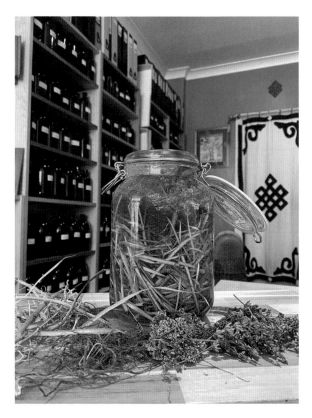

larger amount. I recommend only making a small amount to start with. Just add the quantity of herbs needed to loosely fill the jar. Do not pack the herbs in very tightly otherwise you will not be left with any liquid at the end of the process. Label and date the jar and store it in a dark cupboard for at least 4 weeks. You should check it every so often to make sure the herbs are still properly submerged. Top up with more alcohol if needed and shake it once in a while if you like. Once it is ready, strain it through muslin and bottle it.

Take 5 ml in hot water if needed as occasional pain relief. If you are on any other medication or need regular daily pain relief you should ask for guidance from a trained herbalist. This is so that you can make sure this blend is safe for you and that you are treating the root cause of the pain rather than just masking the symptoms.

Wood Avens 🌿 *Geum urbanum*

'The Blessed Herb.'

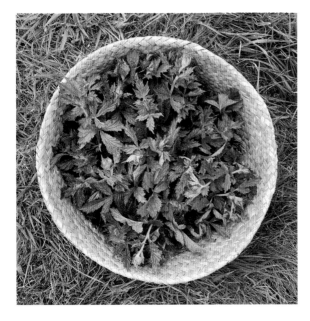

This plant is known as Herb Bennet, or 'The Blessed Herb', because in old times it was believed to ward off evil spirits and venomous beasts. The beautiful trefoil leaf was considered to represent the Holy Trinity, and the five-petalled yellow flower to represent the five wounds of Christ. It was often worn as an amulet and is frequently depicted in decorative architecture dating from towards the end of the thirteenth century.

A common wayside herb, Wood Avens is a very good example of a medicine that has been largely forgotten, pushed aside by seemingly more exciting, exotic alternatives.

Medicinal parts
▷ Aerial parts
▷ Roots

Physiological actions

Summary
▷ Astringent
▷ Styptic
▷ Anti-inflammatory
▷ Carminative (roots)

Physiological virtues

The leaves are gently astringent and styptic. The roots share these properties but are also aromatic, carminative, and febrifuge. At one time the roots were prescribed as a substitute for Peruvian Bark to cure '*agues*', some writers considering it superior for that purpose.

The leaves make a lovely, gentle medicine for diarrhoea, sore throats, and gastric irritation. The roots have a Clove-like aroma, said to be strongest if harvested in March. In fact, the old herbalists set an exact date – 25 March – as the best day to harvest Wood Avens root, provided that the soil was dry. When dried carefully, the root can be helpful to include in capsule formulae for long-standing constipation associated with inflammatory states of the bowel. The root acts as an anti-inflammatory and carminative which relieves griping when prescribed alongside purgatives. Chewing on the whole root can be a helpful first-aid measure for toothache.

Energetics

Wood Avens leaves are astringent; the roots are aromatic, astringent, and slightly bitter. It is a member of the Rose family and so it is not surprising that it brings emotional aspects to its healing properties. Consider it for people experiencing tenacious love and obsession.

In my dispensary

I prescribe the leaves in children's tea blends where we are working to heal an inflamed gut and calm a tendency to a loose stool. I also include the roots as an astringent carminative in a capsule blend to support the bowel.

Historical applications

Wood Avens root was traditionally used for intermittent fever and the '*ague*'. It was a common and effective substitute for *Cinchona officinalis* (Peruvian Bark), which was the source of quinine.

Lyte advises gathering the roots in March, since this is when the scent of Cloves is strongest. He describes it as being hot and dry in the second degree. He wrote that a decoction made with water or wine '*resolveth congealed and clotted blood, and cureth all inward wounds and hurts. And the same decoction cureth outward wounds if they be bathed therewithall. . . . The root dried and taken with wine is good against poison, and against the pain of the guts or bowels.*'

Magical

Wood Avens has a traditional role in exorcism and protection. This may be due to its Christianized links with the Holy Trinity and the five wounds of Christ. The *Ortus Sanitatis*, printed in 1491, states: '*Where the root is in the house, Satan can do nothing and flies from it, wherefore it is blessed before all other herbs, and if a man carries a root about him no venomous beast can harm him.*'

Suggestion for the home apothecary

Dried leaves for teas

Harvest Wood Avens in the spring when the leaves are lush and abundant. Lay them out on trays, and dry in a cool, dark, airy place.

Enjoy in a tea blend with plenty of other herbs. Add more of it if your stool is a bit loose or if you have a sore throat.

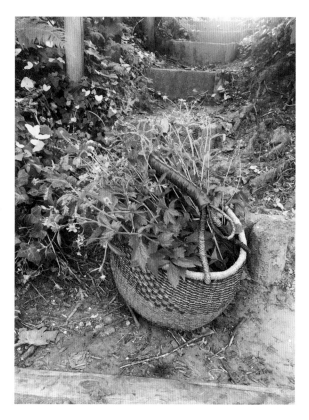

Wormwood   *Artemisia absinthum*

'Wormwood is without sweetness. It stimulates both the digestive and nervous systems.'

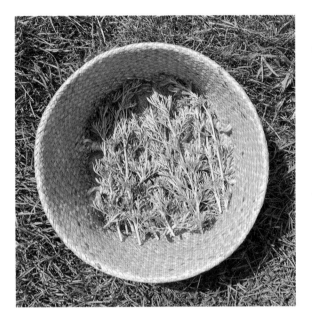

Wormwood is an aromatic bitter. The name 'absinthum' means 'without sweetness'. It is known as '*Wermut*' in German, a word that means 'preserver of the mind'. Wormwood's country names include 'A Hawks Heart', 'Absinthe', or 'A Crown for a King'. It is a key ingredient in the bitter digestives known as Vermouth and Absinthe, the latter being notorious as producing altered states and hallucinations when drunk habitually in large quantities. It is said that the drink Absinthe – or 'The Green Fairy' – was popular with Van Gogh, Picasso, Manet, and Hemingway.

Medicinal parts
▷ Aerial parts

Physiological actions

Summary
- ▷ Bitter
- ▷ Cholagogue
- ▷ Febrifuge
- ▷ Nervine
- ▷ Antispasmodic
- ▷ Anthelmintic

Physiological virtues

Wormwood is an intensely bitter plant. It stimulates the appetite and the secretion of bile while relaxing spasms in the bowels or gallbladder. Its bitter taste activates bitter receptors on the tongue and immediately stimulates the digestion, increasing the secretion of digestive juices and enzymes as well as stomach acid. It can play a helpful role in treating anaemia through its influence on improving stomach acid secretion and better absorption of minerals, including iron. It is anti-inflammatory and can help to bring down a high fever, as it is so cooling to the body.

It is so bitter that, if we taste a fresh leaf, it makes us physically shudder. This reveals its deep impact on the nervous system. It is, in fact, a nervine tonic. It is antispasmodic, relaxant, and antidepressant, and it stimulates cardiac function. In the past it was also prescribed for 'the falling sickness'.

As its common name suggests, Wormwood is an effective anthelmintic. It can be toxic at large or prolonged doses so should be prescribed with care, although its intense bitterness naturally limits its consumption. If making an infusion, choose a weak one (5 g of dried herb in 500 ml of water); in a tincture, do not exceed 3 ml per day. At very low doses Wormwood can be a helpful tonic to our nerves, but at higher doses it can become a depleting influence.

I was taught that Wormwood is traditionally helpful to balance thyroid function, especially in cases of hypothyroidism, but it can act amphoterically. This may be through a direct action on the thyroid gland or it may be through supporting better digestion and absorption. It has been discovered that there are bitter receptors within the thyroid, so this pathway makes equal sense to me. I prescribe it with Kelp and Nettle in my Seaweed capsules.

Wormwood stimulates the uterus. It was prescribed to bring on a delayed period, and in old times compresses were applied during childbirth to speed labour. For this reason, Wormwood should be avoided in pregnancy. The potentially toxic constituent thujone can be passed to infants through breast milk, so it should also be avoided during lactation.

As its name suggests, taken internally it is an anthelmintic and vermifuge. As an external treatment or placed in sachets in cupboards, it is an insect repellent.

Energetics

Wormwood is bitter and cooling. It has a deep influence on the nervous system. It repairs and establishes ordered functioning where this has become disordered or if we feel anxious about it and have lost our trust in it to work properly.

In Tibetan medicine

Wormwood is known as *Tsharbong karpo* [ཚར་བོང་སྐྱ་བོ།]. The medicinal part is the whole plant, including the root. Its taste qualities are bitter-to-hot, with a bitter post-digestive taste and a neutral potency. It is well indicated for

Tripa disorders, treating pharyngitis, lung diseases, and swellings due to heat in the body. It is considered a very versatile medicine, being a rejuvenation medicine and also one that treats kidney diseases. It is good for hot conditions where it is desirable to support the liver and digestion. It should be prescribed with caution in *rLung* and *Pekén* conditions.

In my dispensary

In my clinic I most often prescribe Wormwood as part of a capsule blend for patients who are borderline hypothyroid. It is blended in equal parts with Nettle leaf and Kelp. The size of the capsules that I make are size '0' and the dosage is a maximum of two capsules per day. Each capsule contains just one quarter of a gram of powdered herbs. This blend has made a very significant positive difference to many patients who are able to take it daily over many years without ill effects. The following case illustrates this well.

'Annie' was 70 and came for herbal help because her GP said that she was borderline hypothyroid. She had been through a period of stress over the last few years and felt that this had probably contributed to the situation. She discussed things with her GP, who agreed to monitor her for the time being, but, if things worsened, she advised that Annie should start treatment with thyroxine. Annie was keen to try natural approaches and avoid thyroxine if possible. After going through her case, I prescribed an individually tailored prescription to help support her digestion, which was a little prone to sluggishness, and also to help her nervous system. As well as her tincture, I prescribed two of my seaweed-blend capsules each day. After six months her thyroid function had improved enough to be at the lower end of normal rather than borderline hypothyroid. Annie continues to be well and continues to take her seaweed-blend capsules. Her thyroid function is still checked every so often and remains within a normal range.

I do not reach for Wormwood very often for individual prescription blends, but there are certain cases that call out for its influence. When I do include it, I am not liberal with it, but it is very generous with its virtues. This is one example where I feel that the addition of a small amount of Wormwood in a prescription had a very profound effect:

'Arnie' was an active 70-year-old and had been suffering with a sluggish digestion for most of his life, so much so that he took over-the-counter laxatives daily. In recent years his health had deteriorated, and he was experiencing loss of balance, visual migraines, and daily headaches. On top of this, his energy levels were very low, and he was experiencing a great deal of health anxiety, worrying that there might be something frightening and sinister wrong with his brain or nervous system. We agreed on a complete dietary overhaul, and I prescribed a blend of nervines and digestive and circulation-support-

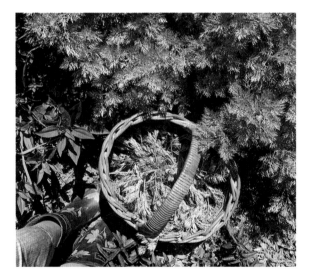

ing herbs. Wormwood was in the prescription in its capacity as liver support and nervine, in particular to help heal Arnie's relationship with his nervous system. It was accompanied by Lemon Balm, Cramp Bark, Skullcap, Passionflower, and Dandelion root.

Within four weeks Arnie was feeling a lot better. He was no longer experiencing any visual disturbance and only had a slight amount of dizziness if he overdid things. He had reduced his need for laxatives and was working on removing his reliance on them completely. Overall, he was feeling a lot more positive and relaxed. He had also found the energy and motivation to restart his daily spiritual practice. A month later he had continued to improve significantly and no longer had any headaches or dizziness. He also had completely ceased using over-the-counter laxatives. Arnie was very happy to be getting out and about more and trusted his nervous system to support him. He loved his new diet and lifestyle and was happy to stick to it in order to look after his body.

Wormwood is also a herb that I consider as a very short-term course when treating proven physical infestations of intestinal worms. I say 'proven' and 'physical' because I am regularly contacted by patients who have been told that they have intestinal parasites that had been diagnosed through energetic means and for which there is no evidence or symptoms. These patients usually have a tendency to health anxiety. Sometimes they have been pursuing 'cleansing' and vermifuge protocols for months before they find their way to my clinic. I find that they often respond better to nourishing and calming herbs, along with support in establishing healthy boundaries. The moral of this story is that when 'parasites' are detected, they are not always physical. A patient may be suffering with a drain on their vital energy due to their life circumstances or unhealthy tendencies within their close relationships.

Historical applications

Hildegard of Bingen knew it as Vermouth. She wrote of making a spring tonic with Wormwood as follows: '*When the vermouth is young and fresh, press the juice and strain it; and then boil wine with a little honey and pour this juice into the wine, so that the taste of the juice predominates over that of the honey wine, and drink it before breakfast from May to October every other day. It suppresses the loins sickness and melancholy in you; it clears the eyes, strengthens the heart, and prevents the lungs from becoming sick; and it warms the stomach and cleans the intestines, providing a good digestion.*'

John Pechey wrote: '*It strengthens the Stomach and Liver, excites the Appetite, opens Obstructions, and cures Diseases that are occasion'd by them, as, the Jaundice, Dropsie, and the like. 'Tis good in long putrid Fevers, it carries off the vitious Humours by Urine, it expels Worms from the Bowels, and preserves Clothes from Moths. The Juice, the distill'd Water, the Syrup, the fixed Salt, and the Oyl of it are used; but the Wine or Beer seems to be the best.*'

Thomas Tusser wrote of Wormwood's insect-repelling and nerve-calming properties in *July's Husbandry*:

'*While Wormwood hath seed get a handful or twaine*
To save in March, to make flea to refraine:
Where chamber is sweeped and Wormwood is strowne,
What saver is better (if physick be true)
For places infected than Wormwood and Rue?
It is a comfort to the hart and braine,
And therefore to have it is not in vaine.'

[Thomas Tusser, *Five Hundredth Pointes of Good Husbandry*, 1577]

Magical

Wormwood is associated with protection, divination, and the development of psychic powers and astral projection. It was carried to protect the bearer against being bewitched and to avoid the biting of sea serpents. It is considered to counteract the effects of poisoning by Hemlock and Toadstools.

It breaks love spells and was also associated with attracting love. This is an old love charm reported in Maud Grieve's *A Modern Herbal*:

'*On St Luke's Day, take Marigold flowers, a sprig of Marjoram, Thyme, and a little Wormwood; dry them before a fire, rub them to powder; then sift it through a fine piece of lawn, and simmer it over a slow fire, adding a small quantity of virgin honey, and vinegar. Anoint yourself with this when you go to bed, saying the following lines three times, and you will dream of your partner that is to be.*

'*St Luke, St Luke, be kind to me,*
In dreams let me my true-love see.'

Suggestion for the home apothecary

Wormwood and Quassia bark nit deterrent rinse

If you have primary-school-age children, you will probably be familiar with the cycles of nit combing that are necessary from time to time. Conventional head-lice treatments are pretty harsh, so this is a gentler way of eradicating them and deterring repeat infections.

Take a handful of Quassia wood chips and decoct gently in a litre of water for 15 minutes. Turn off the heat and add a handful of Wormwood. Leave the herbs in the hot water until it has cooled. Strain, and store any that is not immediately needed in the fridge. Fill a spray bottle with some and keep some in a jug.

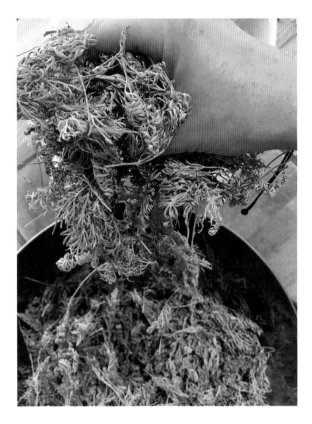

Wash the child's hair with shampoo, rinse, then apply conditioner. Comb the wet, conditioned hair meticulously from root to tip with a nit comb. It will take about 10–15 minutes for short straight hair and over 30 minutes for long and curly hair. Use as much conditioner as you need to make the job easiest. Keep rinsing the nit comb as you work, so that you are not reapplying lice or eggs. Once you have done this, rinse the hair to remove the conditioner, and then apply the Wormwood and Quassia rinse. This herbal rinse should be left in. Every day, before the child goes off to school, mist their dry hair with more of the herbal rinse from a spray bottle. Repeat the combing process every 3 days for at least a fortnight. Check for re-infestation regularly and keep misting daily.

Yarrow ❦ *Achillea millefolium*

The name 'Yarrow' is a corruption of its Anglo-Saxon name, *gearwe*. Homer, in his epic poem *The Iliad*, described how Achilles used it to stem the bleeding of deep wounds during the Trojan War. Yarrow's association with Achilles gives it its Latin binomial: *Achillea millefolium*. The 'Achillea' refers to Achilles and the 'mille-folium' means 'thousand-leaved' – a reference to its deeply incised, feathery leaves. Many of its country names – such as 'Soldier's Woundwort', 'Herba Militaris', 'Carpenter's Weed', 'Staunch Weed', and 'Bloodwort' – allude to its wound-healing properties

   I have been gathering Yarrow and prescribing it to my patients for many years. It is an old herbal friend, with a myriad amazing properties. Yarrow has a signature that indicates that it is a first aid treatment for deep cuts. Some say that the leaves represent a saw, but for me the thought that its leaves look like a saw has never really rung true. I am grateful to herbalist Matthew Wood for sharing his insight about this. He points out that the leaf looks more like a soft feather. This, he says, points to its efficacy in healing cuts that go down 'to the bone', since the leaf is itself 'cut to the bone' (or at least to the midrib).

Medicinal parts
   ▷ Aerial parts
   ▷ Roots

I tend to gather just the flowers; or the roots for toothache.

Physiological actions

Summary
   ▷ Styptic
   ▷ Peripheral circulatory stimulant

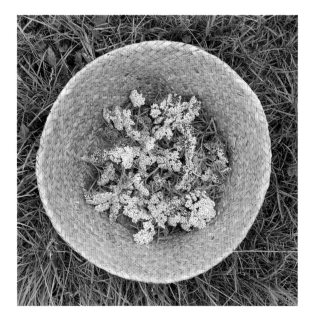

   ▷ Diaphoretic
   ▷ Diuretic
   ▷ Emmenagogue
   ▷ Bitter
   ▷ Anti-inflammatory
   ▷ Antispasmodic

Physiological virtues

I was taught that Yarrow is 'The Master of the Blood' – a reference to its ability to help to balance blood circulation within the body. I like to think that its country name, 'Bloodwort', refers to this.

   Yarrow is a very effective styptic, especially for deep wounds, hence its use on the battlefield or for emergency first aid. It is also a diaphoretic and a peripheral circulatory stimulant. Taking Yarrow internally as a tea or tincture results in an almost immediate sense of improved peripheral circulation, but not in a heating way, like that experienced when you take Chilli or Ginger. Yarrow releases heat to the exterior. In the presence of an acute fever it will work rapidly, but in cases where there has been chronic congestion for many years it will take a bit longer.

I am often asked how Yarrow can be both a peripheral circulatory stimulant and a very effective styptic. While I cannot describe the exact mechanism for this, I totally accept that it is the case. I have seen it many times in practice. Perhaps applying Yarrow directly to a deep cut has not only a direct styptic action, but it also helps to 'take the pressure off' the blood flow to the wound by encouraging a localized dispersal of the blood to the periphery.

In general, when taken internally, Yarrow enlivens the blood and disperses congestion. This property makes it helpful for painful congested menses with large, dark clots.

I often think of Yarrow when faced with a patient who has a hot constitution (*Tripa* in Tibetan medicine) but who requires circulatory support. In these cases, supporting the circulation with herbs such as Ginger and Chilli can be

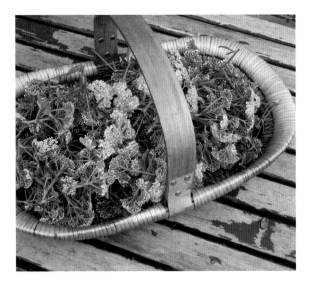

too heating. Yarrow is excellent at allowing that inner heat to be released to the exterior.

When taking the case of a patient, there are two strong signs that point towards a need for Yarrow in their prescription. First, if the tongue shows a central feathery crack with side branches, which looks a little like a Yarrow leaf, take notice. This is a sign that there is deep-seated inflammation in the body and that this is unable to be dispersed due to poor peripheral circulation. The surface of the tongue cracks because the heat is unable to escape to the surface. When a patient takes Yarrow, their inflammation reduces, and they feel better. Over time, the feathery cracking in their tongue lessens too. Second, when taking the pulse, if there is a marked difference in amplitude between the pulses in the two wrists, this is a sign that the blood is 'unbalanced'. I have seen again and again how, after including Yarrow in a patient's main prescription, the pulses have quickly evened up. In these cases, the patient almost always reports a significant increase in their feeling of wellbeing once their pulses are even. Yarrow is, after all, 'The master of the blood'.

In the early days of my practice, I was not always so quick to try Yarrow in a patient's blend when the special signs were there if there did not seem to be any other obvious or 'rational' indication for it. These days I include it straight away, as I am completely convinced by the correlation. My earlier hesitancy has, however, served its purpose, as it has given me the chance to become thoroughly convinced by these very helpful Yarrow signs.

Yarrow is indicated when there is 'heat trapped by cold'. In these cases, things can seem a little puzzling. If you go with some of the symptoms – cold hands and feet, congested menses, and sluggish venous return – you might feel that heating remedies such as Ginger and Chilli are required. However, these patients also have symptoms of deep-seated inflammation – for example, long-standing digestive tract inflammation – so, too heating a formula runs the risk of aggravating the trapped heat. Yarrow is bitter and cooling in nature and is therefore a better choice of circulatory support for patients suffering with an excess of the Fire element. It addresses the heat and releases the periphery. This holds true in both chronic 'heat trapped under cold' patterns and for acute fevers. Yarrow opens the pores and moves the blood to the surface and is especially helpful in eruptive diseases, such as measles and chickenpox.

Although Yarrow is technically 'cooling' in nature, I would still be comfortable prescribing it to someone who has a cold constitution but suffers from heavy, clotted, and congested menses, for which it is a specific. This is because I would blend it with other warming herbs and ask the patient to make appropriate lifestyle and dietary adjustments, such as moving more and reducing their intake of cold or raw foods. It is also worth noting that, although many energetic systems would describe Yarrow as 'cooling' due to its bitterness, others would describe it as warming due to its ability to get things moving.

When thinking about Yarrow, it is helpful to repeat the phrase 'Yarrow is the master of the blood'. In any situation where the distribution of blood is an issue, this can help us to see when Yarrow might be positive. Think of bruises, nosebleeds, venous stasis, congested or painful menses, fibroids, blood-filled cysts, poor peripheral circulation, fever, restlessness, delirium, haemorrhage that requires dispersal, bleeding haemorrhoids, varicose veins, and hypertension.

Yarrow has many other very helpful virtues. It is generally anti-inflammatory, and it is a kidney-supportive herb, always worth considering for patients requiring diuretic support, especially if they also show some of the other indications for Yarrow. It is a bitter and therefore supports the digestion, too. Its antispasmodic properties help to relieve spasms, and its carminative properties can ease bloating and flatulence. Yarrow also helps to reduce coughing and is sedative. In Norway it is traditionally considered to be a cure for rheumatism.

As a topical preparation, it is said to help prevent hair loss, and the roots, chewed, can alleviate toothache. An inhalation can be helpful for hay fever and mild asthma.

Yarrow promotes menstruation, so it should not be taken during pregnancy.

Energetics

Yarrow is bitter, cooling, and stimulating. Some describe it as warming due to its stimulating nature. It is protective, stopping excessive blood loss and the loss of vital energy through exposure to draining relationships. It clears stagnation in our blood and in our lives.

In Tibetan medicine

Although, as far as I am aware, Yarrow is not part of the traditional Tibetan pharmacopoeia, we know it is bitter and therefore is characterized by a predominance of the Air and Water elements. Air and Water together are flowing and encourage movement, especially of the fluids in the body, the blood and the interstitial fluids, for example. I find that Yarrow can be helpful for patients with a combinational imbalance of *Tripa* and *Pekén* when there is heat trapped under cold. Where there is a combination of heat and cold imbalance, it is traditionally considered best to treat the heat first, since that is often the most serious issue, which can flare up quickly. After that is resolved, we can treat the cold. Prescribing cooling but stimulating herbs, such as Yarrow, can be a good strategy – provided, of course, that Yarrow fits the physiological needs of the case too. For patients with a combinational imbalance of *rLung* and *Pekén*, administration of Yarrow should be balanced by warming and nutritious herbs and diet – including herbs such as, for example, Goji (sour and nutritious) and Caraway (warming and nutritious). The Air element within bitter herbs, such as Yarrow, can potentially make *rLung* more pronounced, unless it is balanced by an appropriate stabilizing diet and lifestyle. Occasional intake of Yarrow, such as during a fever or during menstruation, will not be harmful to those with an excess of *rLung*, provided

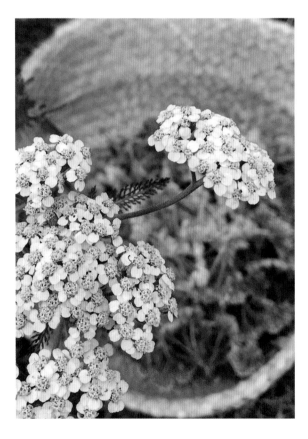

that the lifestyle and diet are appropriate for the constitution of the patient.

In my dispensary

I used to give Yarrow tea to my children as a diaphoretic when they had fevers. They soon learnt that they felt much more comfortable after drinking the tea. I remember that one evening a neighbour knocked on the door to ask if I had any liquid paracetamol for her youngster, who was feverish. I thought that it was odd that she should knock on my door with such a request, but she was new to the village and perhaps she did not know about my work with herbs. I told her that I had never used liquid paracetamol, as I had Yarrow instead, and she was welcome to have some of that. I will never forget the shock on her face. She opted to carry on and knock on another few doors, rather than to try my Yarrow.

In my clinic, I work with Yarrow in tincture, tea, and capsule form, according to the individual case. Here is a typical example where Yarrow was indicated: 'Ellie' was in her early 60s and told me that her circulation was not as good as it used to be. Her feet were always cold, and she had to wear socks in bed. When I took her pulse, I found that the right-hand and left-hand sides were significantly different in amplitude. It was clear to me that Yarrow would be helpful, so I added it to her personalized tincture blend at a rate of one fifth of the total. Four weeks later her pulses were totally even, and she reported that her circulation was much improved. Although her tincture blend contained other herbs to support her digestion and mood, I knew that Yarrow was responsible for this particular aspect of her improvement.

The following case shows Yarrow's ability to disperse blood following injury. I was contacted by a patient who was worried about her grown-up daughter who had sustained a blow to the head, which resulted in concussion. She had been admitted to hospital for a scan, which showed nothing to worry about, so she was discharged. She was in quite a lot of pain, though, and my patient asked me to suggest what she could do to help her daughter. I did not know the daughter and her medical history, so I wanted to suggest topical treatment rather than internal medicine. I immediately had a strong intuition that the daughter should apply a Yarrow compress on the site of the injury and have a Yarrow foot bath twice a day to support the balancing of the blood. My patient had Yarrow to hand and followed my advice. She told me that the effects were noticeable almost immediately, and her daughter quickly felt much more comfortable.

No account of Yarrow would be complete without a description of Yarrow's action when there is a deep cut. This one is from personal experience. I was clearing out some shelves in my old clinic room when I lived and practised in West Dorset. I reached up to pull some items from the top of a high bookshelf without checking exactly what they were. As I pulled them off, a heavy item fell and hit my hand. I looked down and saw that it was actually a paper guillotine, and it had fallen with the blade unsheathed. It had inflicted quite a deep cut on the side of my left index finger. I rushed out into the garden, because I did not want to contaminate my clinic or apothecary stock with my blood. The bleeding was pretty profuse by this time, but I was excited to apply Yarrow and see first-hand its action on a deep cut. I knew exactly where there was a patch of Yarrow in the garden and picked a handful. I scrunched it up and held it firmly onto the cut. I left it in place for about a minute, and then had a peek. The bleeding had already very nearly stopped. I was mightily impressed, I have to say. I avoided going to the emergency department for stitches, and the cut healed with minimal scarring and no infection. In writing this account, I checked and had to look very hard to see any sign of a scar on my hand.

Historical applications

Historical writers were universally in agreement about Yarrow's styptic qualities, whether they are internal or external.

Hildegard of Bingen wrote: '*Whoever is wounded in the inside of the body, whether it came through a knife or an inner injury, should powder yarrow and drink it in warm water.*'

Parkinson wrote: '*Dioscorides saith that his Achillea sodereth or closet bleeding wounds and preserveth them from inflammations . . .*'. He also wrote about Yarrow's other qualities, saying that it '*stayeth the flux of blood in women being applied in a pessary, as also if they sit over a decoction thereof while it is warme, and is drunke against the bloody flux*'. He added that '*The oyle made thereof stayeth the shedding of the haire*', and that '*the roote or the greene leaves chewed in the mouth is said to ease the paines in the teeth.*'

Magical

As well as being a very effective healing herb, Yarrow is a potent protection against evil or harm. Alexander Carmichael included in *Carmina Gadelica* (Vol. II, 1926) some Gaelic incantations to be spoken when picking Yarrow. This is one woman's powerful incantation to draw on Yarrow's powers of protection. It was translated by Kenneth Jackson in *A Celtic Miscellany*, 1951:

> *May I be an island in the sea,*
> *may I be a hill on the land,*
> *may I be a star when the moon wanes,*
> *may I be a staff to the weak one:*
> *I shall wound every man,*
> *no man shall wound me.*

When worn, Yarrow protects; when held in the hand, it stops all fear. Yarrow is said to remove evil and negativity from a person or a place. Yarrow also has the reputation of enabling a person to develop second sight through the opening of psychic channels.

Suggestion for the home apothecary

Yarrow, Peppermint, and Elderflower tea/inhalation

Combine equal parts of Yarrow, Peppermint, and Elderflower to make a tea or inhalation blend that is very helpful for colds and influenza. Keep some ready blended in your medicine cabinet, so that you can take it straight away if you succumb to 'flu.

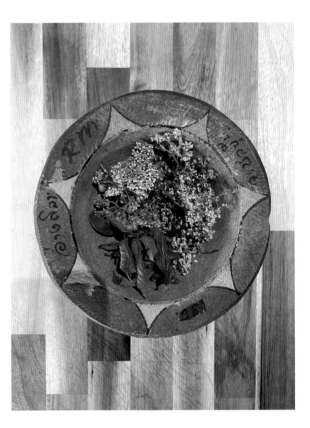

Capsules

Powdered herbs can be encapsulated either as simples or as blends. Empty capsule shells can be purchased online. I always choose non-gelatine-containing versions. The capsules can be filled by hand or with the use of a filling machine. These range from very simple pieces of equipment to highly engineered, sophisticated gadgets.

The capsule dosage depends entirely on the herb or herbs and the individual circumstances of the patient. I very often prescribe 2 size '0' capsules per day – for example, for Turmeric, or Rosehip, which are being taken mostly as a health-promoting supplement. The dose of capsules can be increased to 4 a day in some circumstances, provided it is tolerated. For example, a higher dose may be considered if the patient has an acute urinary-tract infection and is taking herbal diuretics and urinary system support. Another example would be for a patient who is quite low in iron and is taking a blood-building capsule. It may be appropriate to prescribe 4 a day at first in these cases, and then reduce the dose down to 2 per day. With some herbs – such as Marshmallow root, prescribed to protect and soothe an inflamed digestive tract – I quite often prescribe as many as 9 capsules a day for a short time period in cases where the situation is very aggravated. The capsules are spaced out during the day, as 2 before and 1 after each meal. This can (and should) be reduced as the patient responds to holistic treatment measures.

In my dispensary I always work with size '0' capsules. I find that many patients prefer that size; they tell me that they find larger ones (size '00') much more daunting to swallow.

Compresses and fomentations

Compresses and fomentations are water-based herbal preparations, such as infusions, that are applied to the skin. The terms compresses and fomentations are often used interchangeably. In both cases, cloths are dipped in an aqueous extraction of a herb and placed on the body. Compresses are more often a way of describing an application when treating a specific area, such as a burn, wound, or irritation, while a fomentation can also include the situation where the cloths are placed on the body in order to deliver herbal medicine more systemically – for example, the application of diaphoretic herbs via fomentations to the wrists and ankles, or the application of expectorant herbs to the chest by repeatedly applying warm fomentations on the back. Cloths should be replaced frequently, to keep the area covered with warm herb-soaked cloths. Compresses and fomentations are ideal for treating swelling and bruising, as well as cooling fevers.

Creams

Infusions can be incorporated into a cream by emulsifying them with an oil. Alternatively, you can purchase a base cream and add your herbal extraction – either a tincture or an infused oil – into that. Creams are applied at least twice a day, depending on the circumstances. I do not make my own creams for my dispensary, but there is plenty of information about creams online if you are interested in exploring this way of applying herbs.

Decoctions

Harder plant parts, such as roots, twigs, bark, berries, and stems, are more suited to being taken as a decoction. The plant part is simmered in water in a stainless-steel container for up to 30 minutes. A double decoction is made by simmering the herb for a specified time in a specified quantity of water, straining off the liquid, and then adding more water and simmering for a further length of time – usually another 20 minutes. The second simmering is strained and the liquid is added to the first before being stored in a fridge for up to 3 days. Doses are measured out and taken warm at regular intervals throughout the day.

When making a decoction, the various components of the herb are extracted at different rates into the boiling water. With continued boiling, the earlier-extracted and more volatile components may be driven off. The double decoction will preserve the more volatile components, while also gaining access to those constituents that require a longer time of simmering before they are extracted from the herb. Standard quantities are 30 g dried herb or 60 g fresh herb to 750 ml water, which reduces to 500 ml during simmering. A typical dose will be 1–3 cups a day, depending on the situation and the herbs.

Gargles and mouthwashes

Gargles and mouthwashes usually contain astringent herbs, such as Sage, which tighten the mucous membranes of the mouth and throat. The preparation of a gargle or mouthwash is the same as that of an infusion or a decoction. Tinctures can also be suitable if they are diluted with approximately 20 times the amount of hot water.

Glycerites

Glycerites are herbal preparations made by steeping herbs in a mixture of vegetable glycerine and water. Glycerine is a weaker solvent than alcohol for oil-soluble components, but glycerites have a pleasant, sweet taste, are non-alcoholic, and can be a good option for children. Dosage is similar to that described for tinctures, but, as always, it is very dependent on the individual situation. I personally do not work with glycerites in my clinic, preferring to prescribe teas and capsules to those who wish to avoid alcohol. Part of the reason for this is that the shelf life of glycerites is usually much shorter than that of tinctures. However, there is absolutely nothing wrong with glycerites. If you want to work with them, just make a small amount that you know will be used up within a year.

Infused oils

Herbs can be infused into oils and then applied as a treatment to the skin or scalp.

Infusions

Infusions are perhaps the simplest method of taking a herb as a medicine. For a hot infusion, boiling water is poured onto a measured amount of the herb in a lidded cup. This is allowed to steep for 10–20 minutes before the 'tea' is drunk. The steeping process allows the aromatic and volatile components, vitamins, and essences to move out of the herb's tissues into the water.

Infusions are most suited to the soft parts of herbs, such as flowers or leaves, or to soft-stemmed plants like Cleavers (*Galium aparine*). Infusions are typically taken throughout the day, either drunk freely or kept to two or three cupfuls at specified times, for example, before or after meals, depending on the specific action of the herbs and the nature of the illness. The standard quantities used to prepare an infusion are 30 g dried herb or 75 g fresh herb in 500 ml water.

Cold overnight infusions are suitable for mineral-rich spring herbs or herbs rich in mucilage. They are prepared by chopping the fresh or dried herb, covering with cold water, and leaving overnight. Drink a cupful each morning during the spring.

Ointments or balms

Infused oils can be warmed and mixed with a setting agent, such as beeswax. Once the wax has melted, pour the mixture into jars, and leave to set. Ointments and balms are excellent for wounds or burns as they can hold the medicinal herbs in place, keeping the area moist, and preventing infection and scarring. Apply several times a day. Be cautious in cases where it is better to allow good air circulation – for example, in fungal infections.

Pessaries and suppositories

Pessaries and suppositories allow medicinal herbs to come into contact with the tissues of the vagina or the rectum, without being altered by the processes of digestion. Infused herbal oils are set with beeswax or some other setting agent and formed into lozenge shapes by means of a mould. If you choose coconut oil, or a mix with cocoa butter, you will not necessarily need a setting agent, as the carrier medium will be solid at room temperature but will melt when inserted into the body. Alternatively, finely powdered herbs are mixed directly into a carrier oil and formed into lozenge-shaped pellets. An example of the proportions would be a quarter cup of cocoa butter, a quarter cup of coconut oil, melted in a pan, with 2 tbsp of infused herbal olive oil plus 2 tbsp of finely powdered dried herbs stirred in once it is melted. The choice of herbs and the infused herbal oil will depend on the intended action of the suppository or pessary. The mixture is poured into moulds and allowed to set. Store in the refrigerator. These are inserted into either the vagina or the rectum, where they melt to release the medicinal constituents. The herb is readily absorbed into the bloodstream from these areas. It should be noted that herbs administered in this manner will have a generalized effect on the body, as well as a localized influence.

Pills

An alternative to capsules is to mix the powdered herb with a binder, such as honey, and then to roll it into even-sized pills. The pills can be coated with arrowroot powder or some other powder to prevent them from sticking together; they are dried before being stored in an airtight container. Depending on the size of the pills, take 1–6 daily. Chew thoroughly, and sip hot water to help in swallowing them.

Poultices

Fresh, dried, or powdered herbs can be applied to the body to ease pain, in particular nerve or muscle pain, to reduce inflammation, or to promote healing. The herbs are usually chopped, steeped in hot water, and applied to the affected area with a cotton bandage to seal in the heat. Where there is an open wound, some gauze can be placed onto the wound first and the wet herbs applied over the gauze, so that the wound is not irritated. The medical constituents are drawn out of the herbs into the wound or through the skin, to give relief. Herbal poultices are also very effective at drawing pus out of a wound; my personal favourite is Rosemary mixed with brown bread and hot water. For burns, wounds, or irritated skin, fresh mucilaginous herbs such as Comfrey or Marshmallow can be chopped or ground and applied as a poultice without the need for steeping in hot water. Comfrey poultices should not be applied if a wound is dirty, as it promotes such rapid surface healing that the poison could be sealed into the wound. In cases of severe respiratory congestion, a chest poultice can be made with expectorant and antimicrobial herbs such as Thyme or Garlic. You will need enough of either herb to generously cover a muslin cloth laid over the patient's back. Apply and leave in place as a 'sandwich' between layers of muslin or linen cloth. A hot water bottle can be placed over the area to warm it up. Leave in place for 20 minutes at a time, replacing the hot water bottle as needed. Make sure you check for skin irritation and remove the heat or the entire poultice earlier, if necessary.

Powders

Powders are dried powdered herbs that can be stirred into hot water or taken directly on the tongue. Be warned – there is a knack to this. Make sure you do not inhale while the dose of powder is on your tongue. Typical doses are approximately ¼–⅛ tsp per day, depending on the circumstances.

Steam inhalation

Steam inhalation allows the medicinal constituents of herbs to come directly into contact with the respiratory tract. This method is excellent to clear catarrh and relieve sinusitis. Herbs are added to a steaming bowl of water and covered with a cloth. The patient places their head under the cloth and inhales the vapours.

Tinctures

Tinctures are a concentrated extract of a herb in an alcoholic base. The herb is steeped in alcohol for a specified amount of time, often in a weight-to-volume specified ratio. I prefer to make tinctures according to the level of herb added to a standard-sized jar. I loosely fill my jar when aerial parts or flowers are involved, but only approximately one-third full with bark, seeds, or roots. The amounts also vary according to whether the herb is dried or fresh. The strength of alcohol required varies according to the balance of oil-soluble and water-soluble components in the chosen herb, as well as the level of water contained in it. It is important that the final tincture is at least 25% ABV alcohol for it to be shelf stable. Tincturing a dried herb that has mostly water-soluble constituents, such as Goji berry, can be done with 25% ABV, but if the berries are fresh and therefore have a higher water content to start with, then a higher strength, perhaps 50% ABV, will be needed. Herbs with a very high proportion of oil-soluble components, such as resins, will require a very high ABV (90% or 96%) in order to dissolve the resins. Many herbs require a balance between the two and are extracted with around 45% ABV, provided that they are dried to start with. The ABV should be increased if they are fresh. I describe my method of tincture making in detail in my book *Self-Sufficient Herbalism*. Most tinctures last for several years and are prescribed at between just a few drops a day and 5 ml in hot water two or three times a day. Some people prefer to take bitter tinctures in cold water, but I personally always advise my patients to take them in hot water. This is for a number of reasons, including the fact that I am prescribing personalized blends that may be a mixture of bitter and other herbs. Additionally, I feel that taking them in hot water enhances absorption and makes the medicine a little more palatable. In the end, though, like many aspects of herbal medicine, it is a personal choice. Neither option is wrong.

Vinegars

Vinegars are made by steeping herbs in vinegar – usually Apple cider vinegar. They are ideal for those who want to create a shelf-stable product that is non-alcoholic. Vinegars are especially good at extracting minerals from herbs. Once the vinegar has been made, it can be made into an oxymel with the addition of honey.

Adaptogen: helps us to adapt to stress as well as supporting and balancing normal metabolic processes.

Adrenal tonic: supports and balances adrenal function.

Alterative: promotes and restores healthy functioning of body systems in a non-specific way.

Amphoteric: normalizes function of an organ or body system, reducing or stimulating, as needed.

Analgesic: pain-relieving.

Anaphrodisiac: reduces sexual desire.

Anodyne: alleviates pain.

Anthelmintic: removes parasitic worms.

Antiallergenic: reduces the tendency to an allergic response.

Antiandrogenic: blocks or suppresses the action of androgens.

Anticatarrhal: removes catarrh from the body and reduces its formation.

Anticoagulant: thins the blood and lengthens the time taken for clots to form when there is an injury.

Anticonvulsant: prevents seizures or convulsions.

Antidepressant: reduces depressive tendencies.

Antiemetic: prevents nausea and sickness.

Antifungal: treats fungal infections.

Antigalactagogue: reduces lactation.

Antihypercholestaemic: reduces blood cholesterol levels.

Anti-inflammatory: reduces inflammation.

Antilithic: reduces or removes stones that have formed in the body.

Antimicrobial: helps the body to stop microbes from causing disease.

Antiparasitic: removes and deters parasites.

Anti-pruritic: reduces itching.

Antiseptic: prevents the growth of disease-causing micro-organisms.

Antispasmodic: relaxes muscles.

Antisudorific: reduces sweating.

Antitussive: reduces coughing.

Antiviral: acts against infection by viruses.

Aperient: a mild laxative.

Aphrodisiac: stimulates the libido.

Aromatic: contains high levels of fragrant aromatic compounds.

Astringent: causes the contraction, drying, and tightening of tissues.

Bacteriostatic: prevents the growth of bacteria.

Bitter: having a bitter taste, which, in turn, stimulates the bitter receptors in the body.

Blood sugar balancer: helps to normalize blood sugar regulation within the body.

Bone and ligament healer: heals bones and ligaments.

Cardiotonic: supports the healthy function of the heart.

Cardiovascular tonic: having a general tonifying and healing effect on the cardiovascular system.

Carminative: relaxes the smooth muscle within the gut and helps the digestive process.

Cholagogue: stimulates the production and release of bile.

Circulatory stimulant: stimulates the circulation.

Decongestant: relieves nasal and upper respiratory tract congestion.

Demulcent: contains mucilaginous compounds that soothe and heal irritated and inflamed tissues, either by physically coating them or by influencing them in some other way.

Diaphoretic: encourages sweating, so that the body is cooled.

Digestive stimulant: stimulates the digestion.

Diuretic: increases the secretion and elimination of urine.

Emetic: causes nausea and vomiting.

Emmenagogue: having an action on the female reproductive system, stimulating blood flow to the pelvic area, promoting menstruation, and sometimes encouraging uterine contractions.

Expectorant: promotes the release of mucus and phlegm from the respiratory system.

Febrifuge: reduces fever.

Galactagogue: promotes lactation.

Haemostatic: reduces blood flow, stops bleeding.

Hepatic: supports the action of the liver.

Hepato-protective: protects the liver from toxins.

Hormone balancer: promotes healthy balance of reproductive hormones.

Hypnotic: tends to cause sleep.

Hypoglycaemic: reduces blood glucose levels.

Hypotensive: reduces blood pressure.

Immune tonic: supports the healthy action of the immune system.

Insect repellent: repels insects.

Kidney tonic: supports the healthy function of the kidneys and urinary system.

Laxative: promotes bowel movements.

Lymphatic tonic: supports the healthy function of the lymphatic system.

Mucous membrane tonic: supports the health of the mucous membranes in the body.

Musculo-skeletal tonic: supports the health of the musculo-skeletal system.

Narcotic: reduces pain and can affect mood or behaviour.

Nervine: supports the nervous system, either by stimulating or relaxing it or by generally toning and healing the tissues.

Nutritive: nourishes and supports healthy tissues in the body.

Oestrogenic: influences the oestrogen balance within the body.

Peripheral circulatory stimulant: supports the healthy functioning of the peripheral circulation.

Prebiotic: providing a favourable growth medium for beneficial gut bacteria.

Prostate tonic: supports and tonifies the prostate gland.

Purgative: strongly laxative.

Relaxant: promotes relaxation and reduces tension.

Reproductive tonic: supports and tonifies the reproductive system in both males and females.

Sedative: promotes calm and induces sleep.

Sialagogue: promotes the production of saliva.

Stimulant: enlivens the systems of the body.

Styptic: when applied to a wound, causes bleeding to stop.

Sudorific: promotes sweating.

Thyrostatic: reduces the activity of the thyroid gland.

Tonic: supports body tissues, helping them act in a balanced and healthy way.

Urinary system demulcent: soothes and heals inflamed tissues in the urinary system.

Urinary system relaxant: relaxes the smooth muscle in the urinary system.

Urinary system tonic: supports and tonifies the healthy functioning of the urinary system.

Uterine stimulant: stimulates contractions in the uterus.

Uterine tonic: supports healthy functioning of the uterus.

Vasodilator: dilates the blood vessels.

Vermifuge: removes worms.

Vulnerary: heals wounds.

Agrippa, Marcus Vipsanius [63–12 BC]: Roman general, statesman, and architect.

Avicenna (Ibn Sina) [AD 980–1037]: Persian polymath, great physician, astronomer, and philosopher; considered to be the father of early modern medicine.

Bach, Dr Edward [1886–1936]: British doctor and homeopath; developed Bach flower remedies.

Bacon, Francis [1561–1626]: English philosopher and statesman; promoted natural philosophy, in which interconnectedness and spiritual aspects of the natural world were integrated into early scientific method.

Bald's Leechbook [c. AD 900]: Old English medical text; the one surviving copy has a Latin inscription that means: 'Bald owns this book which he ordered Cild to compile'.

Banckes, Richard [active 1523–1546]: *Herball*, known as *Banckes' Herball*; full title is: '*A Boke of the properties of herbes called an herbal: wherunto is added the time ye herbes, floures and sedes shold be gathered to be kept the whole yere, with the vertues of ye herbes when they are stilled; also a generall rule of all maner of herbes drawen out of an auncyent booke of physyck.*'

Barlow, Edith [1929–2023]: Highly skilled and inspiring herbalist; had initially learned herbalism from her grandmother, Susan Meacock; having witnessed her grandmother saving a young boy's life with herbs, put aside ideas of a career in dance to study herbal medicine formally. Worked for many years with herbalist W. Neil Grayson in Rodney Street, Liverpool, and continued to treat patients until shortly before her death aged 93.

Bingen, Hildegard of [1098–1179]: German Benedictine abbess, visionary, composer, and polymath; wrote extensively on herbal medicine, health, and spirituality.

British Flora Medica, The [1845]: Also known as *History of the Medicinal Plants of Great Britain*; authors, Benjamin Barton and Thomas Castle; available to view online via the Wellcome collection.

Bruton-Seal, Julie: Herbalist, craniosacral practitioner, and photographer. Author, with her husband, Matthew Seal, of a number of herbal books, including *Kitchen Medicine* (2010) and *Hedgerow Medicine* (2014).

Caisse, Rene M. [1888–1978]: Canadian nurse, working in the 1920s; met a patient who had survived advanced breast cancer by taking a natural formula given to her by an Objibwa medicine man. Caisse became a firm proponent of the formula's value, renaming it ESSIAC after her own name, spelled backwards.

Carmichael, Alexander [1832–1912]: *Carmina Gadelica* (Vol. II, 1926), a collection of traditional lore, including prayers, charms, incantations, and blessings, gathered in Gaelic-speaking areas of Scotland between 1860 and 1909.

Chaucer, Geoffrey [1340s–1400]: English poet and author, sometimes referred to as the 'father of English literature'. *Canterbury Tales*.

Chöjë Akong Tulku Rinpoché [1940–2013]. Born in Kham in Eastern Tibet; was recognised at age 2 as a reincarnation of the First Akong, Abbot of Dolma Lhakang Monastery near

Chamdo. After a formal education in medicine and religious practice became, while still a teenager, abbot of the monastery. Later went to the monastic university of Shechen Monastery and received transmission of the Kagyu and Nyingma lineages from Kongtrul Rinpoche of Shechen. In 1959, at age 20, fled Tibet, walking over the Himalayas, eventually, against all the odds, reaching safety in India. Travelled to Britain in 1963 and at first lived in Oxford with Trungpa Rinpoché and Chimé Rinpoché; founded the first Buddhist monastery in the West (Samye Ling) in 1967. Was a pioneer in bringing traditional Tibetan Medicine to the West as well as developing a new form of psychotherapy, or mind-training, known as Tara Rokpa Therapy. He returned to Tibet frequently, undertaking charitable work through the organization Rokpa and training many doctors who, on graduation, were able to offer medical treatment in remote villages. Was murdered in 2013 during one of his trips to Tibet. *Taming the Tiger: Tibetan Teachings for Improving Daily Life* (1994); *Restoring the Balance: Sharing Tibetan Wisdom* (2005); *Limitless Compassion: A Way of Life* (2010).

Christopher, Dr John [1909–1983]: Having experienced much illness as a child and seen his adoptive mother suffering with diabetes and dropsy, was inspired to study herbal medicine, after meeting a naturopathic doctor. Developed over 50 popular herbal formulae; founded the School of Natural Healing in Springville, Utah.

Clary, Dr William J.: Personal communication, quoted by Dr John King (*q.v.*), *American Eclectic Dispensatory* (1854).

Colbatch, Sir John [1666–1729]: *The Treatment of Epilepsy by Mistletoe* (1720).

Coles, William [1626–1662]: 'Herbarist'; wrote about the 'signatures, anatomical appropriations and physical vertues of plants'. *Nature's Paradise,* also known as *Adam in Eden* (1657).

Culpeper, Nicholas [1616–1654]: Herbalist, physician, and astrologer; passionate about making herbal medicine available to lay people. Had learned Latin while studying at Cambridge and caused quite a stir by translating the *Pharmaco-poeia Londinensis* from Latin into English, thus breaking the monopoly of knowledge held by the wealthy physicians at the time. *Complete Herball* and *English Physician.*

Culver, Dr: Eighteenth-century physician who popularized the use of Black Root as a laxative.

Dawson, Warren R. [1888–1968]: *A Leechbook or Collection of Medical Recipes of the Fifteenth Century* (1934).

Dioscorides, Pedanius [AD 40–90]: Greek physician, pharmacologist, and botanist. His work as a surgeon with the Roman army allowed him to travel widely and to study medicinal plants and substances from all over the Roman empire. His work, *De Materia Medica,* served as the primary text on pharmacology until the end of the fifteenth century.

Dodoens, Rembert [1517–1585]: Flemish physician and botanist, also known under his Latinized name, Rembertus Dodonaeus; has been called the father of botany. His work, *Den Nieuwen Herbarius* (1533), was translated into English by Henry Lyte (*q.v.*), and published under the title *A New Herball* (1586).

Elizabeth I [1533–1603]: Queen of England and Ireland from 1558 to 1603.

Evelyn, John [1620–1706]: English writer, landowner, gardener, and horticulturist.

Felter, Harvey Wickes [1865–1927]: Pharmacist and leader of the eclectic medical movement. Together with Dr John Uri Lloyd [1849–1936], an eclectic medical practitioner, rewrote and enlarged *King's American Dispensatory* (1905).

Fuller, Thomas [1608–1661]: *The history of the worthies of England who for parts and learning have been eminent in the several counties: together with an historical narrative of the native commodities and rarities in each county*; includes comments and information on the distribution of medicinal herbs (quoted by Maud Grieve, *q.v.*).

Galen (Aelius Galenus) [AD 129–216]: Greek physician, writer, and philosopher; his writings had an enormous influence on medical theory and practice between the Middle Ages and the mid-seventeenth century.

Gattefossé, René-Maurice [1881–1950]: Born and educated in Lyon; joined family perfumery business; inspired formula maker; instrumental in encouraging the development of the French Lavender industry and improving distillation processes. *Le Guide Pratique et Formulaire du Parfumeur Moderne* (1906).

Gerard, John [1545–1612]: Trained as a barber surgeon; had a strong interest in plants, a large garden, and an extensive collection of unusual and exotic plants, many of which were gifted to him by others who had travelled to collect them. *Herball*, or *Generall Historie of Plants*.

Green, Thomas [late eighteenth century to early nineteenth century]: *Universal Herbal: Botanical, Medical, and Agricultural Dictionary. Contains an account of all the known plants in the world arranged according to the Linnaean system. Specifying the uses to which they are, or may be, applied, whether as food, as medicine, or in the arts and manufactures, with the best methods of propagation, and the most recent agricultural improvements* (1816–1820).

Grieve, Maud [1858–1941]: Passionate about herbs and herbal medicine. In the 1900s she and her husband established a nursery in Chalfont St Peter, Buckinghamshire; with the outbreak of the First World War, they transformed it into a herb farm to supply home-produced medicines for the war effort. *A Modern Herbal* (1931) with help and editing from herbalist Hilda Leyel.

Griffiths, Jeremy (DBTh, MIRCH): Founder of The Green Man Herbal Apothecary; has been practising as a registered medical herbalist since 2003; has a truly holistic approach, always seeking to understand and treat the root cause of illness and working with herbs according to their individual natures and temperaments.

Grigson, Geoffrey [1905–1985]: Renowned British poet, writer, editor, critic, anthologist, and naturalist; childhood in rural Cornwall had a significant influence on his poetry and writing. *The Englishman's Flora* (1975).

Haffner, Christopher: Acupuncturist and licensed practitioner of traditional Chinese medicine.

Harington, Sir John [1561–1612]: English courtier, author, and translator, popularly known for being the inventor of the flush toilet. Translated from Italian to English verse the *Regimen sanitatis Salernitanum* [Health regimen of the School of Salernum], a medieval collection of health tips, published as *The English Man's Doctor* (1607).

Hedley, Christopher [1946–2017]: Inspiring herbalist and herbal educator; studied herbal medicine at the UK School of Phytotherapy; made a fellow of the National Institute of Medical Herbalists in 1999. With his wife, Non Shaw, wrote *Herbal Remedies: A Practical Beginner's Guide to Making Effective Remedies in the Kitchen* (1996).

Hemingway, Ernest [1899–1961]: American novelist, short-story writer, and journalist; awarded Nobel Prize in Literature in 1954.

Hippocrates [460–375 BC]: Greek physician, considered to be one of the most outstanding figures in the history of medicine; introduced the systemic classification of diseases, humoural theory, and the use of prognosis and clinical observation.

Hoffman, David: Internationally renowned medical herbalist. Author of numerous books, including *Holistic Herbal: A Safe and Practical Guide to Making and Using Herbal Remedies* (1996), and *Medical Herbalism: The Science and Practice of Herbal Medicine* (2003).

Holmes, Peter: Medical herbalist, essential oil therapist, and Chinese medicine practitioner with over 30 years of extensive education, clinical practice, and teaching experience. Author of several herbal books, including *The Energetics of Western Herbs, Revised and Expanded Edition* (2020).

Homer [c. 8th century BC]: Greek poet, credited with being the author of the *Iliad* and the *Odyssey*.

Howe, Barbara [1922–2015]: Herbalist and tutor at the IRCH; practised from her home in Wilmslow; had a large garden, grew and gathered her own herbs, and made her own medicines.

Hughes, Dr Richard [1836–1902]: Homoeopath, known as 'The Grand Old Man of British homoeopathy'; strongly endorsed Hahnemann's Similia principle, but criticised his other theories, such as the Theory of miasm, the Theory of vital force, and the Doctrine of drug dynamization.

Jackson, Kenneth [1909–1991]: English linguist and translator who specialized in the Celtic languages. *A Celtic Miscellany: Translations from the Celtic Literatures* (1951).

James, Ifanca Hélène [1943–2010]: Medical herbalist; founded her practice, The Herbal Clinic, in Swansea in 1977; worked until 2007 as a tutor for the IRCH.

Johnson, Dr E. Stewart: Pharmacologist and medical practitioner; author of *Sheldon Natural Remedies: Feverfew* (1997).

K'Eogh, John [c. 1681–1754]: Irish Doctor of Divinity and naturalist; chaplain to Baron Kingston at Mitchelstown.

Khenpo Troru Tsenam [1928-2004]: Born in the Derge Kingdom of DhoKhams; became a monk, and was educated in the ritual and profound meditation practices of the Kagyu lineage, then studied medicine, astrology, and poetry at the Katok Monastery in Eastern Tibet. In 1956, took the chair in the monastic university at Troru, becoming known as Khenpo Troru Tsenam. In 1961, during the Cultural Revolution, was imprisoned by the Chinese and spent 10 years in a prison in the Pomi area of Tibet, later receiving a formal apology for his incarceration. After his release, worked tirelessly to restore knowledge and practice of Tibetan Medicine, a subject that was in danger of being lost. Was one of the most outstanding Tibetan medicine scholars of our age, a lineage-holder of the *Yuthok Nyingthik* and all other Tibetan medical teachings. He is believed to have been a reincarnation of the Medicine Buddha.

King, Dr John [1813–1893]: Studied medicine in New York City at Wooster Beach's Reformed Medical College; graduated in 1838; fluent in German and French. Teacher within the Reform school and the Eclectic movement; published, among other works, the *American Eclectic Dispensatory* in 1854, a carefully compiled reference that benefited greatly from his methodical attitude, his passion for the subject, and his ability to translate from French and German. (Revised and expanded edition published in 1905 as *King's American Dispensatory: see* Dr John Uri Lloyd.)

Kloss, Jethro: Pioneered ideas that led to the flourishing natural foods and lifestyle movement we see today. His writing was inspiring, practical, and ground-breaking. *Back to Eden* (1939).

Kress, Henriette: Finnish herbalist and author of herbal books in English, Finnish, and Swedish: maintains and expands an enormously helpful online resource for herbal practitioners known as *Henriette's Herbal Homepage*. *Practical Herbs 1* (2011), *Practical Herbs 2* (2013).

LeSassier, William [1948–2003]: American herbalist and acupuncturist; taught and inspired many of the major herbalists currently practising in the United States, e.g. Matthew Wood (*q.v.*), David Winston, Margi Flynt, and Dina Falconi.

Linnaeus, Carolus [1707–1778]: Swedish botanist, zoologist, taxonomist, and physician; formalised binomial nomenclature.

Lloyd, Dr John Uri [1849–1936]: Pharmacist and leader of the eclectic medical movement. Together with Dr Harvey Wickes Felter [1865–1927], an eclectic medical practitioner, rewrote and enlarged *King's American Dispensatory* (1898).

London Dispensary, The: Founded in 1696 as central means of dispensing medicine to the poor when physicians were treating the patients in their own homes; this model was then replicated in the New York City, Philadelphia, and Boston dispensaries, founded in 1771, 1786, and 1796, respectively. In time, physicians began to treat their patients at the dispensary.

Lyte, Henry [c. 1529–1607]: English Botanist. Translator into English of *Den Nieuwen Herbarius* by Rembert Dodoens (*q.v.*), published under the title *A New Herball* (1586).

Macer Floridus [11th century]: (Alleged pseudonym of Odo de Meung.) French cleric and physician; presumed author of the herbal poem, *De Viribus Herbarum* [On the properties of plants]. The herbal, commonly referred to as the *Macer Floridus*, written in Latin hexameter, presented the medicinal uses of plants. The rhyming verse aided doctors and apothecaries in memorizing medicinal recipes and treatments.

Manet, Edouard [1832–1883]: French modernist painter, pivotal in the transition from Realism to Impressionism.

Mattioli, Pietro Andrea [1501–1577]: Renowned botanist and physician; personal physician to Ferdinand I; prolific commentator on Dioscorides' *De Materia Medica* (*see* Dioscorides).

Mediolano, Johannes de [1050–1100]: Doctor from Salerno. *Regimen Sanitatis Salerni* (of uncertain date, but probably 1235–1311), translated by Sir John Harington and published as *The English Man's Doctor* (1607).

Meyer, H. C. F.: German lay physician living in Pawnee City in the United States; around 1870 began making and selling a patent medicine called 'Meyer's Blood Purifieer', containing Echinacea; was later in correspondence with Dr John King (*q.v.*) and Dr John Uri Lloyd (*q.v.*) regarding the efficacy of his medicine.

Milarepa, Jetson [1052–1135]: Tibetan yogi from Gungthang province of Western Tibet. After a hard childhood trained in black magic to seek revenge on those who had wronged his mother. Later regretted this and spent the rest of his life studying and practising the Buddhist dharma. Received the full transmissions of the Mahamudra teachings from Marpa, who famously asked him to build towers with his bare hands and then tear them down again before finally accepting him as a student. Milarepa (which means 'cotton-clad') spent his life practising these teachings and meditating in isolated mountain retreats. One of his many students, Gampopa [1079–1135], became his main lineage holder.

Mithridates VI Eupator, King [ruler 120–63 BC]: Ruler of the Kingdom of Pontus. Poisoning was a real threat to rulers at this time, and his father had been poisoned at a banquet. Was fascinated by medicine and, when he came to power, researched antitoxins and cultivated immunity to many poisons by ingesting sublethal doses.

Myddfai, Physicians of (in Welsh, *Meddygon Myddfai*): Succession of physicians who lived in Myddfai, Carmarthenshire, Wales. It is said that the original healing lineage was passed to the family via the 'Lady of the Lake', who had appeared from Llyn y Fan Fach in the twelfth century. The medical teachings were passed down through the generations and published by John Pugh as *Meddygon Myddfai* (1861).

Nero [AD 37–68]: 5th emperor of Rome, from AD 54 to 68, notorious for his cruelty and debauchery.

Nicander of Colophon [2nd century BC]: Greek physician, poet, and grammarian.

Paracelsus (Theophrastus von Hohenheim) [c. 1493–1541]: Swiss physician, one of the first scientists to introduce chemistry to medicine.

Parkinson, John [1567–1650]: Great herbalist and botanist, apothecary to James I, and a founding member in 1617 of the Worshipful Society of Apothecaries. *Theatrum Botanicum* (1629).

Pechey, John [1655–1716]: Physician; wrote prolifically on diseases as well as plant virtues and pharmacology. *Compleat Herbal of Physical Plants* (1694).

Picasso, Pablo [1881–1973]: Spanish painter, sculptor, printmaker, ceramicist, and theatre designer, who had enormous influence on twentieth-century art.

Pliny the Elder (Gaius Plinius Secundus) [AD 24–79]: Roman naval and army commander; fascinated by the natural world and natural philosophy. His work, *Naturalis Historia* (AD 70), served as a model for subsequent encyclopaedias.

Russell, Dr Violet [1930s]: Assistant Medical Officer for the London Borough of Kensington; active in working to promote access to abortion among working-class people.

Sappho [c. BC 615–c. 550]: Poet born on the island of Lesbos; ran an academy at Mytilene devoted to the cult of Aphrodite and Eros, for unmarried young women.

Shakespeare, William [1564–1616]: English playwright, poet, and actor. Regarded as the greatest writer in the English language and the world's pre-eminent dramatist.

Stapley, Christina: Prolific herbalist, educator, and author; teaches both historical and modern aspects, always with a practical emphasis; shares her herbal knowledge widely through books, hands-on workshops, and courses.

Stevens, Charles [1504–1564]: French Physician [Charles Etienne]. *L'agriculture, et maison rustique* (1580), with Jean Liebault; English translation, *Maison Rustique, or the Countrey Farme* (1616), by Richard Surfley.

Su Jing: *Tang Materia Medica* (AD 659). Su Jing supervised 23 people in the production of this great work, widely considered to be the first pharmacopaeia in the world.

Tralles, Alexander of [c. AD 525–605]: One of the most eminent physicians in the Byzantine Empire; wrote extensively; his work combined physiologically based prescribing with the use of charms and amulets. *Twelve Books on Medicine.*

Turner, William [1509–1568]: Physician and botanist; supporter of the Reformation; twice had to flee the country, giving him the chance to study European medicine and flora. He wrote in English rather than Latin. *Newe Herball* (1551).

Tusser, Thomas [c. 1524–1580]: English poet and farmer. *Five Hundred Points of Good Husbandry* (1557–1562), a work in rhyming couplets, described a year in the country; it is considered notable for its defence of the concept of land enclosures.

Tutankhamun [c. 1370–1352 BC]: Antepenultimate Pharaoh of the Eighteenth Dynasty, ancient Egypt, reigned from the age of 9 until his death at the age of 19; restored the polytheistic form of religion that had been reformed by his predecessor.

Van Gogh, Vincent [1853–1890]: Dutch Post-Impressionist painter who posthumously became one of the most famous and influential figures in Western art history.

Van Derveer, Dr Lawrence: Eighteenth-century doctor, of Roysfield, New Jersey, credited with the introduction of *Scutellaria* as a remedy for hydrophobia.

Waller, Emily Elizabeth [1863–1932]: Medical herbalist in Congleton; quoted by Maud Grieve (*q.v.*) in *A Modern Herbal* (1931). Grieve and Waller were contemporaries and were both members of NIMH, so would very likely have known each other.

Weiss, Rudolf Fritz [1898–1991]: Considered the leading figure in phytotherapy in Germany. *Die Pflanzenheilkunde in der Ärztlichen Praxis* [*Plant-Based Curative Science in Medical Practice*] (1944); later published as *Herbal Medicine* (1960).

Welsh Botanology, A [1813]: First work to cross-reference the Welsh-language names of plants with their Latin names; author, Rev. Hugh Davies [1739–1821], a cleric and botanist from Anglesey, educated at Peterhouse College, Cambridge.

Wood, Matthew: Graduate of The Scottish School of Herbal Medicine and member of the American Herbalists Guild. Highly experienced practitioner; also draws upon homeopathic principles in his practice. Prolific writer and educator in the field of Western herbal medicine. *The Earthwise Herbal* (2008, 2009).

Wordsworth, William [1770–1850]: English poet, one of the founders of the English Romantic movement in literature.

Name index

Subject index